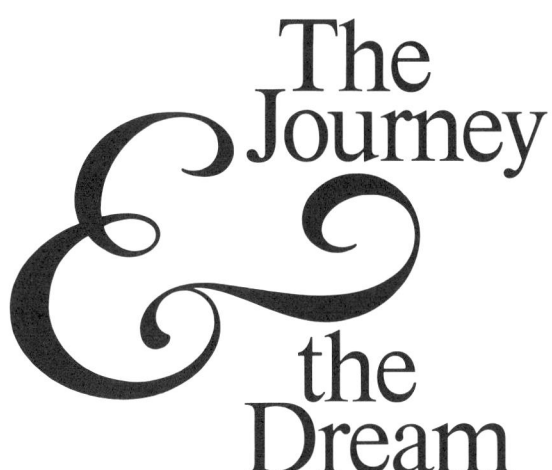

The Journey & the Dream

A History of the American Diabetes Association

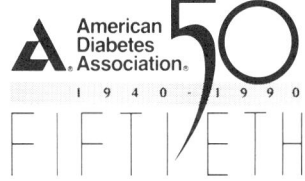

This publication is sponsored by an educational grant from Eli Lilly and Company.

© Copyright 1990 by the American Diabetes Association,® Inc.
ISBN 0-945448-12-0
Printed in the United States of America.

Table of Contents

Acknowledgments v
Preface vii
Chapter One: Beginnings (1937-41) 1
Chapter Two: The War Years (1941-45) 19
Chapter Three: Detecting Diabetes in America
                  (1945-50) 35
Chapter Four: Growth and Reorganization
                  (1950-55) 59
Chapter Five: Expanding Our Reach (1955-60) 83
Chapter Six: Identity Crisis (1960-65) 105
Chapter Seven: Years of Transition (1965-70) 125
Chapter Eight: Planning Becomes Imperative
                  (1970-75) 147
Chapter Nine: Opportunity and Momentum
                  (1975-80) 177
Chapter Ten: A Corporation Emerges (1980-85) .. 215
Chapter Eleven: Fulfilling Our Mission (1985-90) ... 247
Chapter Twelve: American Diabetes Association
                  Affiliates 287
Epilogue: The Journey Continues 321

Appendices
Appendix 1:   ADA Constitution 323
Appendix 2:   ADA Presidents 324
Appendix 3:   ADA Chairmen of the Board 325
Appendix 4:   ADA Executive Directors/Executive
                  Vice Presidents 325
Appendix 5:   First *ADA Forecast* Editorial 325
Appendix 6-A: Report of the Treasurer (1941) 325
         6-B: Report of the Treasurer (1950) 326
Appendix 7-A: Banting Medal Recipients 326
         7-B: Best Medal Recipients 328
         7-C: ADA Award Recipients 329
Appendix 8:   Research Symposia 332
Appendix 9:   ADA Annual Meetings 332
Appendix 10:   Nationwide Comprehensive
                  Long-Range Plan 333

Index 335

ACKNOWLEDGMENTS

The first seven chapters of this book are drawn in large part from material written and assembled by Cecil Striker, M.D., first president of the American Diabetes Association, and Paul F. Erwin, Ph.D., associate professor of American history at the University of Cincinnati. Their meticulous accounting of the formative years of the American Diabetes Association serves as a firm foundation for this text.

"In gratitude for the spirit and labors of those who served through the American Diabetes Association during the past years," wrote the two authors in the dedication of their book in 1970, "presented with pride to the current membership, we salute the past in this volume with a challenge that calls for even greater achievements within the coming decades." Those achievements are ones that will help us realize the dream, the ultimate victory, of a cure for diabetes.

That first history of the American Diabetes Association was never published. In subsequent years, Dorothy Born of the National Service Center staff added material and edited Dr. Striker's and Dr. Erwin's tome. In 1988 and 1989, the book took its final form with contributions from the staff of the American Diabetes Association National Service Center, in particular, Robin Ashlock, Edward Nykwest, Mary T. Linden, Kim Fawcett, Donald Jewler, Janice T. Radak, Susan H. Coughlin, and Caroline A. Stevens.

This book is, of necessity, an informal and anecdotal account of the history of the American Diabetes Association. Nevertheless, every effort has been made to compile a factual account, with balanced interpretations of events and fair characterizations of the individuals involved in various chapters of our history. The book is based on available records and interviews with dozens of people who were on the scene at the time various events occurred. The Association is not responsible for inadvertent errors or omissions.

A draft of the history was distributed at the 1988 ADA Annual Meeting, with a call for comments from all interested parties. The final draft was circulated to a number of reviewers, as well.

Thanks also to those who reviewed either all or sections of this book: Ronald Arky, M.D.; JoAnn Ahern, R.N.; Jean Betschart, R.N., M.N.; Dorothy Born; Charles M. Clark, Jr., M.D.; John A. Colwell, M.D.; Benjamin Greenspoon; Virginia Hanson-Ullom; Barbara Lofquist; Wendell Mayes, Jr.; Lynne Perry; Patricia A. Schultz, R.N., M.S.; and Dorothea Sims.

Finally, a special thanks to Eli Lilly and Company for its generous grant, which made publication of this book possible.

PREFACE

Unlike tuberculosis or the plague, diabetes has not decimated whole populations or dramatically changed the face of history. Yet diabetes is one of humankind's oldest afflictions. While this disease dates back to ancient times, its true nature was not uncovered until the early eighteenth century. The most significant progress in the understanding of diabetes—not including the discovery of insulin—has been achieved only in the last 50 years. The American Diabetes Association (ADA) has been in the forefront of this progress, and as we approach our fiftieth anniversary, it is time to tell our story.

Our purpose in writing this history is to trace the evolution of the American Diabetes Association from its founding to the present. This is also the story of how care and treatment of diabetes have been advanced by the people and programs of the Association. Every attempt has been made to reproduce from the available records evidence of this evolution and the strides—as well as the stumbles—the Association has taken. We believe the record speaks for itself.

"The patient suffering from the syndrome of diabetes mellitus is the reason for the existence of this Association. His medical, social, and economic problems are our problems," declared Cecil Striker, M.D., the first president of the American Diabetes Association, in 1940. With this statement, Dr. Striker set the course the American Diabetes Association would follow. Searching for the way to prevent and cure diabetes, and helping people with diabetes live healthy, productive lives, has always been the mission of the American Diabetes Association.

How well has the Association carried out its mission? What have been its triumphs? Its failures? How are 11 million Americans coping with diabetes today? What is their hope for tomorrow? To answer these questions, we need to look back.

In the late 1930s, the United States was gradually emerging from the Great Depression. Sweeping fiscal reforms and welfare legislation, introduced by President Franklin D. Roosevelt, had fostered growing social consciousness in America. President Roosevelt's message that "the health of the people is a public concern" was just beginning to be understood.

Within the medical profession, there was disagreement about how diabetes should be treated. Yet, to a small group of physicians discussing diabetes at a meeting in 1937, one thing was certain: Insulin was not the whole answer. Among the questions this group debated were:

- Why was the incidence and mortality of diabetes rising steadily—16 years after the discovery of insulin?
- Does insulin cause early vascular deterioration?
- What diet is best?
- Does exercise play a role in diabetes control?

The doctors reached no consensus, but concluded that much more time, study, and discussion should be devoted to this devastating disease.

As a result of these early discussions, a Committee for the Establishment of a National Diabetes Association was formed. Twenty-five physicians met on June 12, 1940, to draft a constitution and bylaws establishing the American Diabetes Association. Looking back at the dreams and aspirations of these physicians, as well as those of the thousands of volunteers who followed, we find an unbroken course of freely given time, talent, love, and devotion. We see how these efforts propelled the American Diabetes Association to the front ranks of voluntary health agencies.

The exchange of ideas among physicians and research scientists was the stimulus for the formation of the American Diabetes Association. At the first Annual Meeting in 1941, attended by 250 physicians, five scientific papers were read. This first professional education program became the foundation for the Scientific Sessions and Postgraduate courses of today. The Scientific Sessions, with an annual attendance of more than 3,000 physicians, research scientists, and health professionals, and the Postgraduate Course enjoy an international reputation.

By the mid-1960s, the incidence of diabetes had tripled compared to the 1940 rate, and the number of new cases continued to climb. Basic research in diabetes was desperately needed. And although the American Diabetes Association was flourishing as a professional society, it did not have the research funds needed to meet this growing challenge. In 1970, after years of debate, the Association was reorganized into a voluntary health agency with a primary goal of funding research.

The Association has grown from a professional society of 250 physicians to a voluntary health agency with a professional membership of more than 9,000 physicians, scientists, nurses, dietitians, and educators, in addition to a lay membership of 255,000. From an initial start-up budget of $1,500 in 1940, the Association's annual budget grew to more than $30 million in the mid-1980s, and it continues to grow. The Association's first publications—*Abstracts*, distributed to physician members only, and a pocket-sized digest, *ADA Forecast*, for the individual with diabetes—have grown in number, as well as reputation and prestige. Today's publications include two research journals, one clinical practice journal, one bimonthly publication for primary-care physicians, one monthly patient-education magazine, and one quarterly newsletter for people who live with diabetes, plus a host of books, pamphlets, and other materials. The annual circulation of all the publications exceeds six million copies.

Most important, the care and treatment available to people with diabetes has improved tremendously. Early and accurate diagnosis, improved medications and delivery systems, new technologies in blood-testing techniques, and improved knowledge of nutrition and the role of exercise have revolutionized diabetes management, particularly in the last decade. But all this is not enough. There is an impatience and a frustration shared by all those affected by diabetes to realize their dream: a cure for diabetes. "Other dread diseases have been conquered. Why not diabetes?" they ask. And so, the mission goes forward. The journey continues.

Dorothy M. Born
1988

Chapter One
Beginnings
1937-41

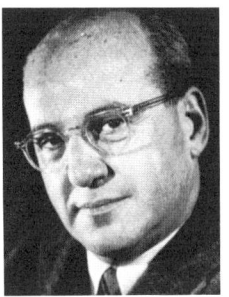

ADA PRESIDENT
Cecil Striker, M.D.
(1940-41)

Since ancient times, diabetes had meant slow death by starvation. But in 1921, the picture changed dramatically. Suddenly, with the discovery of insulin, diabetes was no longer a fatal disease. For the first time in history, people with diabetes were given the hope of living a near-to-normal life. The discovery of insulin in 1921-22 by Frederick G. Banting, M.D., and then student assistant Charles H. Best remains one of the greatest achievements in the history of modern medicine. And accordingly, Dr. Banting was awarded the Nobel Prize in Physiology and Medicine in 1923.

In 1936, protamine insulin came into use. A mixture of regular insulin and protamine (obtained from salmon sperm), protamine insulin was developed by Hans C. Hagedorn, M.D., and associates in Copenhagen and enthusiastically embraced by clinicians in the United States and Canada. This "new" insulin had numerous advantages over the old "ordinary" insulin. Protamine insulin acted more slowly and continuously than regular insulin, and many people using the new insulin could decrease the number of injections they took; some could even control their diabetes with one injection a day. They also could tolerate a greater range of carbohydrates in their diet, and hypoglycemic reactions occurred less often.

For a while, it seemed that the riddle of diabetes had been solved. Life expectancy for people with diabetes increased, thanks largely to insulin. Researchers began to turn their attention to other dread diseases. Yet as physicians observed their patients on insulin over periods of five to ten years, some of the early euphoria faded. Miraculous as insulin was in extending life, it became increasingly apparent that insulin was not the whole answer. The incidence of diabetes and diabetes-related deaths rose steadily, as did the number of amputations due to diabetic gangrene. Arteriosclerosis and cardiovascular disease were recognized as complications of diabetes.

In 1937, 16 years after the discovery of insulin, many physicians were skeptical of its effectiveness, many were unfamiliar with its proper use, and some even refused to prescribe it. It was estimated then that approximately 750,000 people in the United States had diabetes and that several million more had the disease but did not know it. There was a scarcity of reliable information, not only for people with diabetes, but also for the physicians and health professionals treating them and for the general public.

It was recognized that diabetes was somehow linked to heredity. It was also recognized that there was more than one kind of diabetes, but there was confusion as to how many kinds. One classification used was "insulin reactive." Diabetes in children and adolescents was considered insulin reactive because insulin acted powerfully and quickly on the blood glucose.

There was confusion about which diet was best for people with diabetes. Before insulin came into use, the only known method of treatment for diabetes was the "starvation" diet, engineered by Frederick Allen, M.D., of Harvard, and later by Elliott P. Joslin, M.D., of Boston. The diet allowed an adult less than 800 calories a day. (The usual calorie count for women is about 1,500 a day; for men, 2,000-2,500.) People with diabetes on the starvation diet were allowed only enough calories to keep their urine from showing sugar. They became extremely emaciated and were often too weak to leave their beds.

With the introduction of insulin came numerous "diabetic diets." A high-fat, low-carbohydrate diet was popular for a while, as was a high-carbohydrate diet.

By the late 1930s, it was becoming increasingly clear that questions about diabetes treatment could be answered only through greater physician study and the exchange of ideas.

The Beginnings

At a meeting of the American College of Physicians in New Orleans in 1937, a small group of physicians interested in diabetes gathered over lunch. Their discussions revealed the uncertainties about how diabetes should be treated. The physicians questioned what constituted good control of the disease, how and when insulin should be given, which diet was appropriate, and if exercise was really a factor in control. They felt a great need to share experiences, to talk, to listen, and to learn from one another. They lamented, too, the lack of opportunity to discuss diabetes at regular medical meetings that included greater numbers of their colleagues.

For two years, the physicians mulled over the idea of an organization devoted strictly to diabetes. Was there a real need? How could such an organization be developed? Who should participate? What would be the minimum requirements for starting such an organization? Cecil Striker, M.D., of Cincinnati, and Herman O. Mosenthal, M.D., of New York City, kept the idea alive through correspondence. In 1939, Dr. Mosenthal wrote, "For a national diabetes association I believe there are three requirements: . . . leadership, a definite program, and monetary resources."

Across the country, the problems of diabetes treatment, as well as the often fearful perceptions of diabetes by employers and insurance companies, had brought physicians and public health officers together in local diabetes societies. By enlisting the cooperation of such societies in New York City, Philadelphia, Detroit, Cincinnati, and Rochester, New York, sufficient interest was kindled to form a national organization.

Each society was asked to send delegates to participate in a meeting of the Committee for the Establishment of a National Diabetes Association at the Hotel Statler in Cleveland, Ohio, on April 2, 1940. The meeting was attended by 12 physicians: Cecil Striker (chairman); Herman O. Mosenthal (secretary); Samuel S. Altshuler, William S. Reveno, Laurence F. Segar, and George C. Thosteson, of Detroit; Joseph T. Beardwood, Jr., of Philadelphia; Charles F. Bolduan, of New York; C.B.F. Gibbs, of Rochester, New York; Louis B. Owens and J. L. Tuechter of Cincinnati; and Frederick W. Williams, of New York City.

In his opening remarks, Dr. Striker said that more than a year had been devoted to planning for the meeting and bringing together physicians who supported the idea of a national diabetes association. The need for

Remembrances Of Times Past: The 1920s

Leona Scheidler of Hamilton, Montana, wrote about her more than 60 years with diabetes in the "Reflections" column of *Diabetes Forecast,* August 1987. She considers herself "one of the lucky ones."

In May 1927, Leona Scheidler was 19 years old and weighed 78 pounds. She could

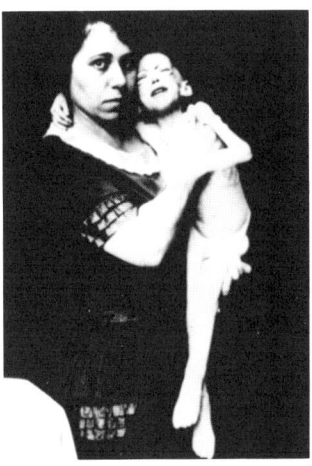

The effects of diabetes and the starvation diet of the pre-insulin era. Photo courtesy of the Joslin Diabetes Center.

not stand alone and her vision was blurred. Diagnosed as having diabetes, she took her first shot of insulin (U20) in an Ann Arbor, Michigan, hospital on May 15, 1927.

Leona stayed in the hospital for nearly a month, recovering her health and strength and learning how to manage her diabetes. She felt lucky to have

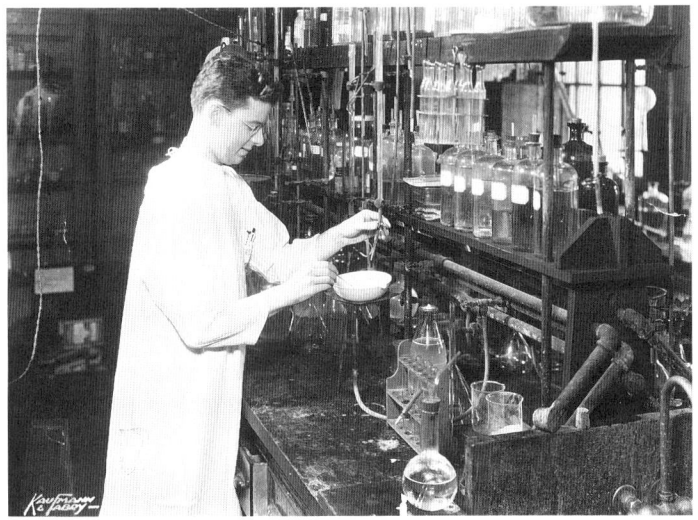

This young researcher, Randall G. Sprague, was one of the first Americans with diabetes to receive insulin therapy in the early 1920s. He began his research in the early 1930s and, in 1953, would become the twelfth President of the American Diabetes Association.

such an association, he said, was obvious: In 1940, the mortality rate of people with diabetes was approximately equal to that of people with tuberculosis, but the number of people with diabetes far exceeded the number of people with tuberculosis. Dr. Striker noted that there had been an invitation to join forces with the Tuberculosis Association. Members of the Tuberculosis Association felt that the establishment of a new organization would drain funds from their efforts. In the economic climate of the times, this was a cause of some concern. However, after deliberation, the delegates decided to reject this offer because the group felt that the problems of diabetes were too urgent: Diabetes needed its own forum.

Each member present was called upon to speak either for or against the formation of a national diabetes organization. All but one spoke in favor.

Charles F. Bolduan, M.D., assistant health commissioner of New York City, and an ardent supporter of the idea of a national diabetes association from the beginning, suggested that in order to be effective the organization should:

- Publish a report (monthly, bimonthly, or quarterly) of diabetes-related activities throughout the country.

- Make press releases available to the local diabetes societies for distribution to the local media, and maintain a file of information on all aspects of dia-

a doctor who "was way ahead of his time in dealing with diabetes. Unfortunately, he followed the nutritional thinking of the day, which said that someone with diabetes could not tolerate carbohydrates. He prescribed a high-fat diet," Leona said.

"At every meal, I had 30 grams of butter and 100 grams of whipping cream. Each week I ate a quart of whipping cream," she recalled. "I used a teaspoon to eat my vegetables, which were swimming in butter." Her doctor told her not to drain the fat from bacon, but to eat it.

Leona was allowed no bread, no milk, and no starchy foods. She was allowed a serving of fruit, 60 grams of meat, and some vegetables each day. For a snack, Leona ate agar, "which looks a little like fish scales. I put it in hot water with a little food coloring and saccharin, the only nonsugar sweetener available. The agar hardened like gelatin. With whipped cream on top, my snack was complete."

Diet wasn't the only ordeal; diabetes care was difficult as well. She used Benedict's solution to test her urine, four or more times a day. "I measured one inch of this blue liquid in a test tube and put in five drops of urine. I placed the test tube in a tin cup of water, which I boiled for five minutes. If there was no sugar, the solution stayed blue."

She took four injections a day. Her syringes were glass, with stainless steel needles. "They were heavy and needed to be boiled after each use, along with the syringes," Leona recalled. "I kept a fine wire to put into the needles to unclog them. But even that did not always help. Everything I needed to do was very time-consuming."

betes so that the association could supply authoritative information to newspapers upon request.

- Assist local groups in the organization of meetings on diabetes, and make films, slides, posters, leaflets, and perhaps speakers available to them.
- Prepare leaflets, both for physicians and for the public.
- Assist local and state groups in securing legislation favorable to people with diabetes.
- Subsidize clinical, laboratory, statistical, and sociological research by competent investigators.
- Study the problem of supplying insulin and prostheses to people with diabetes.
- Organize, in cooperation with local groups, studies to determine the prevalence of diabetes in various age, sex, and other groups.
- Encourage the establishment of summer camps for children with diabetes and assist with organization and management.
- Enlist the support of insurance companies and foundations in the diabetes work carried on by the association and its affiliates.

Dr. Bolduan's suggestions stemmed from his experience with the New York Diabetes Association, which was carrying out most of these activities at that time. His recommendations were unanimously accepted, and it is interesting to note that most of these quickly became key ADA programs that continue to thrive.

The vote to establish a national diabetes association passed unanimously. Dr. Striker, as chairman, appointed three committees. Each committee was asked to draft a report for the next meeting. These reports were to address: 1) purpose and scope of the organization, 2) constitution and bylaws, and 3) funding. Dr. Mosenthal suggested that the association be known as "American" rather than "National" so as not to exclude the many interested Canadian physicians—there being no similar organization in Canada. In this way, the Association would also pay tribute to the country where insulin was discovered. His suggestion was readily accepted, and the American Diabetes Association was born.

Laying The Foundation

In the spring of 1940, Hitler's armies marched across

The Discovery of Insulin

The discovery of insulin is one of the most dramatic events in medical history. Insulin would save millions of lives throughout the world.

In the early years of the twentieth century, researchers such as George Ludwig Zuelzer, M.D., in Germany, E. L. Scott, M.D., in the United States, and N.C. Paulesco, M.D., in Rumania, realized that diabetes was linked to the "internal secretion" of the pancreas and came close to isolating the substance.

In 1921, Frederick Banting, M.D., a Canadian surgeon, had

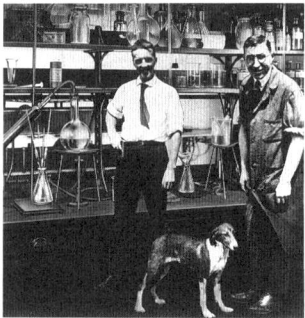

Student assistant Charles H. Best (left) with Dr. Frederick Banting, August 1921, superimposed on photo of their laboratory.

an idea for obtaining the pancreatic extract. Although skeptical, J.J.R. Macleod, professor of physiology at the University of Toronto, provided Dr. Banting with laboratory space at the University and assigned him a student assistant—Charles H. Best. Best had just completed the University's physiology and biochemistry course.

In May 1921, Banting and Best began their search for the pancreatic substance that would be safe and effective in the treatment of diabetes. Through the summer, they tried numerous experiments and eventually produced an extract that reduced blood-glu-

Europe. In the United States, the mood was isolationist; Americans hoped that war would not reach their shores. Franklin Roosevelt was elected to an unprecedented third term as president of the United States. That same year, penicillin was developed and subsequently saved the lives of thousands of civilians and soldiers during World War II.

The times were not the most favorable for launching a new enterprise, but the founders of the American Diabetes Association were undeterred. On June 11,

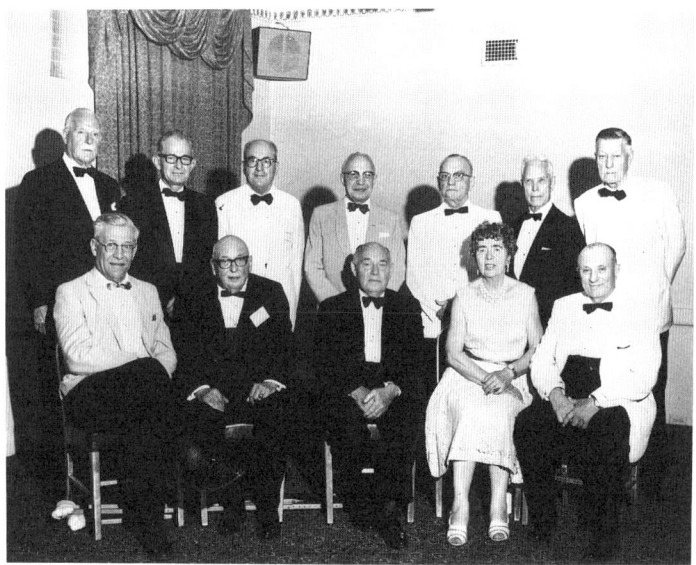

Founders of the American Diabetes Association. Seated, left to right, Frederick W. Williams, M.D.; J. West Mitchell, M.D.; Edward Tolstoi, M.D.; Mrs. Charles F. Bolduan; and George E. Anderson, M.D. Standing, left to right, Beverly Chew Smith, M.D.; George C. Thosteson, M.D.; Cecil Striker, M.D.; William S. Reveno, M.D.; Paul F. Polentz, M.D.; C.B.F. Gibbs, M.D.; and Joseph T. Beardwood, Jr., M.D.

1940, the group met in New York City at Schrafft's Restaurant at 46th Street and Fifth Avenue. By this time, their number had grown from 12 to 26. Those founding physicians include: Cecil Striker (chairman), of Cincinnati; I. Arthur Mirsky and Willard Wallenstein, of Cincinnati; Sidney Adler and Samuel S. Altshuler, of Detroit; Herman O. Mosenthal (secretary), Benjamin I. Ashe, Charles F. Bolduan, Frank B. Cross, Beechman J. Delatour, George E. Anderson, Herbert Pollack, Philipp J.R. Schmahl, Ralph Scott, Beverly Chew Smith, Edward Tolstoi, and Frederick W. Williams, of New York City. From Pennsylvania: George F. Stoney, Erie; Anna O. Stephens, Laurelton;

cose levels in dogs whose pancreases had been removed.

"We made dogs diabetic by taking out pancreases," wrote Dr. Best. "The dogs reacted like a child with diabetes. Very severe. They lived only a week or ten days. Then we began to experiment with extracts from pancreases. The dogs got well and frisked about the laboratory and stayed alive as long as we gave them insulin."

Banting and Best reported the results of their studies in November 1921. The first published report of their findings appeared in December 1921 in the *American Journal of Physiology*.

Banting and Best were joined in their research by biochemist James B. Collip, who had been recruited by Macleod. In a matter of weeks, Collip came up with a formula for purifying the extract and making it a usable product. This purified version of the "internal secretion" of the pancreas—eventually called insulin—made control of diabetes clinically possible.

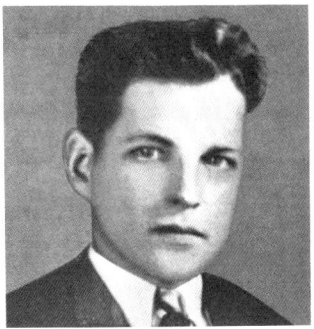

Leonard Thompson, the first person to receive an injection of insulin, January 11, 1922.

On January 11, 1922, the first patient was treated, but not until after the insulin was tested by Banting and Best. "We gave each other good, big

Joseph T. Beardwood, Jr., Philadelphia; Joseph H. Barach, Pittsburgh; Paul F. Polentz, Scranton; J. West Mitchell, Sewickley; and Belford C. Blaine, Joseph N. Ganim, and Charles M. Levin, whose cities are unrecorded. Two doctors who helped in the founding of the Association but who did not attend the June 1940 meeting were E.S. Dillon, of Philadelphia, and William Muhlberg, of Cincinnati, of whom Dr. Striker said, "Without their counsel, work, and inexhaustible enthusiasm, ADA might never have been established."

William Muhlberg, M.D., served as treasurer of the Association from 1940 to 1948. As the medical director of the Union Life Insurance Company of Cincinnati, he procured for the fledgling organization its first corporate contribution—$500—from his employer. Eli Lilly and Company followed with a gift of $1,000 a year for the first three years. These two contributions comprised the Association's budget. Coming on the heels of the Great Depression, these contributions reflected favorably on the integrity of the founders, the esteem with which they were regarded, and the generosity of American industry toward the advancement of a worthy cause.

At that first meeting, a tentative Constitution and Bylaws were presented and adopted, pending legal approval. The Constitution was written by E.H.L. Corwin, Ph.D., secretary of the New York Academy of Medicine and an active member of the New York Diabetes Association. After the founders adopted the Constitution and it had passed through the appropriate legal scrutiny, the American Diabetes Association was formally incorporated in Ohio as a nonprofit organization. The date was August 28, 1940.

The Constitution (Appendix 1) clearly states the founders' vision of the American Diabetes Association: its purpose and objectives, political structure, committees, meetings, and membership.

It is clear from the Constitution that the Association was conceived as an elite professional organization of physicians, identified as "active" members. In the early years, members paid $2 annual dues. Membership requirements were stringent; new applications, as well as requests for reinstatement, had to be approved by the Executive Committee.

Although the Constitution also provided for associate, honorary, and corporate members, the founders limited the scope of these memberships considerably for nearly 30 years. In fact, after hearing a report in 1942 that associate membership (non-physician health professionals) had reached 23, the Board of Trustees

injections first, and it was safe," recalled Dr. Best. The first patient to receive insulin was a 14-year-old boy, Leonard Thompson. Thompson, a Canadian, had suffered from "severe" diabetes for two years, and was surviving on the "starvation" diet prescribed for diabetics at the time. Insulin saved his life.

In the spring of 1922, Banting, Best, and Collip "lost" the formula for insulin and were unable to make any more. How could they have lost the formula? The members of the group did not keep clear records. They were performing delicate procedures with crude equipment, inexact temperatures, unclear methods, and chemical unknowns.

Through the spring of 1922, Banting, Best, and Collip worked frantically to reproduce the formula. They eventually succeeded. A patent on the insulin-making process was applied for in the names of Best and Collip, who immediately assigned the patent to the University of Toronto.

On May 3, 1922, Macleod, speaking for Banting, Best, Collip, and himself, announced that the group had isolated and purified an extract of the "internal secretion" of the pancreas. But the team at Toronto could only make very small amounts of insulin. Connaught Laboratories, in Toronto, was able to make a small amount of insulin. But the Eli Lilly Company, of Indianapolis, Indiana, in a special agreement with the University of Toronto, was the first to produce insulin commercially.

In 1923, the Nobel Prize in Physiology and Medicine was awarded to the discoverers of insulin. But the award was given to Banting and Macleod, not Banting and Best. Macleod's being named a discov-

agreed "not to actively seek associate members." It was not until 1970 that these positions were relaxed.

The Constitution also provided for the annual appointment of committees by the president (Article VI). The three standing committees were nominating, finance, and membership. (The committees are a good indicator of the Association's modest needs at that time.) It was also stipulated that special committees with any particular purpose could be appointed by the president with the approval of the Council, which was the forerunner of today's Board of Directors. Over the years, the number of national committees grew; this growth in the number of committees is cyclical and varies with the Association's needs. Although committees can slow the administrative process, over the years they have provided a democratic forum in which the voices of many are heard, thus enriching the scope of the Association's work.

To allow for the growth and development of the American Diabetes Association, the Constitution stated that Bylaws may be altered, amended, or repealed by a two-thirds vote of the members of the Council. This provision (Article VIII) has been invoked many times over the years. In fact, scarcely a year has passed in which there has not been some amendment to the Bylaws.

With the Constitution and Bylaws approved, the members proceeded to the election of officers. Because he had been the primary force in the founding of the Association, Cecil Striker, M.D., was elected president by acclamation. Other officers selected were First Vice-President Herman O. Mosenthal, M.D.; Second Vice-President Joseph T. Beardwood, Jr., M.D.; Secretary Samuel S. Altshuler, M.D.; and Treasurer William Muhlberg, M.D.

Because of his outstanding contributions to the study of diabetes, Elliott P. Joslin, M.D., a senior figure in the field of diabetes at home and abroad, was invited to become honorary president. Frederick G. Banting, M.D., and Charles H. Best, M.D., were also named honorary presidents.

Councilors (Council members) elected were Joseph H. Barach, M.D., of Pittsburgh; Edward Dillon, M.D., of Philadelphia; Seale Harris, M.D., of Birmingham; Henry John, M.D, of Cleveland; Lewis H. Newburgh, M.D., of Ann Arbor; Louis B. Owens, M.D, of Cincinnati; James E. Paullin, M.D. of Atlanta; W.D. Sansum, M.D., of Santa Barbara; James. R. Scott, M.D., of New York City; H. Clare Shepardson, M.D., of San Francisco; Russell M. Wilder,

erer of insulin caused some controversy. He had been away on vacation throughout the discovery period and did not participate in the actual research, while Best, who had worked with Banting from the beginning of the project, received no prize. Collip, who developed a clinically safe and usable form of insulin, also received no prize. However, Banting shared his half of the prize with Best, while Macleod shared his portion with Collip.

Coping With Diabetes In The 1930s
Looking back at nearly 60 years with diabetes, Luise Degraffenried of Bartlesville, Oklahoma, remembered the early symptoms of type I diabetes.

"I was tired, hurting, urinating often, and not gaining any weight," she said. But her parents believed she was growing taller and that everything was normal.

In 1932, Luise became extremely ill. Her parents took her to the family doctor, who gave her "some thick, sweet 'pick me up' and sent us home."

Luise became comatose several days later and was taken to Children's Mercy Hospital in Kansas City, Missouri. "I awoke from the coma and was told I had been asleep for three days," Luise recalled. "I didn't know where I was nor where my parents were. The nurse told me I was in the hospital and had diabetes."

Each day, Luise was taught to check her urine sugar. She used an alcohol lamp to boil 5 cc of Benedict's solution with drops of urine. While Luise was learning about insulin injections, diet instructions, and testing her urine for sugar and ketones (all by Dr. Elliott P. Joslin's method), her mother

M.D., of Rochester, Minnesota; Frederick W. Williams, M.D., of New York City; and R.T. Woodyatt, M.D., of Chicago.

ADA Goes Into Action

On December 7, 1940, one year before the bombing of Pearl Harbor, the new officers met to plan for the first Annual Meeting and to discuss how best to introduce the new organization to medical societies and individual physicians. They could not decide whether to approach the American College of Physicians (ACP), which had been the spawning ground for the idea, or the larger and more prestigious American Medical Association (AMA).

The matter was settled rather fortuitously when Dr. Striker met with Dr. Morris Fishbein, editor of the *Journal of the American Medical Association (JAMA)*, to acquaint him with the plans for the new association. Dr. Fishbein was most enthusiastic, saying, "There is a real need for such an organization, and its formation is long overdue." He readily agreed to announce the formation of the American Diabetes Association in *JAMA*, thus giving it the unofficial blessing of the AMA. Heartened by Dr. Fishbein's cooperation, Dr. Striker asked his advice on a location for the first Annual Meeting. Without hesitation, Dr. Fishbein suggested that the American Diabetes Association hold its meeting Sunday, June 1, 1941, in Cleveland, Ohio—one day before the opening of the annual AMA Convention. This, he said, would ensure the American Diabetes Association a larger audience and would simplify the arrangements. Dr. Striker and the ADA officers eagerly accepted this offer.

In the meantime, formal announcements of the founding of the American Diabetes Association appeared in *JAMA*, as well as the *Archives of Internal Medicine*, *Science*, the *Annals of Internal Medicine*, and the *Journal of the Canadian Medical Association*, as well as many local medical publications throughout the United States and Canada. By February 1941, invitations to join the new association were mailed to more than 1,200 physicians in the United States and Canada. On May 9, invitations were extended to a group of 275 surgeons. This latter list was prepared by Beverly Chew Smith, M.D., a leading surgeon and diabetes specialist in New York City. In 1985, Dr. Smith recalled that he had been shocked by the high numbers of diabetic amputees that he saw during his residency and internship. It was this experience, he said, that led him to devote a major part of his practice to this prob-

also had to come to the hospital daily for instructions about diabetes care.

"I boiled my syringes in a pan and then kept them in alcohol," Luise said. She eventually got a porcelain sterilizer. Although it was very small, the sterilizer "was better than the pan and alcohol." Luise used regular and protamine zinc insulin, but had problems with insulin reactions. She said she often passed out and had to be taken back to the hospital.

Meal planning was also difficult. "Everything I ate was weighed on a scale," Luise said. "Mother made bread out of thrice-washed bran flakes. If I was hungry, I ate sauerkraut boiled three times (with changes of water each time). This was bulk food." Luise also remembered having gluten bread, using mineral oil to fry eggs, making candy with agar, and using saccharin.

At school, Luise's teachers couldn't tell when she was having a hypoglycemic reaction. "One day in high school I slept through three hours of school and my fourth hour teacher finally realized I had a problem," she said. Nonetheless, Luise graduated from high school in 1939. These were Depression years. With the help of the school nurse, the vocational rehabilitation program sent Luise to college.

"I wanted to be a registered nurse but no college would accept me because of diabetes," she recalled. A doctor who had treated Luise often recommended that she become a medical technologist. Luise applied, but again was rejected because of diabetes. Luise said the doctor convinced St. Luke's Hospital in Kansas City to accept her for an internship. Luise graduated in April 1943 and passed her national registry in October 1943.

lem. This was the Association's first membership drive; as a result of this effort, 400 applications were received. All who applied and were accepted in 1941 became charter members of the American Diabetes Association.

The first Annual Meeting of the American Diabetes Association was held June 1, 1941, in Cleveland, at the Hotel Hollenden. Approximately 250 ADA members attended. The issues addressed and resolved were few compared with today's ADA meetings, but they were issues that answered the basic needs of the time: setting the amount of dues, publishing a scientific journal, and establishing relationships with other associations and groups. According to the minutes, the Council decided to:

- Set dues at $2 per year for associate members—the same amount as active members;

- Appoint one committee to investigate publishing a journal and another to work on cooperative ventures with The American Dietetic Association;

- Commend the Metropolitan Life Insurance Company for its offer to develop a public diabetes education campaign; and

- Accept a $500 grant from the Union Life Insurance Company of Cincinnati, for the purpose of publishing the proceedings of the first Annual Meeting.

Dr. Striker's introductory remarks outlined the purpose of the new association and its immediate concerns. "The patient suffering from the syndrome of diabetes mellitus is the reason for the existence of this Association. His medical, social, and economic problems are our problems. Since he represents one of a group, consisting of almost three-quarters of a million similar individuals, the enormity of these problems becomes obvious. Since the incidence of diabetes and the mortality from this disease are increasing in spite of modern developments in medicine and surgery, a concerted attack on diabetes is essential. Hence, it is fitting that an organization should exist where both formal and informal examination of these problems can be made by individuals coming together from all parts of the country. For this reason we have opened our membership to all medical specialties. The association will be a forum for the interchange of ideas, it will foster discussion, help to alleviate problems, and promote the welfare of the patient. The areas of immediate concern facing us are: tables of uniform food

The First American To Receive Insulin

James Havens, Jr., was the first person in the United States to receive insulin. Along with his doctor, John Williams of Rochester, New York, Havens was part of an exciting time in medical history.

Before May 3, 1922, a diagnosis of diabetes was usually a death sentence. Doctors could only watch helplessly as their patients sickened, slipped into comas, and died. The only treatment—near starvation—merely managed to prolong the patient's life for a few more years of suffering.

Everything changed when J.J.R. Macleod, M.D., made his dramatic announcement in the spring of 1922. He and three colleagues at the University of

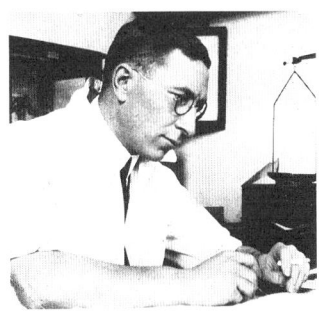

Frederick Banting, M.D.

Toronto—Frederick Banting, M.D., biochemist James Collip, and student assistant Charles Best—had succeeded in isolating and purifying an extract of the "internal secretion" of the pancreas. The men called their discovery "isletin," but it was soon known far and wide as "insulin": a Latin derivative of the word "island."

At first, only small amounts of insulin could be produced. Its quality was uneven; its purity was questionable.

None of that mattered to James Havens, Jr. At 22, he

analysis and dietary procedures, various therapeutic agents, the rising mortality from diabetes, education of the laity, and postgraduate training of the physician."

Charles H. Best, M.D., of Toronto delivered the keynote address. As the co-discoverer of insulin, an eminent figure in the field of medicine and diabetes, and a hearty supporter of the new organization, his presence added luster and distinction to the occasion. (Dr. Frederick Banting, knighted in 1934, died in 1941 on his way to the United Kingdom. The plane he was in crashed in Newfoundland, and Banting died before help arrived.)

Elliott P. Joslin, M.D., delivered the first Banting Memorial Address. At the time, Dr. Joslin had reserva-

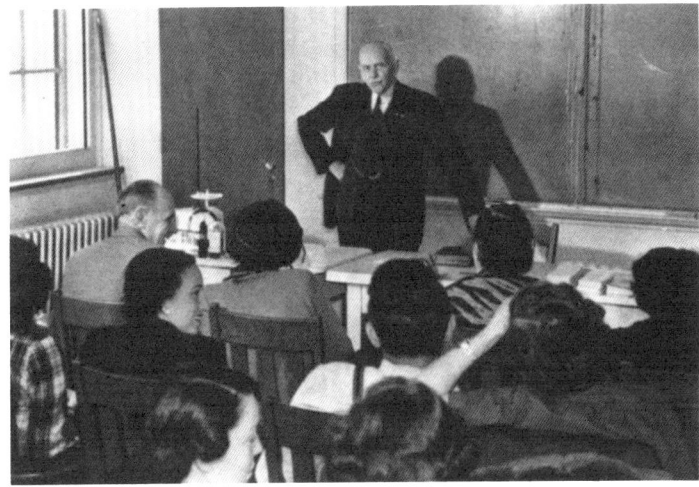

Elliott P. Joslin, M.D., founder of what today is the Joslin Diabetes Center.

tions about the idea of a national diabetes association. However, his address, "Diabetes, Yesterday, Today and Tomorrow," was especially well received and he joined the cause. Thereafter, he became a staunch supporter, ardent worker, and respected member of the American Diabetes Association. He served as an honorary president from 1940 until his death in 1962.

Five medical and scientific papers were also presented at this meeting. The topics reflected the stage of research and treatment of diabetes 20 years after the discovery of insulin.

"The Prevention of Diabetes," by Charles H. Best, M.D., and R.E. Haist, M.D., Toronto, Canada, presented a visionary idea, saying, "Early diagnosis is a clinical problem about which much needs to be done . . . . We do not see diabetes until most of the islet

weighed 73½ pounds and lived on 820 calories a day. He was dying; he knew it, and so did Dr. Williams.

Dr. Williams had doubts about insulin, but was willing to try anything to save Havens. In desperation, he went to Toronto and personally asked Dr. Banting for some insulin.

There was none. But Banting promised Dr. Williams some soon, and in May 1922, a small vial of the precious elixir found its way across the Canadian border to Rochester. A Pullman porter secretly carried it past customs, aboard a Canadian National Railroad train from Toronto. Arrangements had been made.

Dr. Williams gave Havens the first injection on May 21, 1922. It didn't work.

Dr. Williams sent for Dr. Banting, who went to Rochester and himself examined Havens. Dr. Banting recommended larger doses of insulin, which Dr. Williams administered.

A day later, Havens' urine was free of sugar. Within two weeks, he was out of bed and walking. From then on, a regular supply of insulin rode with Pullman porters across the border. On occasion, even bootleggers were used to carry the precious cargo.

The first few months were difficult for Havens. The insulin was sometimes unreliable; the injections were painful. By July, Dr. Williams thought Havens was heading for a coma. There were adverse reactions to injections, and Havens' tolerance for the extreme pain of the injections was stretched to the breaking point.

Havens hung on grimly, and in August, when quality insulin began to be produced in Rochester, the worst was suddenly over. Havens improved immediately. His life, which seemed

cells have been injured . . . . This is not a very satisfactory state of affairs. It would appear that one of the great problems for clinicians and experimentalists is to attempt, perhaps by entirely new means, a way to detect the patients who are on the verge of diabetes."

Other scientific papers presented were "The Etiology of Diabetic Acidosis;" "Comments on Nutritional Requirements" (a summary report on the findings of the Committee on Food and Nutrition of the federal government's National Research Council); "Standards of Diabetic Therapy;" and "Avoidance of Degenerative Lesions in Diabetes Mellitus."

From its very beginning, the Association was interested in encouraging the formation of local diabetes organizations. "This implies the necessity of setting up a central office which can act as a clearing house for all problems pertaining to diabetes, so that any group or individual can obtain authentic information concerning diabetes," said Dr. Striker in his presidential address. Indeed, during this first meeting, the Council voted to help "local communities desiring to start a local or state diabetic council" by having the Association "act as a clearing house" of information.

When plans were made for the second Annual Meeting, all agreed that the Banting lecture had been an outstanding success, and, along with Dr. Best's keynote address, had made the meeting an historical medical occasion. By unanimous vote, the Banting Memorial Lecture was established as an annual event, a custom that prevails to this day and is acknowledged as the highlight of the ADA annual Scientific Sessions.

Preserving The Record

The founders of the American Diabetes Association were aware of the importance of publications to a medical society. They were convinced that the Association would change the course of medical history, and they wanted to make sure that these events were properly recorded. It is not surprising, then, that the recommendations of the first Publications Committee called for the publication of the *Proceedings*, financed by the grant from Union Life Insurance Company mentioned earlier, and *Diabetes Abstracts*, a quarterly review of scientific papers, underwritten by a gift from Eli Lilly and Company and edited by Franklin B. Peck, M.D., Eli Lilly's medical director. Within 18 months of its inception, the Association had launched both publications.

The *Proceedings*, published from 1941 to 1950, became the chronicle of the early years of the American

over a few months earlier, had only just begun.

Havens went on to become a celebrated graphic artist. His specialty was woodcuts; he was elected to the National Academy of Design. He married, and fathered two children. For the rest of his life, Havens remained on insulin, and controlled his diet faithfully. In 1960, he died of cancer at the age of 59.

Dr. Williams—the man who saved Havens' young life in 1922—became chief of medicine at Rochester's Highland Hospital. He remained there for more than 30 years, and is credited with starting the first complete unit for the study of metabolic diseases, chiefly diabetes, in the United States. Strangely, Dr. Williams is best remembered today for his expertise with trees, and his pioneering work in the area of milk refrigeration.

Edison: Discovery Of A Different Sort

While in his thirties, inventor Thomas Alva Edison made a discovery he wasn't especially pleased with—he had diabetes.

Edison diagnosed his own case after testing his urine for sugar. He viewed his diabetes as simply another challenge to conquer and successfully treated himself with his own peculiar diet for many years. Not until he was in his eighties was he persuaded to seek medical treatment from several physicians, including Dr. Elliott P. Joslin.

Edison's personal and dietary habits were unusual. He led a very active life, often working around the clock and sleeping as little as four hours a night. He followed a diet that had been used by male members of his family for genera-

Diabetes Association. Its pages reveal the gradual evolution of the Association and its influence on the treatment and understanding of diabetes and its complications during those years. The *Proceedings* cost $1.69 per copy; ADA members were charged only $1.50. Renewal bills were enclosed in members' copies, and this move elicited a 78-percent response, which delighted members of the Council. In addition, free copies were sent to libraries throughout the country. *Proceedings* and *Diabetes Abstracts* were the voice of the Association until 1952, when they were combined and published as the journal *Diabetes*.

Dr. Striker's office in the Provident Bank Building in Cincinnati became the Association's administrative headquarters. The Association allocated $35 per month for salary, stationery, and postage to Ellen Williams, Dr. Striker's secretary. Obviously, much of the work in those first years was performed by volunteers.

Diabetes: A Medical Specialty?

From the founding of the American Diabetes Association, many members expressed the desire that diabetes be classified as a medical subspecialty. They believed this would add prestige to the organization in the eyes of medical professionals and the public. The Council sent a formal request to the Board of Internal Medicine early in 1941. But an official communication received from the Board in December 1941 stated, "After careful deliberation the Board of Internal Medicine voted unanimously to discourage the subspecialty in diabetes." It was the Board's position that while endocrinology might well be qualified as a subspecialty of internal medicine, diabetes was not. The Council was disappointed, and although subsequent requests were made, none were accepted.

(The term "diabetologist," as used today, designates a physician who limits his or her practice to the treatment of diabetes. This individual may or may not be certified by the Board of Internal Medicine in endocrinology and metabolism. However, a physician who is board certified in the subspecialty of endocrinology and metabolism must have had advanced training in diabetes mellitus.)

Duty Calls

On December 7, 1941, Japan bombed Pearl Harbor. This event signalled America's entry into World War II and changed the lives of all Americans. The war could have had a disastrous effect on ADA leadership. How-

tions. The diet—originally conceived in the 16th century—consisted mainly of milk, herring, and green vegetables. By adhering strictly to this sparse diet (low in both calories and carbohydrates), Edison managed his diabetes alone for a half century and did not require insulin until his later years.

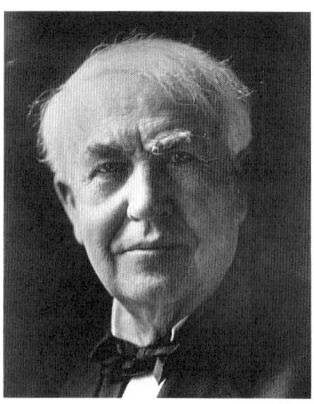

Thomas Alva Edison Photograph courtesy of the Joslin Diabetes Center.

Despite frequent bouts with illness in old age, Edison would invariably recover and return to work. He was 84 when he finally died on October 18, 1931. Cause of death was toxic kidney disease—a possible complication of his diabetes.

ever, the Association's Constitution wisely provided for the orderly succession of officers. Dr. Cecil Striker, the Association's first president, served for one year, then became secretary in 1941, a post he held until 1947. As 1941 drew to a close, ADA members and Americans nationwide prepared to do their part for the war effort.

Pieces Of The Puzzle:
What We Knew About Diabetes

1941

June 1, 1941, marks the date of the first Annual Meeting of the American Diabetes Association. At that meeting, Elliott P. Joslin, M.D., summarizes the state of knowledge about diabetes in his Banting Memorial Address.

"Early statistics of diabetes are inaccurate. Most of the patients lived short lives and died of tuberculosis. But the contrast between diabetic statistics of yesterday and today are sufficiently great, even if yesterday only goes back to between 1898 and 1914, and today includes 1937 to March 1940.

"In the former period, the average duration of diabetes for 326 fatal cases was 4.9 years and the average age of death was 44.5 years. In a recent period, duration has risen to 12.5 years and age at death to 64.8 years, for 927 fatal cases. So few children now die that, in terms of life expectancy, a diabetic child of 10 years first seen by me has an outlook of 40 additional years.

"In the early period, coma claimed 63 percent and in the recent period 3.6 percent. In 1900, diabetes ranked 27th as a cause of death, but eighth in 1939.

"We all recognize that we physicians are much nearer in agreement [about diet] than ever before. A simple, measured diet in terms of bread (3 slices), oranges (3), 5 and 10 percent carbohydrate vegetables (4 portions), milk and 20 percent cream, and cereal (one portion, 30 grams) gives a basis of carbohydrate, 150 grams. I confess that more than ever I believe in a moderate restriction of carbohydrate, not the terrible restriction which was discarded.

"Practically everyone recognizes the values of protamine zinc insulin in protecting the patient. Unquestionably we are on the verge of new insulins. My only fear is that insulins only a trifle better than those now available will confound the general practitioner who really is responsible for the treatment of most of the diabetics in the country. Better our present insulins than the introduction of another insulin only 10 percent superior. . . .

"Education is implied in all that has gone before, because education is necessary for a knowledge of the diet and an understanding of the use of insulin and in the interpretation of reported tests of urine and blood. I never find a diabetic who knows too much . . . . The treatment for most diabetes is simple, and doctors should be encouraged to carry it on.

"Tomorrow's treatment: There must be something like an antidiabetic hormone. Which one of you will discover it?"

At that same meeting, physicians discuss standards of therapy for people with diabetes. One topic of debate is blood-glucose control. Some physicians claim that hyperglycemia is harmless and even beneficial in the absence of glycosuria, or sugar in the urine.

"We do not believe that a hyperglycemia up to 0.20 percent is particularly harmful to a diabetic, provided the urine is sugar free," says ADA President Herman O. Mosenthal, M.D., (1941-42). "The satisfactory control of diabetes should include an adequate deposit of glycogen in the liver, muscles and other tissues, . . . freedom from acidosis, . . . and no dehydration. All these can be accomplished in the presence of hyperglycemia. A high blood sugar, without concurrent glycosuria, is in all probability, of no significance."

Other physicians, such as Dr. Elliott Joslin and his associates, and Dr. Frederick Allen, disagree. They argue that allowing blood sugar to rise above so-called normal levels is dangerous, because, to paraphrase Dr. Joslin:

1) It is an abnormal state.

2) A high blood sugar stimulates insulin secretion and allows no opportunity for rest such as the pancreas of a healthy person enjoys between meals and at night.

3) Hyperglycemia contributes to "a lack of normal tissue repair and resistance to infection, predisposes to degenerative phenomena in arteries and nerves, and leads to weakness, weariness, and impotence, although we freely admit that positive proof is lacking that all these harmful effects are due to hyperglycemia per se." (Dr. Joslin, as quoted by Dr. Mosenthal during the 1941 meeting.)

Julian D. Boyd, M.D., Robert L. Jackson, M.D., and James H. Allen, M.D., write in the first *Proceedings* about the importance of good diabetes control and the need to extend diabetes care beyond insulin therapy alone.

"Though insulin had made it easy for the patient with diabetes to survive, therapy with insulin had such a broad zone of safety that its use tends to encourage a policy of laissez-faire on the part of the physician and the patient . . . The effects of poor control of diabetes are cumulative and terminate in serious complications or sequelae which lead to impaired function or to death.

"A physiologic level of control is one which would avoid any degree of hyper- or hypoglycemia or glycosuria, and which would conserve the sugar handling function in maximal degrees. Presumably if one could accomplish this, all conceivable disturbances of the body due to diabetes would be avoided. Through suitable nutritional guidance and the proper administration of insulin one can work toward an approximation of that state."

The Association does not issue nutritional guidelines for people with diabetes. However, physicians discuss the May 1941 meeting of the Committee on Food and Nutrition, part of the federal government's National Research Council, which had been set up by the National Defense Advisory Commission. The committee's recommendations are: 3,000 calories for men, 2,500 for women, and 3,800 for adolescent boys. (No recommendations were noted for adolescent girls.)

"The 3,000 calories may seem a little high to some of us who have been feeding patients weighed diets," says Russell M. Wilder, M.D. "Some of us feel that a lower caloric intake [of 2,700 calories] is desirable in the treatment of diabetes and feel that our patients are quite as able to carry on with less than with more calories."

The government's Committee on Food and Nutrition gives no attention to the amount of dietary carbohydrate and fat, though both are topics of discussion by physicians attending the Association's first Annual Meeting.

Chapter Two
The War Years
1941-45

ADA PRESIDENTS

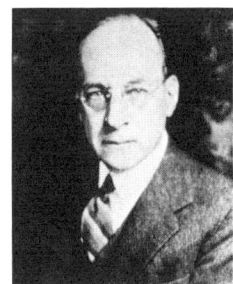 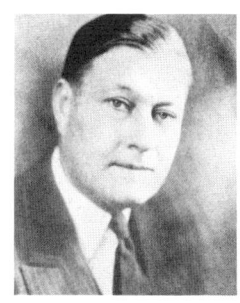 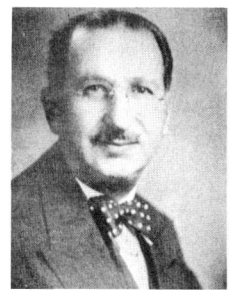

Herman O. Mosenthal, M.D. (1941-42)   Joseph T. Beardwood, Jr., M.D. (1942-44)   Joseph H. Barach, M.D. (1944-46)

With the bombing of Pearl Harbor, young men by the thousands rushed to join the armed services. While men went to war, women went to work in the factories. There were shortages of everyday items; food, clothing, and gasoline were rationed. Travel was curtailed, and priority for supplies was given to the military. President Franklin D. Roosevelt imposed wage and price controls and declared a state of emergency.

All of these events had an effect upon the newly formed American Diabetes Association. Travel restrictions curtailed meetings; paper shortages threatened the new publications; and most important, diminished insulin production and food rationing endangered the health of people with diabetes. Many of the Association's plans and activities had to be postponed, even though they had barely begun.

In June 1942, 200 physicians gathered at Hadden Hall Hotel in Atlantic City for the Association's second Annual Meeting. Attendance was lower than it had been at the previous year's meeting because some members had already joined the armed services. In his opening remarks, incoming ADA President Herman O. Mosenthal, M.D., (1941-42) noted:

"This meeting takes place while the clouds of war are hanging over us .... What have we to do with the all-out effort? Should we not discontinue our activities for the duration? This is easily answered, for we, to whom the medical supervision and guidance of close to three-quarters of a million diabetics is entrusted, should without let-up strive to free them of restrictions, handicaps and complicating diseases, so that they will . . . take their place in communal activities and do their bit in the battle program.

"At present there is no greater issue, national or individual, than winning this war and it is clear that our Association, by bettering and simplifying the treatment of diabetes, and by defining and promoting the employability of diabetics, is rendering a distinct service to diabetics, to our country, and to humanity."

At these early ADA meetings, there were many tributes and accolades to Drs. Banting and Best, the co-discoverers of insulin. As mentioned earlier, both men were made honorary presidents of the Association. Because of Dr. Banting's untimely death in 1941, tributes to his memory became even more numerous. Dr. Striker had a gavel carved from the branch of an oak tree that grew at Dr. Banting's birthplace. As the outgoing president at the second Annual Meeting, he presented the gavel to his successor, Dr. Mosenthal, saying, "This gavel seems a fitting memorial to the person to whom we owe the very existence of this organization." The passing of the memorial gavel remains a tradition at the Annual Meeting Banquet.

Another significant event at this meeting was the secretary's announcement that income tax exemption had been granted to the Association as of January 14, 1942, by the commissioner of Internal Revenue. The Association was advised that any contributions made to the Association would be tax deductible. In addition, the Association was exempted from employment taxes. Bequests, legacies, and property willed to the Association, or for ADA use, were declared deductible in estimating the net value of an estate for state tax purposes.

It was inevitable that the war would bring the Association into close contact with other branches of the federal government. One of the first such contacts was initiated by Federal Security Administrator Paul D. McNutt. As liaison for the War Department, he requested a list of Association members so that he could verify qualified physicians, should they be needed in the war effort. Quackery in medicine was prevalent in the 1940s, and the field of diabetes was no exception. J.J. Durrett, M.D., director, Medical Advisory Division of the Federal Trade Commission, requested that the Association provide him with names of some of its members to assist in prosecuting the manufacturers of diabetic remedies making illegitimate claims. Several members served as expert court witnesses, and Dr. Durrett acknowledged that this cooperation facilitated prosecution in a number of cases.

In the early days of the war, fear of air raids and invasions were daily concerns. "War and the Diabetic," a paper presented by Joseph T. Beardwood, Jr., M.D., at the second Annual Meeting in 1942, described the particular perils facing people with diabetes in the event of a wartime disaster. Dr. Beardwood encouraged each community to arrange for "several depots of insulin that could be tapped by the diabetics in that community if their usual center of supply were destroyed."

Concerns about potential shortages of insulin and needles were taken to the U.S. War Production Board. Fears had been allayed somewhat when the board responded in August 1941, "So far as we can foresee, the supplies of insulin will be adequate to take care of civilian demand in the U.S. This is also true of needles and syringes. While there are shortages, we recognize the extreme importance of these to diabetics, and we have been reassured that supplies are obtainable and will remain so."

In England, the government provided insulin, syringes, and food to people with diabetes. However, there was a serious problem in recognizing people with diabetes among the injured. "Identification of diabetics in a crisis," Dr. Joseph Beardwood declared, "is mandatory." Dr. Striker initiated a system of identification tags so that in the event of a catastrophe in the United States, people with diabetes would receive prompt and appropriate medical treatment. It was expected that this program would be implemented by local governments. But while there was an exchange of correspondence between the American Diabetes Association and the Office of Civilian Defense, no action was taken. Ultimately, identifications tags were provided by Eli Lilly and Company.

Not all countries were as fortunate as England and the United States in being able to provide diabetes supplies. In September, 1942, ADA Secretary Cecil Striker, M.D., received a desperate communication from Juan A. Pons, M.D., chief of medical services, Presbyterian Hospital in Puerto Rico: "Due to circumstances beyond our control all shipments of insulin have been stopped and our supply is nearly gone. Only the most needy are given insulin and we are seeing many cases of acidosis. We find ourselves back to the early twenties as far as treatment is concerned; 4,000 diabetics depend upon you. Can you help? If you have any suggestions these will be valuable. Use of air mail in replying will be appreciated." The Association apprised the National Institutes of Health of the situation, then contacted insulin manufacturers. An emergency shipment of insulin was sent to the Presbyterian Hospital. This was enough to sustain people with diabetes in Puerto Rico until the normal lines of shipping were resumed.

To help provide physicians and health professionals with information about the diabetic emergencies of hypoglycemia and acidosis, the American Diabetes Association contacted the American Red Cross. The Red Cross agreed to include diabetes information in its first-aid manual, which was widely distributed during the war. Further arrangements for emergency care of people with diabetes in the event of a civilian catastrophe were made with the American Hospital Association and the American Catholic Hospital Association. Emergency diabetes-care notices appeared in their respective journals.

The war efforts of the American Diabetes Association were recognized in 1944, when the Association was elected to the National Health Council (NHC), an organization that coordinates all information concerning health activities. For the Association to be able, so early in its existence, to meet the standards of the NHC was widely regarded as a credit to the vision and management of the initial ADA officers. Membership in the prestigious NHC continues to this day.

Diabetes In The Armed Services

Diabetes was one of the conditions listed in the United States "Mobilization Regulations" as making an applicant nonacceptable for induction into the armed forces. If the condition were discovered before induction, diabetes prevented the applicant from entering the military services. However, if diabetes was discovered after the individual had entered the services, the soldier or officer would be admitted to a hospital for study and treatment. Then the medical officer would decide whether to discharge the patient or to allow him to return to duty.

During 1942, 1,160 members of the Army in the continental United States were treated for diabetes. Of that number, 256, or 22 percent, were returned to duty. In the Navy, during 1942, 336 men with diabetes were treated; 89, or 26 percent were returned to duty.

"From the standpoint of the diabetic, if his assignment is made intelligently, he will be better off in the Service than in civilian life," said Samuel S. Altshuler, M.D., in June 1944 at the fourth Annual Meeting. "As a civilian, it is not always possible for a diabetic to arrange for daily urine examinations or periodic blood sugar tests. For financial reasons, or because of inability to absent himself from his work, the patient does not ordinarily consult his physician as regularly as the doctor would like. . . .

"The diabetic in the Army would undoubtedly receive more nearly ideal attention than he would in civilian life. For one thing, the discipline practiced in the armed services would also apply to the diabetic officer or soldier in following orders for maintenance of dietary and insulin routines,

Despite The Storm, A Time Of Growth

Because of wartime travel restrictions, the ADA Annual Meetings of 1943-45 were cancelled. The Council, empowered to act for the Association, held two meetings per year, and an extraordinary amount of work was carried out by mail and telephone.

In 1943, ADA President Joseph T. Beardwood, Jr., M.D., (1942-44) summarized the work of the Council: "Many of our activities this year have been in the field of public health or social service care of diabetes." In a prophetic vein, he went on to say that he felt a lay group, rather than a professional association, could have better handled the problems the Association encountered. "No group of patients have a greater right to organize and protect their interests than diabetics," he said. "I am firmly convinced that many of the things we tried to do which have met with discouraging delays would easily have been handled by an active and aggressive lay organization." It would be more than 20 years before the American Diabetes Association included lay members on a national level.

During the war years, the Association published an average of eight scientific papers per year. Those not delivered at a meeting due to wartime restrictions were published in the *Proceedings*, which were sent to all members, giving them an opportunity to read both the papers and discussions.

In 1943, the Publications Committee agreed that, henceforth, editorials that appeared in *Diabetes Abstracts* be noncontroversial, with material reflecting the established policy of the American Diabetes Association. The Publications Committee report, signed by committee Chairman I. Arthur Mirsky, M.D., went on to say that more than 100 requests for copies of *Diabetes Abstracts* had been received during the year, indicating a growing interest in the publication.

The rapid growth and development of the Association in its first five years can be measured by the number of committees formed to address the issues of that time. In 1940, there were three committees. By 1945, that number had more than tripled.

One of the new committees, the Committee on Foundation of Local Societies, was directed to develop the Association's philosophy toward local diabetes societies. "It was the decision of the committee that local associations must be independent, and bound to the American Diabetes Association only from the point of view of community of purpose and inspirational guidance. These local associations could be affiliated with

personal hygiene, and frequent examinations of urine and blood. . . .

"With the diabetes well controlled, as it would be under these circumstances, the risk to the Government should be no greater with the diabetic than it is with the nondiabetic."

Not all physicians agreed with Dr. Altschuler. "Is it necessary," questioned Morris Margolin, M.D., "to entail the risk for the patient and for the government that might result in increasing pensions, and so on, just to get diabetics into the armed services? Wouldn't it be wiser to leave them out altogether?"

By the end of 1943, 13 million men and women had undergone physical examinations for induction into the military. Of that number, about 5,500 were rejected for glycosuria (sugar in the urine) and 15,500 for diabetes.

the international aspect of the ADA by being accepted as an affiliate of the American Diabetes Association," wrote committee Chairman George E. Anderson, M.D., in the 1945 *Proceedings*.

In its report, the committee estimated that a total of 62 possible affiliates could be formed and that "with these in place and an appropriate relationship to the ADA, the lot of the diabetic would be vastly improved." The report emphasized that the national organization should do everything possible to assist these groups.

A prospectus prepared by the Committee on Foundation of Local Societies outlined step-by-step procedures for local groups to use in establishing diabetes societies, each of which would be modeled after the national organization. The prospectus provided for the establishment of a "clinical society," incorporated in the state as a nonprofit membership organization, as well as the selection of officers and the election of a board of directors.

Once a clinical society was established, the prospectus called for a parallel "lay society." "Membership in this society would naturally spring from among the patients of the members of the clinical society," stated the prospectus. It should be noted that when the Association was founded, some diabetes societies were already in existence. To some in these organizations, the establishment of a national diabetes association was seen as an unwelcome intrusion into their established territories.

Membership, A Continuing Concern

Quality and control of membership were almost obsessions in the early years of the Association. In 1944, a Committee on Standards For Admission to Membership was appointed. Its report one year later testifies to the elitism that was prevalent at that time. Membership, the report said, should consist of the following categories:

1) Active, open to any member of the medical profession (physician) in good standing, whose interests are or will be mostly in the fields of diabetes or metabolism;

2) Fellowships, open only to members of a specialty board; applicant must have been a member of the Association for at least a period of two years, and have demonstrated qualifications, i.e., teaching diabetes, connected with a recognized diabetes clinic for a period of at least five years, or have contributed to diabetes literature;

3) Honorary Fellowship, or "Master," to be conferred by the Council upon individuals who have an outstanding reputation in the field of diabetes (election to such a position was to be limited); and

4) Associate, open to nonphysician health professionals (mainly dietitians at that time).

The report concluded, "It is the consensus of this committee that from now on a more definite and accurate control and survey be made of all new members." This was not to discourage applications, but to assure that all applications be "passed upon by a proper committee, and reviewed by an admissions committee."

By 1945, total membership had risen to 769, with each state as well as Canada and England represented. This increase occurred in spite of the war and an increase in dues from $2 to $10.

The Council was convinced that insurance companies should become the backbone of the Corporate Membership, because it was in the companies' best interests. In 1942, letters sent to more than 200 corporations yielded 16 corporate members—all insurance companies—enrolled at $50 per year. William Muhlberg, M.D., of Union Life Insurance Company of Cincinnati, and chairman of ADA's Committee on Corporate Membership, said in his report that he felt this was a rather meager response. "The medical directors of insurance companies were for the most part very favorably impressed, but failed to convince their executive officers. In general, the executive officers of insurance companies are not particularly interested in public health or preventive medicine, their chief concern being in the financial and agency branches of the business.

"Strangely enough," his report continued, "it is the medical departments, through favorable mortality experience, that are contributing funds for practically all of the so-called dividends of the mutual companies and profits of the stock companies. It would seem logical to encourage further financial benefits by promoting health activities from which the insurance companies are unquestionably the beneficiaries. There appears, however, to exist a fear that a corporate membership in the ADA would open the way for appeals for contributions from other similar organizations."

By 1945, there were 24 corporate memberships held by insurance companies—a 50 percent increase in three years.

Assuring An Adequate Supply Of Insulin

Though World War II brought a diminished production of bottled insulin, good planning assured most Americans with diabetes of a sufficient supply, according to George H. A. Clowes, Ph.D., director emeritus of the

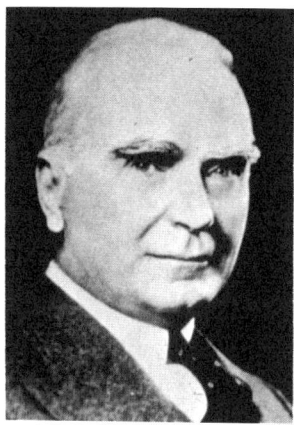

George Henry A. Clowes, Ph.D.

Eli Lilly Research Laboratories. At his Banting Memorial Address at the June 1947 Annual Meeting of the American Diabetes Association, Dr. Clowes talked about insulin during the war years.

"Fortunately, it was realized at an early stage in the development of insulin that in order to safeguard the diabetic, who was dependent for his very existence on an adequate daily supply of insulin, it would be necessary to build up very large reserves to guard against the possibility of a serious catastrophe in the insulin plant or some interference with the supply of pancreas. . . .

"It was very fortunate that large reserves had been built up and maintained during the years preceding World War II. With the advent of the Office of Price Administration (OPA), with every effort concentrated on providing adequate supplies of beef and pork for the armed forces and with restrictions placed on prices, it did not pay the packers to save pancreas and other glands, and their production was consequently greatly curtailed. Furthermore, the very extensive black market operations resulted in a complete loss of pancreas and other glands, since black market operators were concerned only with the production of meat, which could be sold at a high price, and as a rule they had no facilities for the freezing and storage of glands, even had they been interested in saving them. This meant that during the war period and a considerable part of the postwar period our reserves of pancreas and insulin were reduced. President Truman and members of his cabinet were aware of this situation and in announcing

A Story Of Syringes
Dorothea Sims of South Burlington, Vermont, remembers well the difficulties in using glass syringes in the 1940s. "We accepted glass syringes because that's the way it was. We lived in an area where the water was very hard, and eventually, after all that boiling, there would be a cloudy calcium film that rendered the syringe useless. But the greatest hardships were on vacations, which in our family were usually on a sailboat or hiking. This entailed boiling syringes in a rocking sailboat or persuading the 'Mom and Pop general

store' in some small town to let me use their back burner.

"I still have the stainless steel tube with a rubber stopper in which the syringe was stored in alcohol. The rubber stopper always leaked in my knapsack or purse. The greatest skill was required to sharpen the needles on my husband's Arkansas oil stone," she said.

Interestingly enough, the change from the use of the glass syringe to the disposable syringe took time. By necessity, technology had accelerated during World War II, when penicillin required a disposable syringe for use in field hospitals. The syringe used for penicillin was the forerunner of today's plastic disposable insulin syringe, differing in only one respect: The penicillin was sealed into the syringe. The design was refined after the war, and when new plastics became available around 1950, the contemporary disposable syringe with its very fine needle was marketed. When the disposable syringes were first offered, there was no great rush to buy them. Many people seemed wedded to the glass syringe and were reluctant—at least initially—to change.

Dorothea Sims, however, had no objections. "There was no resistance on my part when the plastic syringes with their exquisitely sharp needles became available. The only problem with them was that they seemed very extravagant and, if you were on a trip, they took up quite a lot of space in your luggage, especially if you were on multiple injections," she said. "It took about a decade for health professionals to realize that with minimal precautions, the syringes could be reused several times. This is now well documented and widely practiced."

the discontinuance of OPA controls on meat, the President made special reference to the necessity of reestablishing conditions under which glands would be saved in adequate amount for the production of insulin and other important hormones.

"It will, I know, be of great interest . . . to know that, from the day on which the OPA control was discontinued and the price of glands was raised to a point at which it was profitable for the packer to collect them, our reserves of pancreas and insulin have increased . . . . From the estimated kill of livestock there should be an ample amount of pancreas to meet all insulin needs," concluded Dr. Clowes.

Setting Standards

One issue of great importance—and some controversy—in the early 1940s concerned insulin syringes. To gather information and opinions on all the syringes in use, the Committee on Insulin Syringe Unification surveyed the membership in 1943-44. Its findings revealed that a rather diverse group of syringes were in use:

- 1 cubic centimeter (cc) syringes graduated in units for use with U10 and U20 insulins;

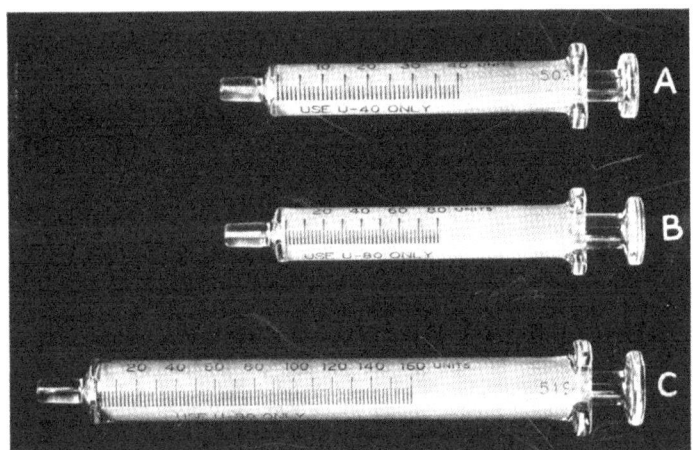

"The American Diabetes Association has designed, approved, and endorsed a new type of insulin syringe. In the past, much confusion and considerable danger has been created because of the multiple types and kinds of insulin syringes offered for sale to the users of insulin," wrote Lester J. Palmer, M.D., in the January 1949 issue of *ADA Forecast*. Dr. Palmer was the chairman of the Committee for the Standardization of the Insulin Syringe and later ADA president.

Life Abroad: Diabetes During The War

During World War II, most Americans with diabetes were kept well-supplied with insulin and other necessities. They received supplementary allowances of rationed food, though they had to turn in their sugar ration, as law prescribed.

Abroad, life was far different, especially in occupied or conquered lands.

Eva Saxl—Czech-born and later a naturalized American—fled her homeland when the Germans invaded. Along with her husband, Victor, she found her way to Shanghai, China, in June 1940.

Shortly thereafter, Eva began experiencing rapid weight loss, constant thirst, and insomnia. A Chinese doctor soon confirmed that she suffered from "the sugar water disease"—diabetes.

"At first, insulin was readily available in Shanghai," Eva Saxl later wrote. But on December 7, 1941, Shanghai was attacked, along with Pearl Harbor. The city fell to the Japanese a day later.

"We diabetics and our families ran around buying up all available supplies of insulin," Eva Saxl recalled. "One Chinese friend secured 18 bottles and generously offered to share them with me, but he died after the first injection." The liquid had been contaminated.

"I bought what I could and paid fantastic prices, up to 10 U.S. dollars for 100 units," said Victor Saxl. "Not any greenback would be accepted; it had to comply with rigid requirements. The money had to be almost new, or better still, just 'out of the oven' without spots or ugly-looking marks from folding; it had to be crisp. If this rigid test was not met, you could not consider it as a 10

- 1 cc syringes graduated in units for use with U20 and U40 insulins;
- 1 cc syringes graduated in units for use with U40 and U80 insulins;
- 2 cc syringes graduated to 80 units for use with U40 protamine zinc insulin;
- 2 cc syringes graduated to 80 units and 160 units for use with U40 and U80 protamine zinc insulin;
- 2 cc syringes graduated in tenths of a cc and minims (a minim is the smallest liquid measure, 1/60 fluid dram, or about a drop);
- 1 cc tuberculin type syringes graduated in hundredths of a cc; and
- 1 cc tuberculin type syringes graduated in tenths of a cc.

Dual calibrations (two different scales, one on each side of the syringe) on many of the syringes and the variety of insulins available served as obstacles to many people with diabetes in getting the insulin dose recommended by their doctor. The most common error occurred when the insulin dose was read on the wrong side of the scale. The most dangerous error occurred when a syringe graduated in ccs or minims was used, misread or miscalculated, and too large a dose of insulin was taken. In addition, instructions on administering insulin were not standardized, and were often haphazard.

As a result of the syringe survey, the Committee on Insulin Syringe Unification recommended that the Association: 1) adopt a standard insulin syringe; 2) limit syringes to U40 and U80 insulin; 3) establish uniform scales for both syringes; and 4) ask manufacturers to promote the use of a "standard" syringe, if and when one is adopted. (It was not until 1949, that Becton Dickinson began production of the standard insulin syringe recommended by the American Diabetes Association. Since then, the Association has continued to work with manufacturers. In 1973, ADA's Committee on Materials and Therapeutic Agents published new specifications. These were adopted universally by all syringe manufacturers.)

The hope that a single daily injection of protamine zinc insulin would be sufficient to control blood-glucose levels in nearly all people with diabetes was not realized. There were many investigations into mixtures of protamine zinc insulin and unmodified insulin, and

THE WAR YEARS

THE OUTLOOK FOR DIABETES IN THE 1940'S

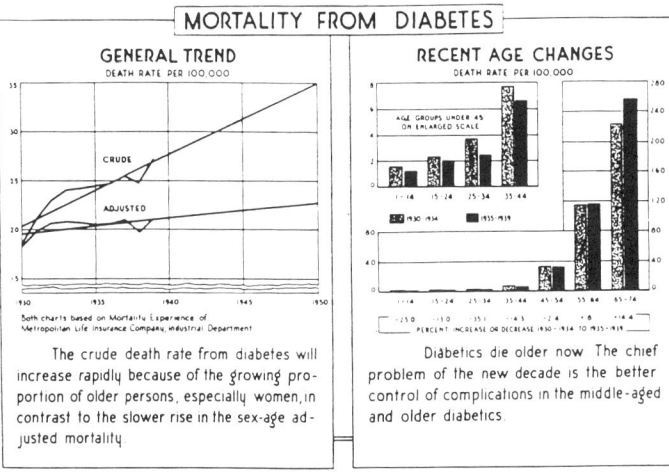

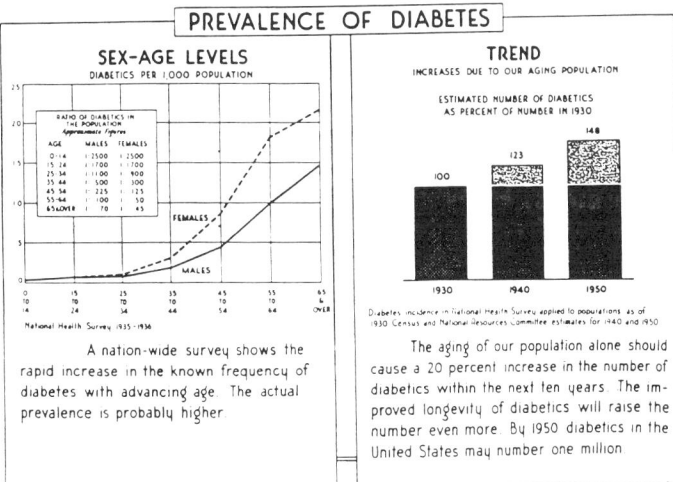

The George F. Baker Clinic of the New England Deaconness Hospital in Boston, Massachusetts, and the Metropolitan Life Insurance Company prepared a series of charts about diabetes, which were shown in 1940 at the American Medical Association and other meetings.

dollar bill; it would be accepted only at a discount of from 3 to 15 percent."

Soon, even black market insulin disappeared, although people were happy to pay for it with one-ounce gold bars. There was no way to get insulin from the International Red Cross.

"To preserve our dwindling stocks, Eva Saxl wrote, "we insulin-dependent diabetics went on carbohydrate-free diets—moderate starvation diets—and injected the least amount of insulin possible. We tried quantities of different Chinese herbs, and I took three entire bottles of German-made Synthalin."

To keep his wife from panicking, Victor Saxl secretly refilled her insulin bottles with water and milk powder, "to make me believe that I had more 'life' left," wrote Eva.

Early in 1943, Victor met with a group of local doctors; he pleaded with them to help him manufacture insulin. They refused, but offered Victor any medical books that referred to the making of insulin. After finding a lab and some primitive equipment, Victor set to work, using rabbits as test subjects.

Eva, meanwhile, became a familiar face at the Seymour Road slaughterhouse in Shanghai. She recalls arriving most days at 5 a.m. "to snatch up the fresh pancreas after any large animal had been slaughtered. We mostly got water buffalo and pig pancreas."

From these raw materials, and through painstaking trial and error, Victor eventually produced a crude but effective brown insulin.

The batches were very small, but they checked out well about half the time. Mr. and Mrs. Saxl shared their treasure with as many other many clinicians made their own modifications in attempt to find a mixture that would provide effective diabetes control.

A report by the Committee on Insulin Syringe Unification showed that there were a number of insulin preparations on the market: unmodified insulin of amorphous origin; unmodified insulin made from zinc insulin crystals; protamine zinc insulin; and globin insulin with zinc. The committee recognized the limitations of each of these preparations and the difficulties involved in mixing them in a syringe. The report emphasized the need for an immediate-acting insulin with "an effect between unmodified and protamine zinc." Such an insulin would make more than one injection a day unnecessary. Needles were not as fine nor as painless as they are today, and there was considerable demand for a single daily injection of insulin, particularly among parents of children with diabetes. The committee recommended that to avoid further confusion the introduction of new insulins be discouraged unless they provided definite advantages over those already on the market.

One of the basic patents on insulin was due to expire in December 1941. Thereafter, it would be possible for any manufacturer to make and sell insulin. From the beginning, The Committee on Insulin of the University of Toronto had zealously controlled the manufacture and distribution of insulin in the United States. The primary concern of the patent holders was to make sure that people with diabetes were provided with safe insulin. The systems of control then in effect did not require the U.S. Food and Drug Administration (FDA) to examine insulin samples for quality. Therefore, the Association acted to encourage Congress to amend the Food, Drug, and Cosmetic Act and require testing and certification of insulin.

Despite Congress's preoccupation with the war, the legislation was deemed very important and was handled speedily. Introduced by Representative Clarence F. Lea on December 14th, 1941, it was presented two days later on the floor of the House. "Mr. Speaker I ask unanimous consent for the immediate consideration of this bill providing for the certification of batches of drugs composed wholly or partly of insulin," said Representative Lea. In explaining the purpose of the bill, he said, "Control of insulin quality by the University of Toronto has been most considerable. That control has been on a non-profit, humane, and scientific basis. It required that all manufacturers comply with standards set up by the Committee on Insulin in order

people as possible. They saved many lives, and no one died from lack of insulin after Saxl developed his formula.

The homemade insulin production continued for three years, until liberation. After the war, the couple left Shanghai aboard a U.S. troop ship and landed safely in San Francisco.

When Eva Saxl wrote her account in the January 1978 issue of the International Diabetes Federation Bulletin, *she had lived with diabetes for 37 years.*

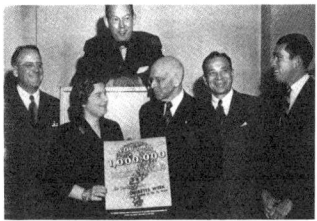

Mrs. Eva Saxl holds the 1950 Diabetes Week poster. Around her are the complete cast of a special half-hour radio show, starring Fred Allen, that was broadcast over the Mutual Network on Friday, November 10, 1950. (left to right) Edward L. Bortz, M.D., past president of the American Medical Association; radio host Fred Allen; Elliott P. Joslin, M.D., honorary president of the American Diabetes Association; Herbert Pollack, M.D., secretary, Committee on Therapeutic Nutrition, National Research Council; and Bill Talbert, famed tennis champion.

to engage in the manufacture and sale of the drug. Control was through ownership of the patent right. When the patent expires, present control will cease and the quality and strength of insulin, so important for users, will be jeopardized. The effect of insulin is such that injury and death may result from taking either too much or too little. Under the amendment to the Food, Drug, and Cosmetic Act, every batch of insulin would be submitted to tests to assure freedom from infection, and purity and strength.''

The bill passed in the House on December 18 and in the Senate the next day. It was signed into law by the president on December 22, just nine days after it was introduced. (By 1953, after more than 10 years of insulin certification, only two batches submitted for testing by the FDA were not certified. This type of control continues to protect insulin users today.)

Also at that time, there was general agreement that there should be standards of treatment for diabetes clinics. However, upon investigation, the Association's Committee on Clinics found that the methods of individual physicians differed in any given clinic and that it would be impossible to formulate standards or regulations. The committee did provide guidelines for minimum requirements in diabetes outpatient clinics. The committee suggested: 1) operating all clinics on a strict appointment schedule to provide adequate patient attention; 2) establishing a social service department in each clinic so that follow-up care of patients would be available; 3) providing laboratory facilities at each clinic for immediate urine analysis, instruction in dietetics, and instruction in insulin administration; and 4) providing additional laboratory facilities for blood-sugar and blood chemistry testing.

With regard to hospital administration, the committee recommended: 1) instruction for nurses in insulin administration, collection of urine specimens, and recognition and treatment of hypoglycemia and acidosis; 2) provision for urine analysis; 3) assured availability of hospital beds; 4) preparation of an outline for a nursing course in diabetes; and 5) production of manuals for establishing and conducting a diabetes clinic for a hospital metabolic unit.

Pieces Of The Puzzle:
What We Knew About Diabetes

1942

ADA members continue to discuss the important role that carbohydrates may play in the diet of people with diabetes. At a round table discussion in June, during the second Annual Meeting at Atlantic City, New Jersey, Dr. Herman O. Mosenthal, chairman of the meeting, poses this question: "What is the optimal distribution of carbohydrates in the meals throughout the day?"

The discussion includes this recollection by Edward Tolstoi, M.D., of New York:

"About 15 years ago we had an opportunity to study the chemical processes of two arctic explorers who were fed exclusively meat for the duration of one year. The diet, as you see, was principally of proteins and fat, and at the end of that time both men were tested with glucose for their tolerance . . . and both responded with a typical diabetic curve, and one with glycosuria (sugar in the urine) as well.

"After the test, both men were placed on an ordinary so-called diet containing a mixture of proteins, fats, and carbohydrates, and two weeks later a repetition of the glucose tolerance curve revealed configurations which approximated those of normal . . . we felt that the improvement in tolerance was due to the ingestion of carbohydrate."

Among the physicians present are Elliott P. Joslin and Charles H. Best, co-discoverer of insulin.

1943

Most of the papers delivered at the third Annual Meeting echo one great concern: World War II.

In his paper, "Some Effects of the War on British Diabetics," R.D. Lawrence, M.D., observes:

"The actual effect of the shock and strain of raids has been in my experience very slight in the many thousands of diabetics I have seen continuously in London. Morale remained high, insulin dosage much the same even in patients who were 'blasted' and rendered homeless, with a few exceptions. Shock and nerve strain are said to aggravate diabetes but I was surprised to note little effect . . . . There was a large increase in gangrene in the cold London winter of 1940-41 from chilling of feet in the cold and damp shelters night after night."

Dr. Elliott P. Joslin notes that the theory that trauma alone can cause diabetes has steadily lost support with increasing knowledge of the nature of diabetes. Evidence shows that trauma can indirectly activate or accelerate the appearance of diabetes in people who are hereditarily predisposed to the disease, especially if the trauma is accompanied by infection, lack of exercise, weight gain, or overeating. Dr. Joslin comments that age, race, positive heredity, and most important, obesity, are predisposing factors in the development of diabetes.

A point system of rationing is instituted on March 1, 1943, under the direction of the Office of Price Administration (OPA).

"As point rationing was extended to include a broad range of meats, fats and processed foods, it became evident that certain groups would require special consideration," according to the October 16, 1943 issue of the *Journal of the American Medical Association (JAMA)*. "Prominent among these were hospitals and those sick individuals whose illness demands rationed foods in amounts greater than that provided by their points . . . .

"Provisions for patients with diabetes mellitus may need to include per week not more than: meat, including fish and poultry, 64 ounces; bacon, 8 ounces; butter or margarine, 16 ounces; other fats and oils, 7 ounces; eggs, 7; milk, adults, 7 pints; milk, children to age 16, 7 quarts; fruits and vegetables, 72 ounces.

"To be eligible to receive any supplementary allowances of rationed foods, the patient with diabetes mellitus must surrender his sugar ration," according to *JAMA*.

1944

Experiments with new insulin mixtures continue. Drs. Franklin B. Peck and John S. Schecter of the Eli Lilly Research Laboratories report on their two-year study of more than 150 patients with diabetes. Their report, while not final, states that after trying many insulin mixtures, conclusions were difficult to draw.

"In the face of such widespread variability in total content as well as distribution . . . of one of the most fundamental factors governing the requirement of patients for insulin—the basic food load—it seems very doubtful that any one standardized modification will ever be capable of providing in a single daily injection the much desired 24-hour control of blood-sugar levels of patients having diabetes of all grades of severity."

Also in 1944, researchers noted that when obese people over the age of 40 are first diagnosed with diabetes, the treatment of choice is dietary restriction. When the diet is restricted to the point of weight loss, elimination of sugar in the urine, and production of blood-glucose levels in the normal to near-normal range, there may be a remarkable return in tolerance for carbohydrates.

1945

More is learned about the relationship between diabetes and heredity. A long-term study by two Canadian physicians—L.S. Penrose, M.D., and E.M. Watson, M.D.—reveals new information and confirms some long-held theories. Among the findings:

- Pairs of brothers and pairs of sisters with diabetes occur much more frequently than brother-sister pairs.

- Parents can be transmitters of diabetes although they themselves are not known to be affected. In the study, such cases are "almost equal in number to those where the parent is known to be affected . . ."

- There is a slight tendency revealed for transmission of diabetes through a like-sexed parent to offspring than for an unlike-sexed parent.

ADA members continue to express concern about the seriousness of retinopathy. "The frequency of its occurrence is increasing steadily in the general run of diabetic patients and especially in the younger age group," said Henry P. Wagener, M.D., at the fifth Annual Meeting in 1945. "It becomes increasingly apparent that something inherent in the diabetes is responsible for the development of the retinopathy. Yet no specific factor has been proved to be accountable and hence preventable or removable."

"There had been a progressive improvement in the treatment of diabetic coma with a continued lowering of the mortality rate," said ADA President Joseph H. Barach, M.D., (1944-46) at the same meeting. "Joslin's mortality rate in a series of more than 100 cases in 1945 . . . was less than 2 percent, whereas in 1914 it was 63.7 percent."

Chapter Three
Detecting Diabetes In America 1945-50

ADA PRESIDENTS

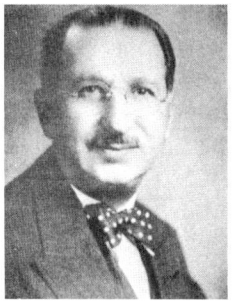

Joseph H. Barach, M.D.
(1944-1946)

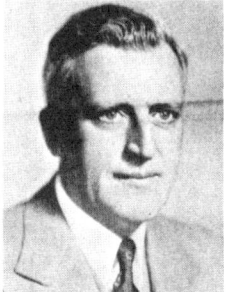

Russell M. Wilder, M.D.
(1946-47)

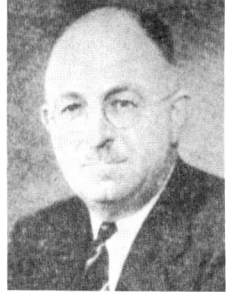

Edward S. Dillon, M.D.
(1947-48)

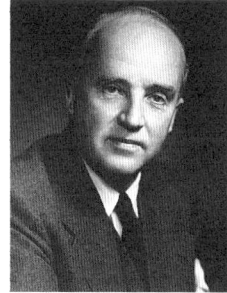

Charles H. Best, M.D.
(1948-49)

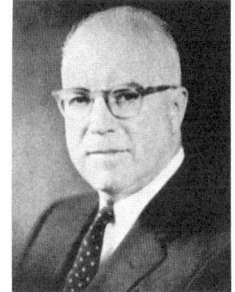

Howard F. Root, M.D.
(1949-50)

In August 1945, the war finally came to an end. There was general rejoicing across the country as men and women returned from distant battlefields. Wartime restrictions were eased, but shortages persisted: Electrical equipment, automobiles, and housing were scarce. As the euphoria of peace faded, it was replaced by a sense of impatience and urgency. People were anxious to get on with lives interrupted by the war. This mood carried over to the councilors of the Association, who were eager to move forward with programs and activities that had been delayed for five years.

Important for the growth of the Association, particularly in its public education programs, was the need for accurate statistics. ADA leaders suspected that while diabetes was often the primary cause of death, it was frequently recorded merely as a contributing cause on the death certificate. Only with accurate statistics could the extent and seriousness of diabetes be documented.

ADA's Committee on Statistical Investigation, established in 1943, was charged with collecting statistics for publication in *Diabetes Abstracts*. The statistics covered current mortality (rate of death from diabetes) in the United States, England, Wales, and Canada, and were based on the then-existing "International List of Causes of Death." Significant morbidity statistics on diabetes were also gathered at this time. (Morbidity refers to the rate of disease or proportion of diseased persons in a given area.)

In 1900, diabetes as a cause of death in the United States ranked twenty-seventh; by 1945, it had advanced to eighth place. Recognizing the magnitude of the problem, the United States Public Health Service conducted the first prevalence study to determine the number of cases of diabetes in a given population. The town of Oxford, Massachusetts, was chosen as the site of the study because of the suitable composition of its population—it was considered to be a "typical" American town. A total of 3,516 individuals were tested for diabetes; this group represented 70.6 percent of the town's population of 4,983.

Diagnostic procedures included post-prandial (after-meal) blood and urine analyses, and, in some cases, standard or modified glucose tolerance tests. Seventy cases of diabetes were found; forty had been previously diagnosed; and thirty were newly discovered. This represented approximately 2 percent of the sample, and assuming the same prevalence rate among the 1,497 untested residents, the actual rate was 1.7 percent of the population. Researchers concluded that for every four known cases of diabetes, there were three undiagnosed cases. This ratio of previously undiagnosed to known cases indicated a prevalence in the United States higher than previously reported by the National Health Survey. From the Oxford Study, Dr. Elliott Joslin estimated there were one million people with undiagnosed diabetes in the United States.

Finding those one million people and gathering comprehensive statistics about diabetes would be two major quests of the Association during this time.

The Discovery Of Insulin Commemorated

In September 1946, the Association accepted an invitation from the University of Toronto to participate in a ceremony commemorating the twenty-fifth anniversary

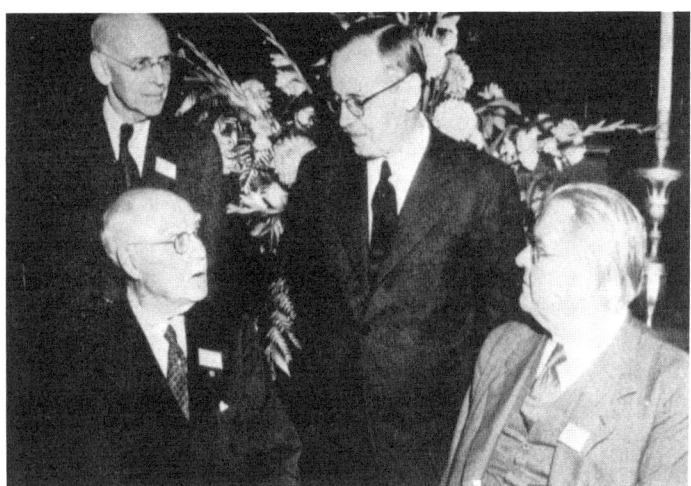

At the 25th Anniversary Discovery of Insulin Celebration sponsored by Eli Lilly and Company in Indianapolis, Indiana, September 23, 1946. Left to right, Elliott P. Joslin, M.D. (standing); J. K. Lilly, Sr.; Bernardo Houssay, M.D.; and Hans C. Hagedorn, M.D.

of the discovery of insulin. The Council's decision to hold the American Diabetes Association's scientific meeting in Toronto at the same time was well rewarded. This first post-war gathering included a large audience of well-known physicians and scientists from Canada, England, Argentina, Denmark, and the United States.

"These anniversary exercises commemorate one of the landmarks in the history of medicine," said Sydney Smith, president of the University of Toronto, in his welcoming address. "If Sir Frederick Banting were with us today, his message I am sure would be that we should carry aloft the torch he held with such distinction and benefaction for mankind."

Premier George Drew, of Ontario, quoted from the Cameron Lecture given by Dr. Banting in Edinburgh in 1929: "It is not within the power of the properly constituted human mind to be satisfied. Progress would cease if this were the case. The greatest joy in life is to accomplish."

Premier Drew went on to say, "Since that day 25 years ago, when first doctors and then laymen, marveled at the discovery of insulin, there has been startling and dramatic evidence of the results of highly trained specialized brains . . . . Minds that can produce insulin and penicillin, and can produce the equally beneficial and destructive elements connected with atomic power, can do almost anything if they have a clear objective purpose. The job of everyone here today is to match those achievements with the science of human relationships, and bring to all people the same clear purpose that culminated in the research we commemorate today.''

ADA President Joseph H. Barach, M.D., (1944-46), then provided a brief description of the Association. ''We are a group of almost 1,000 medical men and allied scientists from many countries, bound together with a sole aim and common cause, to see that diabetes the world over is treated at the highest level of efficiency, in the light of ever-changing knowledge and methods. We realize our responsibility to the over one million diabetics on this continent who have three to four million close relatives and ten million good friends, concerned with their welfare. We cannot stop doing everything possible for this population. To do this, we meet regularly to pry into each other's experience and return to our homes and offices to share this information with our colleagues, so that they can apply it with full benefit to the patient.''

Of Drs. Banting and Best, Dr. Barach said, ''When insulin was discovered, and you had it in the palm of your hand to do with as you liked, when the world would have enriched you with gold beyond dreams of avarice, you insisted that insulin be made available to everyone who might need it, at a minimum cost, and without material profit to yourselves . . . . You gave insulin to mankind, a finished product . . . . You have lived up to the human ideal, that man is indeed his brother's keeper, and for that we honor you today.''

In a special ceremony at the commemorative dinner, Dr. Barach noted that it was a custom of the American Diabetes Association to award the Banting Medal annually to a physician or scientist who has made a significant contribution to diabetes. ''On this happy occasion, and because of the many distinguished guests gathered here, we are departing from our usual custom and are awarding five medals. I am in somewhat of a quandary,'' he said, ''as to the order in which to present these medals, inasmuch as the work of each recipient is equally important, so I have chosen to present them in the order of those who have traveled the greatest distance.''

Dr. Barach presented the Banting Medals to:

The Banting Memorial Medal
The American Diabetes Association bestowed its highest honor on Frederick Banting, M.D., by establishing the Banting Memorial Medal. The bronze medal, bearing the likeness of Sir Frederick Banting, is given annually to a scientist, researcher, or physician of outstanding merit.

The idea of a Banting Memorial Medal was conceived by Joseph H. Barach, M.D., and approved at the Council meeting on February 19, 1944. The Association's highest scientific award, the medal would be presented at the Annual Meeting by the ADA president, after consultation with the Executive Committee.

The Banting Memorial Medal is engraved with the recipient's name and the words: The American Diabetes Association Founded 1940. The medal was awarded retroactively to lecturers and outgoing ADA Presidents from 1941 to 1945 for their contributions to the cause of fighting diabetes.

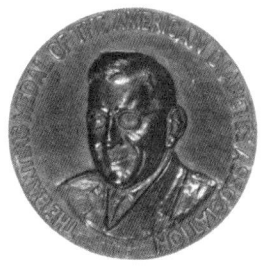

The Banting Medal

- Bernardo Houssay of Buenos Aires, Argentina, for his work on the relation between the pituitary glands of internal secretion and diabetes;

- Hans C. Hagedorn of Copenhagen, Denmark, for his work with protamine zinc insulin;

- R. D. Lawrence of London, "an outstanding authority on diabetes, whose scientific and humanitarian accomplishments are too many to enumerate, and who during the blitz of London stood by the diabetics of England providing and planning for them and seeing them through the war," according to Dr. Barach;

- Eugene Opie who 20 years before the discovery of insulin had written, "Where diabetes is the result of pancreatic disease, injury to the islands of the Langerhans is responsible for the disturbances of carbohydrate metabolism, since that influence which the normal pancreas exerts upon the assimilation of sugar is a function of these structures. There are lesions in the islands of Langerhans in 87 percent of diabetes mellitus," acccording to Dr. Opie; and

- Sydney Smith, president of the University of Toronto, "to serve as a perpetual reminder of the world's great indebtedness to this institution and its service to humankind," according to Dr. Barach.

Twenty-six scientific papers were read at this meeting, eight of which were devoted to some aspect of insulin. Many of these papers included tributes to the discoverers of insulin, Drs. Banting and Best.

Introducing: *ADA Forecast*

Excerpts from the 1947 presidential address of ADA President Russell M. Wilder, M.D., (1946-47) give the first hint of the philosophical struggle that lay ahead for the Association. "We have arrived at a fork in the road. One way to advance would be the training of a highly selected body of physicians, or the other, not so well marked, may take us over rougher territory. Specialist societies have made significant contributions to the medical profession, but can also narrow vision from the forest of general medical experience, to a few small trees. Societies that set the highest standards for admission may sharply circumscribe their effectiveness by their own eliteness. By elevating the standards of medical practice the needs of many may be neglected.

"This places a great responsibility on those of us experienced in diabetes to spread our knowledge to the

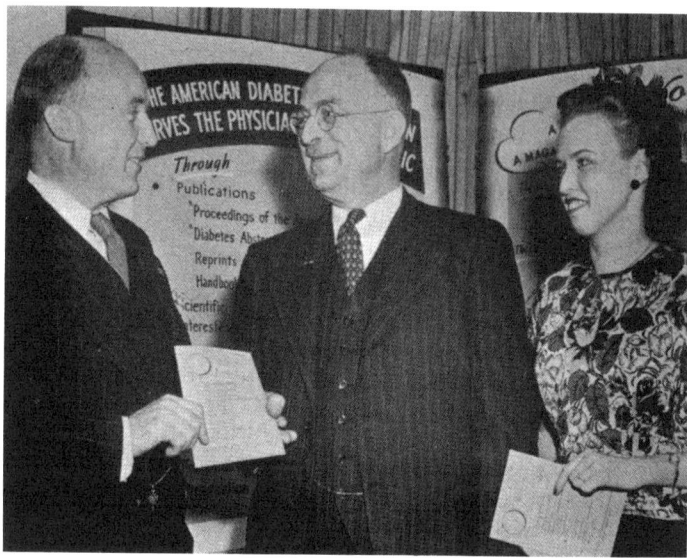

ADA President Edward S. Dillon, M.D., (center) presents the first copy of *ADA Forecast* to ADA Vice President Charles H. Best, M.D., co-discoverer of insulin. Ceremonies were held on December 12, 1947, at the Hotel Russell in New York City. Helen Schildknecht, of Brooklyn, later received her copy to symbolize "the bestowal of the magazine on the million-plus diabetics in the United States and Canada."

Diabetes Detection Drive: The Beginning

The first Diabetes Detection Drive was a direct result of the landmark Oxford Study of 1945. That study revealed three undiagnosed diabetes victims for every four known to have the disease. By 1947, Dr. Elliott P. Joslin estimated that there were one million people in the country with undetected diabetes.

The American Diabetes Association was determined to find those unknowns. At a June 1948 meeting in Chicago, the ADA Council approved a year-round Diabetes Detection Drive (D.D.D.) and targeted December 6-12, 1948, as the first National Diabetes Week.

Its objectives were set forth in the September 1948 issue of *ADA Forecast*: "To find the million unknown diabetics in the United States and Canada and to guide these as well as the many diabetics now forgotten to their physicians for effective treatment."

entire medical community. The questions, shall we remain a select body of professionals or shall we reach out to the general practitioner and the laity, become academic. Through our local organizations, we do reach the local physician and the laity, and through our summer camps the child with diabetes.

"Now we propose to publish a quarterly magazine addressed to the general practitioner and the patient. The magazine will provide, in the simplest terms possible, direction for the management of diabetes. We want to educate the physician in early recognition, diagnosis, and the importance of medical supervision. The diabetic population of the U.S. is estimated at one million, 400,000 of whom require insulin. We can expect support also from our friends in Canada and England in this venture."

Thus, *ADA Forecast* was launched in 1948 with an anonymous gift of $100,000 spread over a three-year period. Elizabeth Mullann was selected as the first editor. She had been the editor of *Diabetic News*, the quarterly newsletter of the Philadelphia Metabolic Association. About 53,000 sample copies and 60,000 descriptive subscription blanks were distributed to physicians, pharmacists, and clinics. The subscription

The magazine called on all its readers to join the cause. In an editorial titled "Calling All Volunteers . . . for D.D.D.," it appealed to the lay readership in strong terms.

"Here is a job which needs your help, too!," the editor wrote. "I am sure that all of you are civic-minded and have been waiting for an opportunity to demonstrate your enthusiasm. Serve as a volunteer worker!"

For the first Diabetes Detection Drive, the rallying cry was "Find them! Teach them! Treat them!" These six words summarized the threefold objective of the Association's call to physicians for coordinated action on behalf of all Americans with diabetes. The words dominated an exhibit prepared by the ADA's Committee on Education that was shown at meetings of national, state, and local medical societies throughout 1948 and 1949. In this way, the Diabetes Detection Drive was first brought to the attention of the medical profession and other interested groups.

As the first National Diabetes Week approached, other groups threw their support behind Diabetes Week, including the American Medical Association, the American Pharmaceutical Association, and various federal health agencies.

Diabetes Week was an outstanding success. Dr. Howard F. Root, chairman of the event, reported "a more successful initiation than we had anticipated." Through the American Diabetes Association, free materials were distributed for potentially carrying out nearly 500,000 urine tests. Around the country, the numbers were impressive: 27,000 tested in Miami, Florida; 38,000 in Dayton, Ohio. The U.S. Public Health Service distributed price was $2 per year for six issues.

In its early days, *Forecast* looked something like *Reader's Digest*. It measured about 5 by 7 inches and had about 30 pages an issue. (In 1974, *ADA Forecast* became *Diabetes Forecast*; in addition to changing its name, the magazine changed its format and size, measuring about 8 by 11 inches. *Forecast* has been in continuous publication since 1948.) A copy of the first editorial (Appendix 5) directed to the physician defines the purpose and audience of the magazine at that time.

Diabetes Detection Efforts

The findings of the Oxford Study, and estimations of one million people with undiagnosed diabetes in the United States, led the Council to pass the following resolution:

"*Whereas*, the number of latent and undiscovered diabetic patients in the U.S. and Canada, has become a matter of growing concern to the members of the American Diabetes Association; and

"*Whereas*, recent surveys by the U. S. Public Health Service and others have disclosed the probable

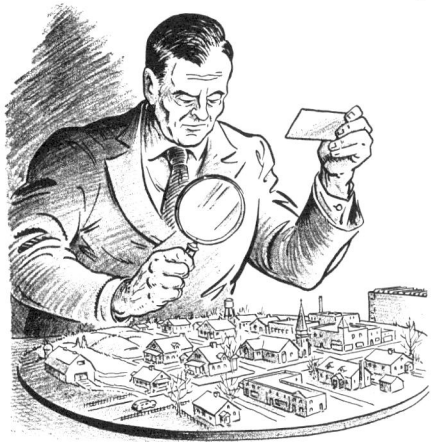

existence of a million or more such hidden cases of diabetes, the Council of the ADA at its meeting in Chicago, June 18, 1948, directs President Charles H. Best to appoint a committee on diabetes detection to undertake the formulation of specific steps to promote the early discovery and prompt treatment of the millions of unknown diabetics in the U.S. and Canada."

Dr. Best issued a challenge to the Committee on Diabetes Detection: "Find the Million Hidden Diabetics." It is interesting to note that this figure of one million rose steadily between 1948 and the early 1980s, when the slogan became, "Find the Five Million" (unknown people with diabetes).

The committee launched a national public aware-

22,000 diabetes radio spots to 1,704 stations during the week. There was heavy publicity in newspapers and over the airwaves.

ADA affiliates played a major role. In the New York City area, for example, the local affiliate established four detection centers, each staffed and run by 60 laymen who served as receptionists, secretaries, and technicians alongside their physicians, who conducted the free tests as members of the Clinical Society.

The success of Diabetes Week assured that it would become an annual event. In 1949, the second Diabetes Week was held October 10-16. Its theme was, "Save A Life: Find An Undiagnosed Diabetic."

Executive Director J. Richard Connelly wrote a story in the November 1950 issue of *ADA Forecast* that reflected the achievements of the Diabetes Detection Drive in three short years.

He said: "The work of organizing Diabetes Week has grown by leaps and bounds, and so have the results. It is estimated that approximately 150,000 people were tested for sugar in the urine during the first (Diabetes) Week in 1948, whereas about a million tested in 1949.

"Today, with the third annual Week upon us, we can report that it is going to be the largest and most effective campaign yet launched. Hundreds of new communities are being brought into the program by local Diabetes Associations affiliated with the ADA or by Committees on Diabetes within state or county medical societies."

In the decades since then, Diabetes Week has grown to become National Diabetes Month.

ness campaign, established National Diabetes Week (December 6-12, 1948), and prepared an exhibit, first shown at the 1948 meeting of the American Medical Association. Dr. Best asked each ADA member to secure 20 subscriptions to the new *ADA Forecast* in order to get the magazine on a sound financial footing and to bring it to the attention of physicians and the laity. Some 22,000 radio spots were distributed to more than 1,700 stations. In addition, the American Medical Association sponsored a coast-to-coast broadcast on diabetes during National Diabetes Week.

The Committee on Detection recommended a twofold program to bring about early diagnosis and treatment for asymptomatic diabetes: an annual urine test for everyone and a blood-sugar test to follow every positive urine test. This ambitious program was augmented by the preparation of a *Handbook for Physicians* printed with assistance from the U. S. Public Health Service (USPHS) and made available to physicians at a nominal charge. Subsequent printing and distribution of the handbook were provided by E.R. Squibb and Sons, whose detail men (salesmen) distributed the book throughout the country. Medical practitioners were urged to make urinalysis routine for all patients and any patients' relatives who might be at risk.

The Council allocated $8,000 to fund the first National Diabetes Week campaign, which was so successful that in 1949, the committee asked for and received $12,000. For this initial campaign, it was necessary to open a temporary office in Boston with a full-time secretary from July 15 to November 15. By 1949, 44 states and nearly 700 communities had participated in National Diabetes Week, and approximately one million people had been screened. Excerpts from a summary of committee records show that the response of the medical community was more than gratifying; public interest and the cooperation of newspapers and magazines indicated wide acceptance of the drive. Newspaper clippings totaled 4,000 and generated approximately 40,000 articles published.

"Diabetes Week was organized to celebrate the first anniversary of the publication of *ADA Forecast*," said ADA Executive Director J. Richard Connelly. "The program, organized and controlled by physicians concerned with detection, could never have succeeded without the enthusiastic aid of thousands of lay volunteers, and who better, than those with diabetes?

"Diabetes Week is a giving week in which physicians all across the country, working through medical

Living With Diabetes: The 1940s

In 1947, William Janz was 10 years old and scared. He was thin and getting thinner. "I had eaten so much food that I should have resembled a balloon, but this balloon had no air in it," he remembered.

"I was so hungry that I'd eat food out of the pan on the stove, yet I was losing weight. I drank water as if we were going to run out of it," he said.

Janz had diabetes. He was hospitalized in May 1947. He still remembers the room number—423A—as his "address" at St. Joseph's Hospital in Milwaukee, Wisconsin.

"What I remember about that address is watching children play, learning how to inject myself with insulin, and learning how to weigh food," Janz said. "My incredible mother must have had a 500-gram headache until years later, when we were told we could stop weighing everything in the diet."

For Janz, the worst part of life with diabetes during the 1940s was canned peas. "Dietitians maintained peas were an important vegetable, and I must have eaten hundreds of thousands of grams of this important vegetable," he recalled. "Dietitians have changed their minds so much about diet that these days people with diabetes are permitted to eat even things that taste good, most of which were outlawed when I was young," Janz said. "I don't mind that, but some things I can't forgive. Like carloads of canned peas."

Besides diet, Janz has seen great improvement in all areas of diabetes treatment since the 1940s. Then, he suffered many

societies and local Diabetes Associations, using volunteer time, energy, and skill, organized an intensive drive to detect, diagnose, and treat as many hidden diabetics as possible. No one was asked for a financial contribution; they were asked only to cooperate, to be tested for diabetes, and the test was entirely free."

Educating The Public

During 1945 and 1946, the national office received and answered about 2,000 requests for general diabetes information. (The number of requests rose steadily until it reached 50,000 annually in 1974, then settled at approximately 25,000 by 1980, as local affiliates and chapters grew rapidly and took over much of this role. By 1989, requests had risen considerably, totaling more than 65,000 a year.)

The Secretary's Report of 1946 suggested that a central clearinghouse of educational material for the laity be established. It was recommended that a committee be appointed to study this question and develop literature that could be used in answering these requests. With the publication of *ADA Forecast* in 1948, this problem was somewhat alleviated, as reprints of articles from the magazine became available. The reprint library became the backbone of the Association's patient education program. There were several attempts over the years by new staff and volunteers to discontinue the reprints and provide more basic information, the assumption being that people could turn to their doctors for more specific information. But these proposals were consistently overruled. People with diabetes wanted specific answers to their questions, and the style and content of the reprints satisfied this need, with the doctor speaking to the patient from the printed page.

In 1949, the USPHS produced an educational film, "The Story of Wendy Hill," for use by local diabetes societies, community councils, community chests, local and state health departments, insurance companies, and public libraries. The live-action, color film was one of the first educational films made about diabetes. It was about 20 minutes long and outlined the symptoms, diagnosis, and treatment of diabetes in the story of a young, small-town wife (Wendy), her family, her physician, and some of the townspeople. The film also debunked myths about diabetes, presented guidelines for living a normal life while coping with diabetes, and discussed insulin therapy. ("The Story of Wendy Hill," a Warner News Inc. production, was presented by the Federal Security Agency, the United States Pub-

times from insulin shock, but not lately. "As a result of blood tests every day, and using the insulin pump, I haven't suffered ... many horrendous shocks recently," he said.

"Diabetes is never easy to live with, but it's a lot easier to live with than it used to be," Janz concluded.

"Just think of all the kids with diabetes who don't have to eat canned peas."

William Janz is a columnist with the Milwaukee Sentinel. *In 1987, he marked his 40th year with diabetes.*

Finding Employment
Employment discrimination continues to be a problem facing many people with diabetes. But things were far worse 40 years ago, before laws and diabetes awareness vastly improved job prospects.

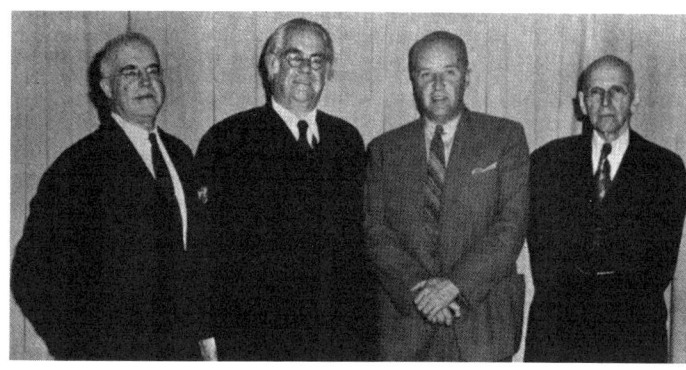

Speakers at a public meeting held in Boston, October 10, 1949, during Diabetes Week. Left to right, ADA President Howard F. Root, M.D.; Hans C. Hagedorn, M.D., discoverer of protamine insulin; Charles H. Best, M.D., co-discoverer of insulin; and ADA Honorary President Elliott P. Joslin, M.D.

lic Health Service, and the American Diabetes Association. The film was produced by Alfred Butterfield, directed by Joseph E. Henabery, and photographed by William O. Steiner.)

In 1950, the Education Committee appointed a Subcommittee on Health Information to make recommendations to the Council on the development and dissemination of information to the public. After a survey of existing materials distributed by insurance companies, it was recommended that the American Diabetes Association develop an inexpensive, basic information piece for wide distribution to respond to the many inquiries the Association received. This effort yielded the booklet, "Facts About Diabetes," which was published in 1950 and distributed until 1975, when it was replaced with the pamphlet, "What You Need to Know About Diabetes."

During the years 1946 to 1950, the Committee on Education became a standing committee. Its primary activity was public education. While a need for patient education was perceived at this time, it was not until 1972 that a patient education committee was appointed.

Fair Employment And Insurance

The concern for fair employment and insurance for people with diabetes has been an ongoing issue in ADA history. In 1948, a newly established Committee on the Employment of Diabetics began to study attitudes of federal and state agencies, large and small businesses, and insurance companies toward the em-

Ironically, it was World War II that first opened many doors to people with diabetes. Disqualified from military service, they ably filled many jobs in industry that were previously closed to them. "To coin a phrase, the war was 'the ill wind that blew the diabetic good'," wrote Claire V. Rider in a 1952 issue of *ADA Forecast*.

It was easier then for people with diabetes to find work with smaller firms than with larger concerns that usually required a physical examination before hiring new employees. Several major firms—such as Metropolitan Life Insurance—slowly adopted more progressive attitudes towards workers with diabetes. Louis I. Dublin, second vice-president and statistician for Metropolitan Life, reflected the changing views when he wrote in the March 1950 issue of *Forecast*:

"I have seen the changes in the health and efficiency of our diabetic employees. There are 92 known diabetics in our active working force at the Home Office. In three out of every five the attendance record is average or better. Our diabetic employees are valuable and experienced workers. The average length of service is 24 years, and about six years since the discovery of the disease. The period of service with diabetes is one-fourth of their working life with the Company.

". . . The diabetic should strive to do better than his fellow worker, because he not only benefits himself, but also helps to break down the prejudice against the employment of diabetics, and thus makes it easier for other diabetics to get and hold jobs," said Dublin.

The federal government was an early leader in the campaign to secure fair employment of people with diabetes. It found that companies having a payroll of 400 people or less did not require a physical examination, and therefore would hire a person with diabetes solely on his or her ability to perform the job. Larger firms, such as the Metropolitan Life Insurance Company and Con Edison of New York, required a pre-employment physical examination. An individual who developed diabetes while employed by a large firm was usually retained and provided proper medical supervision.

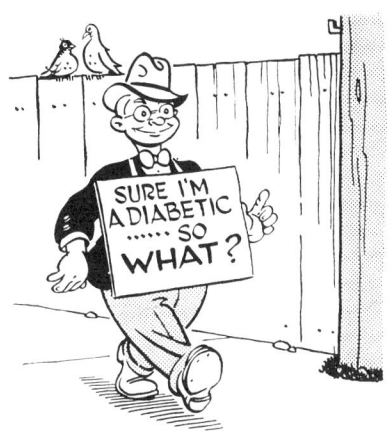

The committee made several suggestions for helping to prevent otherwise able-bodied people from losing out on employment opportunities simply because they had diabetes. Suggestions included:

- Introducing an ADA-designed physical examination form, which would eliminate certain unfair criteria for employment;

- Distributing a manual for employment agencies and prospective employers;

- Establishing night clinics so that workers with diabetes could receive medical attention with minimal disruption to work schedules;

- Conducting statistical studies on the prevalence of disability due to diabetes and the prognosis for the younger versus the older person with diabetes;

- Organizing pressure groups to help see that employers give fair consideration to the person with diabetes;

- Educating workers with diabetes to recognize their limitations, if they exist, as well as encourage them to remain under medical supervision;

ment opportunities for those with diabetes. As early as 1941, the U.S. Civil Service Commission issued a policy statement that, for its time, was unprecedented. In part, the statement read:

"Diabetics who have achieved a reasonable control of the condition are eligible for federal employment with proper placement. Proper placement will be based on the severity of the condition and the medication required for control. Diabetics can more readily maintain a stable control if they are not subject to rotating shifts, or work which requires irregular heavy physical demands. Diabetics should be under the guidance of a clinic or personal physician and should report periodically for physical examination and medical evaluation."

The U.S. government adhered closely to the Civil Service Commission's stated policy. In the immediate postwar years, most state governments and private-sector employers lagged far behind the federal position.

By the early 1950s, the Civil Service Commission was able to publish a list of over 1,200 government positions open to those with diabetes. They were still barred from jobs requiring the operation of a motor vehicle or any moving machinery; they were not allowed to work above ground level in any federal facility.

Much work remained before people with diabetes would even approach equity in the workplace. But the small steps taken in the postwar years would lead to the significant advances that followed.

- Enlisting the help of labor unions and employment agencies; and

- Compiling records of major industries' attitudes with regard to employing people with diabetes.

Medical directors of the Public Health Service Rehabilitation Service and the Industrial Hygiene Foundation reportedly favored this approach as a good way to relax management attitudes toward people with diabetes.

In an article, "Industry and Diabetes," published in *ADA Forecast* in November 1949, John J. Poutas, M.D., medical director of Lever Brothers, wrote, "All diabetics should be clearly told that an individual need not be physically perfect to be capable of employment, provided he is able to meet the demands of the job without endangering himself or his fellow workers.

"Some physicians, and most diabetics are convinced that diabetes does not constitute a vocational impairment. Whatever the truth of the matter, the fact remains that diabetes at present is regarded as a handicap to employment and insurance. It is not only our function, but our duty, as representatives of the diabetics of America to determine the facts, and no longer talk in generalities. We will then be able to furnish accurate information to labor and industry, and guide young diabetics in their choice of vocations so that they will not meet an insurmountable obstacle when they embark on their chosen life's work. The presentation of our case to industry, labor, life insurance companies, and employment agencies has been woefully neglected and is in dire need of forceful promotion."

The formulation of an official policy on employment came three years later and was published in *Diabetes* (Vol. 1:4, 1952) as follows: "It is the philosophy of the American Diabetes Association that controlled diabetics are good, employable risks. They should not be classed with the physically handicapped or crippled, for they are capable of performing a full day's work to satisfaction despite their diabetes." This statement included nine suggested standards detailed for both the employee with diabetes and the employer. This policy prevailed until 1972, when it was revised to correspond to new knowledge of diabetes.

Providing people with diabetes adequate insurance at fair prices was a serious concern. Prior to 1940, it was considered unsafe to offer life insurance to people with diabetes under any condition, according to a 1949 *ADA Forecast* article, "Insurance and Diabetes," written by R. D. Montgomery, M.D., medical officer of

Testing The Exchange Lists
In 1947, Frances O. Hazzard was in the class of interns at New York Hospital/Cornell Medical Center that pilot-tested the proposed *Exchange Lists* in the hospital's nutrition clinic. In 1948, Ms. Hazzard began working at the Veterans Administration Center in Biloxi, Mississippi.

The VA hospital provided therapeutic diet service in the dining room for ambulatory patients from the nearby Old Soldier's Home. Ms. Hazzard's supervisor allowed her to use the proposed *Exchange Lists* to recalculate the menus for these men, many of whom had multiple nutrition problems and health conditions.

"They intensely resented the severe limitations diabetes made regarding food and beverage intake," Ms. Hazzard said. The dietitians worked with the patients in planning new menus, and many of the men were happy at the options offered.

However, many chose to ignore their diabetes and did not eat at the "therapeutic diet" tables. As a result, Ms. Hazzard said, "There were frequent admissions to the emergency room over weekends and holidays due to noncompliance."

As news spread about the new menus, an increasing number of men asked to join the therapeutic diet group. Compliance improved, even when the men went on furlough or were out socializing over the weekend in local restaurants and bars. The men made wiser food choices.

When the chief of dietetic services of the Veterans Administration came to inspect the department, Ms. Hazzard recalled that her supervisor "was a bit concerned that we had made these adjustments before the exchanges had

Manufacturer's Life Insurance Company of Toronto.

"Shortly thereafter, one large insurance company decided that people with diabetes under good control could be insured under certain conditions. This decision had a tremendous impact on the lives of people with diabetes at that time. When the decision was made, however, insurance companies had no comprehensive data on the mortality rate of people with diabetes. As people with diabetes lived longer and developed complications, more information became available and premiums on life insurance rose," wrote Dr. Montgomery.

Assembling accurate statistics on the incidence of diabetes in the United States did not come easily. In 1950, the Association sent a letter to chief of the National Office of Vital Statistics (NOVS), H. L. Dunn, M.D., asking that all deaths due to diabetes be tabulated in detail, whether or not they were assigned as such under the "International List of Causes."

As a follow-up to this letter, ADA Executive Director J. Richard Connelly and John Reed, M.D., also from the Association, visited Dr. Dunn. While Dr. Dunn was sympathetic to the reasons behind the Association's request, he said he could make no commitment to carry it out because of recent governmental budget cuts. He did suggest that a 10-percent sample could be collected along these lines, but he made no promises.

This particular issue, which occupied much time and energy in the early years of the Association, was never resolved with NOVS. Sample statistics were gathered from various sources, particularly insurance companies, and later from the Center for Health Statistics.

In spite of the early difficulties in gathering comprehensive statistics about diabetes, by 1950, employee group life insurance became generally available, and people with diabetes were gradually admitted to these plans.

Spreading The Word About Good Nutrition
Nutrition had been recognized as the cornerstone of diabetes treatment since 1797, when London physician John Rollo reported on the treatment of diabetes by restricted diet. Yet in the 1940s, it was the consensus of the ADA physicians that medical students were graduating with only the barest background in nutrition.

In an effort to bring some order to the plethora of existing theories on the diabetic diet, a Committee on

been officially adopted into our policies and procedures." However, Ms. Hazzard said, the inspector "was pleased with our innovations and made no mention of our variance in her report."

Ms. Hazzard lives in Shreveport, Louisiana, and is active in the ADA Louisiana Affiliate.

More Exchange List Testing
Barbara Lofquist learned how to calculate a diabetic diet when she was a dietetics major in college, 1941 to 1942. It was, she recalled, a complicated calculation. In 1943, Ms. Lofquist served her dietetic internship at the University of Michigan Hospital, and from 1943 to 1950, Ms. Lofquist worked as a dietitian in two hospitals.

"I was aware," she said, "that each hospital had its own system of calculating diabetic diets. Each was complicated. Each required the person to weigh all foods. There was little encouragement to eat out. The scale would have to go along!" She noted that snacks were not included in meal plans—people with diabetes were supposed to eat three meals a day, on time.

In those days, people with diabetes typically followed a diet that restricted carbohydrates, was fairly high in protein, and was very high in fat. "Our usual pattern was to provide 40 percent of the calories from carbohydrate, 20 percent from protein, and 40 percent from fat—much different from the current 50 to 60 percent carbohydrate, 12 to 20 percent protein, and 30 percent fat," Ms. Lofquist said.

The *Exchange Lists*, first published in 1950, "were a real

Teaching Dietetics to Medical Students was appointed. Committee members agreed that medical students needed to be taught what diet therapy could accomplish in treating people who not only had diabetes, but other diseases as well. In 1946, the committee submitted an outline covering suggested principles of nutritional education in medical schools.

In 1947, the Council assigned the Committee on Food Values the task of defining carbohydrates and their use in the diabetic diet. This information would be used to prepare a table of American foods with starch and sugar values. After two years of deliberation

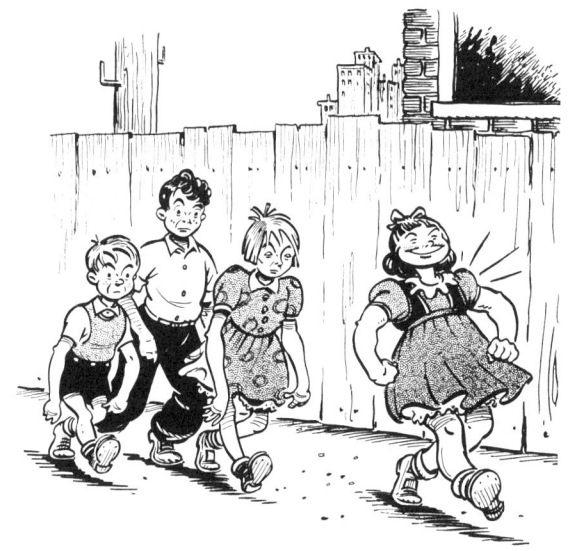

The girl in front eats a healthy diet. From dietary guidelines listed in "Food and Health" by Russell M. Wilder, M.D., in the March 1948 *ADA Forecast*.

and review of the information available from the Department of Agriculture and the United Nations Committee on Calorie Value of Food, it was concluded that a redefinition of "carbohydrate" was necessary.

A year later, at the 1948 Annual Meeting, the committee stated: "The ADA is a body of physicians whose influence is considerable, and is fully competent to define carbohydrate from the standpoint of human nutrition. Such a definition would go a long way to clarify a confused situation and give needed support to the campaign for re-analysis of the carbohydrate value of American foods." Additionally, the committee recommended that the American Diabetes Association prepare a list of American foods giving the glycogenic value of carbohydrate; these values would be tentative,

blessing to diabetics and to the health professionals who calculated the meal plans and taught the patients," Ms. Lofquist said. "It meant learning a new system of meal planning, but it was easy, and there were so many more foods than earlier lists had offered." Ms. Lofquist said that dietitians quickly adopted the "new system."

The importance of the more complete lists of foods available to most people with diabetes was apparent, Ms. Lofquist said, from the number of inquiries dietitians had been receiving. People wanted to know if they could eat certain foods, and if so, how much and how often.

"One very angry young man walked into my office one day and threw his list from a nearby hospital on my desk. 'I can't eat this stuff,' he said. I asked what he would like. 'Bagel,' he said. I wrote the exchange for a bagel on his list and asked what else he would like to eat. He said, 'I guess that's all,' picked up his *Exchange Lists*, and walked away happy. One food, which he'd neglected to ask the hospital dietitian about, made all the difference. He thought the ADA was wonderful," Ms. Lofquist recalled.

From 1943 to 1969, Barbara Lofquist was a hospital dietitian, working with patients and with an outpatient diabetic dining room for those who came for medical check-ups. Ms. Lofquist lives in Detroit, Michigan, and is active in the ADA Michigan Affiliate.

pending the time when better data became available.

In 1949, William H. Olmsted, M.D., chairman of the Committee on Food Values, presented a paper at the ADA's Scientific Sessions entitled, "The Available Carbohydrate of Fruits and Vegetables," based on the committee's findings. That same year, a joint committee of representatives for the American Diabetes Association, The American Dietetic Association, and the diabetes branch of the USPHS took the following action: 1) prepared a revision of the tables of food values based on the carbohydrate content of fruits and vegetables as proposed by Dr. Olmsted; 2) arranged foods into six groups of units, or exchanges, with specified amounts of food in each group having equivalent food values; 3) prepared a set of ready-made diets, four for adults and two for children, to serve as the basis of management in "average" cases of diabetes; and 4) adopted a simple method of calculating diabetic diets using the *Exchange Lists*.

The *Exchange Lists for Meal Planning* revolutionized meal planning and preparation for people with diabetes, eliminating the tedious weighing and measuring of foods for each and every meal. Published in 1950, it

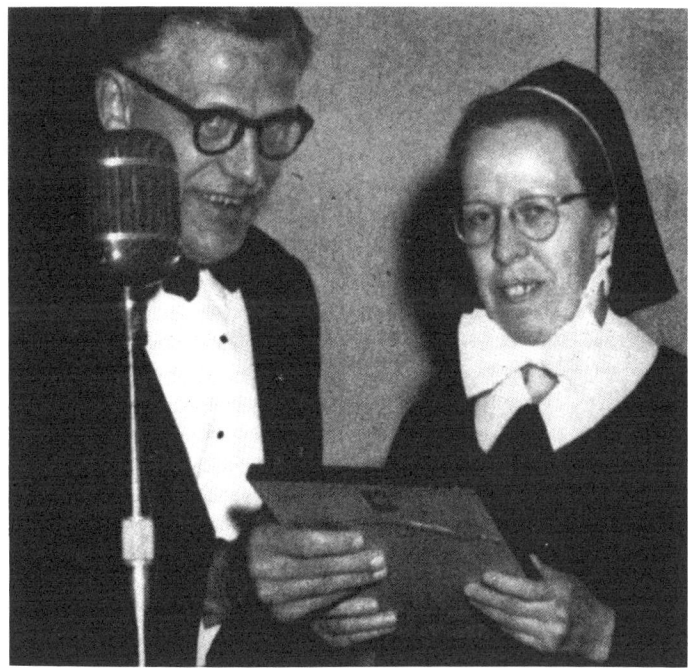

Maude Behrman, *ADA Forecast* food editor, described the proposed *Exchange Lists* in the July 1948 issue of *ADA Forecast*. Here, Frederick W. Williams, M.D., editor in chief, presents her with a citation for her many years of valuable dietery instruction for the magazine.

quickly became the meal planning method of choice for people with diabetes. Other systems have been developed over the years, but the *Exchange Lists* remain the most widely used. The American Diabetes Association maintains a joint copyright on the *Exchange Lists* with The American Dietetic Association.

Also in 1950, the Association set up a committee to serve as an evaluating team for commercial (special) foods for people with diabetes, as well as insulin syringes, and home testing equipment. The Committee on Scientific Evaluation was appointed to take the place of the former Committee on Nostrums. (A nostrum is an agent used to restore health, for example, a medicine.)

After lengthy consultations with American Medical Association (AMA) officials and legal counsel, it was deemed inadvisable for the American Diabetes Association to continue evaluating foods, pharmaceutical preparations, or equipment. Accordingly, the Executive Committee drafted the following resolution:

"*Whereas*: The ADA does not have a laboratory or other facilities for testing and evaluating foods, pharmaceutical preparations, or equipment; and

"*Whereas*, the American Medical Association and the U.S. Government have adequate facilities for evaluation procedures, therefore be it

"*Resolved*, that the ADA not accept foods, pharmaceutical preparations or equipment, or any other items for evaluation or acceptance, and withdraw endorsements of all items previously submitted."

The Council passed this resolution, and thereafter the Committee on Scientific Evaluation served merely as a clearinghouse, through which requests for such evaluations were channeled to the appropriate departments of the AMA or the federal government. This policy is still in effect today.

The Birth Of The Affiliates

When the Association formally began in 1940, other diabetes professional societies were already in existence around the country. Such groups had developed in New York, Boston, Philadelphia, Cleveland, and Los Angeles, for example. Some already had lay members and had already gone into public fund raising.

Should the American Diabetes Association expand its base to include lay people with diabetes? Should the Association remain a small, elite group of specialized physicians and scientists? These were two of the most controversial and complex questions facing the membership and went to the very core of the Association's

Camping In Times Past
One of the most successful, best known, and oldest ADA programs is the summer camping program for children with diabetes. Several diabetes camps actually predated the Association. The first was established in 1925 in Michigan

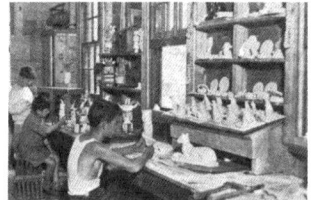

Camp Ho Mita Koda, located in the woods about 25 miles east of Cleveland, Ohio.

by Leonard F. C. Wendt, M.D., and began with four campers. The campers lodged in a private cottage with an adult who also had diabetes. As the camp grew, other arrangements became necessary, and the Red Cross loaned the group a camp at Brighton, Michigan, for four consecutive seasons. It later became known as the Grace Hospital Diabetic Camp. A second camp, Ho Mita Koda, was established near Novelty, Ohio, in 1929 by Henry John, M.D. A third camp, the Clara Barton Birthplace Camp for girls, started in 1932, was established by Dr. Elliott P. Joslin and his associates at the George F. Baker Clinic of the New England Deaconess Hospital in Boston, Massachusetts. It is located in North Oxford, Massachusetts. (Dr. Joslin had started camping programs as early as 1925 in Maine.) Medical supervision at the Clara Barton Birthplace Camp was provided by Priscilla White, M.D.

In 1936, Camp Firefly, the Pennsylvania Camp for Diabetic Children, was started by a small group of diabetes specialists and was sponsored by the Philadelphia Metabolic Association. During the same season, the New York Diabetes Association opened a camp and 32 children attended.

The Washington Diabetic Camp for Children was started in 1937 at the Christ Child Society Farms for Convalescent Children in Rockville, Maryland. The camp was directed by Drs. Samuel Benjamin, K. Hammond Mish, and E. Clarence Rice, all of the Georgetown University School of Medicine. Mary Davis, a dietitian of the Georgetown University Hospital, assisted in running the camp.

Mary B. Olney, M.D., long active on ADA camping committees, established Bearskin Meadow Camp in Kings Canyon National Park, California, in 1938.

Other early camps include the University of California Diabetic Childrens' Camp (1938); the Virginia Mason Clinic's Camp Banting (1938); and Mary Foley Camp in Rochester, Minnesota (1939). By 1948, the number of camps future existence and philosophy.

In 1945, ADA's Committee on the Foundation of Local Societies prepared a prospectus that outlined step-by-step procedures for use by local groups in establishing a diabetes society, each of which would be a facsimile of the national organization. The prospectus provided for the establishment of a clinical society with membership from the medical and scientific professions. The society would be incorporated in the state as a nonprofit membership organization.

The pages of the newly-published *ADA Forecast* became an important platform for pro-laity, pro-affiliate forces. In the very first issue (January 1948), John A. Reed, M.D., wrote about the affiliate movement in an article titled "A Great Forward Movement for the Diabetic."

He wrote: "Could not the diabetics of any community gather together not only for education, but even to have an old-fashioned presbyterian testimonial meeting for raising their spirits by hearing others tell of their own experiences?"

Dr. Reed concluded with the hope that "future officers of the Association will lend their support to this endeavor. No single undertaking by the American Diabetes Association will bring so much benefit to so many as this one enterprise."

In his 1948 president's address, Edward S. Dillon, M.D., offered words of support to the 13 ADA affiliates and to the 33 other local societies then in the process of formation. "We hope that a large number of these [societies] will obtain affiliate status in the near future," he said.

George E. Anderson, M.D., 1945 chairman of the Committee on the Foundation of Local Societies, was another strong supporter of lay societies and their incorporation into ADA. Writing in the February 1948 issue of *ADA Forecast*, he stated: "The Council of the American Diabetes Association is embarking on the basis of a new public health concept: Give the interested layman a chance to fight the disease on a parity with the doctor and unhampered by an over-zealous parental supervision by the medical profession.

"There are in process of formation all over the United States and in parts of Canada local diabetes associations, each a separate membership corporation formed in accordance with a carefully conceived plan established by the Council of the national association. Every new local organization will embody two parallel self-governing groups, a clinical society and a lay society of the corporation . . . . The lay society will be

had grown to 13.

Established in 1947 and located in Montgomery, Alabama, Camp Seale Harris was one of the first camps in the deep South to be sponsored by an ADA affiliate. The camp's founders had several goals. They hoped to help the campers become independent and self-reliant and to show them that they were not alone in living with diabetes. They also wanted to help the children learn the best possible diabetes care, to help the children keep their blood-glucose levels as close to normal as possible. This was no small task in 1947—methods for testing were primitive.

"Perhaps the biggest change in camping has been in the means we have to get blood-sugar levels as close to normal as possible," said Samuel Eichold, M.D., professor emeritus of internal medicine at the University of South Alabama in Mobile. He recounted some of his experiences with Camp Seale Harris in the June 1988 issue of *Diabetes Forecast*. In 1981, Dr. Eichold won the American Diabetes Association's Outstanding Contribution to Camping and Diabetes Award.

"Daily insulin doses were based on urine tests. Campers would test when they got up in the morning and before each meal," Dr. Eichold recalled. There were no blood-glucose meters in the 1940s and 1950s.

"Urine testing never worked very well, even under the best circumstances. Campers would forget to test, samples would spill, and containers were not always correctly labelled. Even worse was the limited value of urine testing, which shows sugar only after levels have risen significantly," he noted.

"Because of our crude meth-

made up exclusively of laymen with a lay governing board and lay officers. No physician will be eligible for membership in the lay society.

"The lay society will interest itself in the spreading of knowledge and literature to the diabetic and to potential diabetics. The lay society will take unto itself the ways and means of establishing and actually running summer camps for diabetic children and convalescent or vacation resorts for diabetic adults. It will take up the cudgels to shape public opinion in order to dispel the present unwarranted discrimination against diabetics in the world of business. The lay society will meet the challenge of the physician by pitching the balls thrown in by the professional group, which alone surely would pitch a losing game," said Dr. Anderson.

The internal structure of the new affiliates reflected the ongoing debate within the Association concerning lay members versus a purely professional society. The formula of clinical and lay societies remained in effect for a generation. While not the complete integration that some had advocated, it nevertheless represented a victory for those ADA members who saw the need for inclusion of lay members if the affiliates were to flourish.

Ten Years Of Progress

In his president's address in 1950, Howard F. Root, M.D., summed up the accomplishments of the Association's first 10 years: "At the end of our first year we had 480 members and today we have 1,400. Our affiliate associations number 28 and many applications are pending. We have three successful publications, *Diabetes Abstracts*, *Proceedings*, and the *ADA Forecast*. Our public awareness program through National Diabetes Detection Week has discovered thousands of unknown diabetics and brought them under medical supervision," he said.

There had been other changes as well. The Council had appointed a full-time executive director, J. Richard Connelly, on August 1, 1949. Mr. Connelly came from the Medical Society of the District of Columbia, with an extensive background in organizational work. He would be responsible to the Executive Committee and the Council for all the activities of the Association, including the *ADA Forecast*.

Rising rents, steady growth, and diminished space had been chronic problems faced by the Association. From the original location in Dr. Striker's Cincinnati office (1941-49), headquarters became three concurrent locations for about a year. Administration was handled

ods of testing, low blood sugar was all too common. Back then, the infirmary was always full of campers receiving intravenous glucose to treat insulin reactions," Dr. Eichold continued. "High blood sugar was also common. Because high blood sugar can cause excessive urination, bed wetting was almost epidemic in the early days of diabetes camps."

"In 1947, we still saw children whose growth was severely impaired because they hadn't been receiving proper insulin therapy."

There was a clear need for more camps for children with diabetes. In 1948, Dr. Henry John, chairman of the Committee on Camps, noted in a report that "while ADA had made a good start, the number of camps in use are not adequate for the needs of the country. Greater publicity, backing by local societies, and community support would all help in promoting the program."

Dr. John emphasized the need for a central clearinghouse for information on how to organize a camp, what the physical setup should be, and what staff was needed. And he made this important point: "Children come to camp to enjoy a summer vacation, and camp must not be an extension of a hospital service, where a child is constantly reminded of his or her diabetes. The medical aspect is important but is only half of the issue. It must be kept in the background, but balanced and integrated into the whole camping experience. This requires well-trained staff counselors. In addition, the American Camping Association is inspecting camps more closely year by year, and standards have to be high."

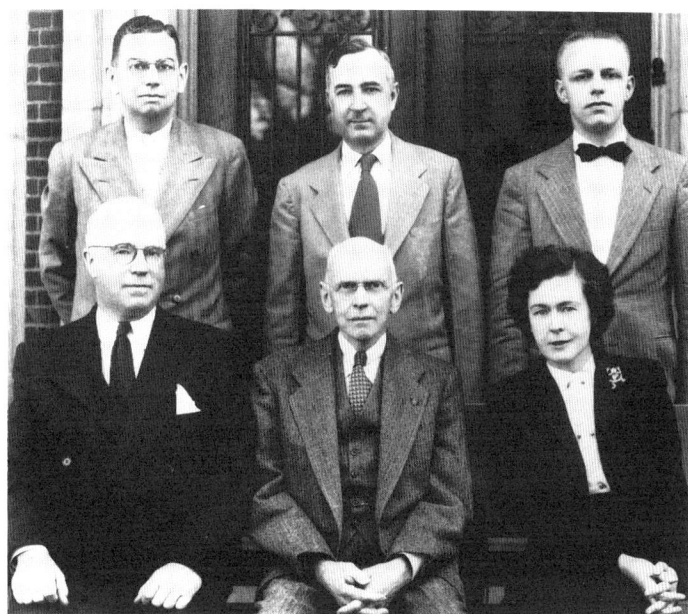

Among the world's most renowned diabetes specialists are (clockwise), from bottom center: Drs. Elliott P. Joslin; Howard F. Root; Allen P. Joslin; Alexander Marble; Robert F. Bradley; and Priscilla White. This group, plus Leo P. Krall (not pictured), were "diabetes pioneers" at the Joslin Clinic.

at 1 Nevens Street in Brooklyn; Diabetes Detection activities were coordinated from Boston; and the editorial offices were in Philadelphia. In 1950, these three offices were consolidated at 11 West 42nd Street. (This was the first of five locations the Association would occupy in New York City. In 1954, headquarters was moved to 1 East 46th Street; in 1964, to 18 East 48th Street; in 1974, to 600 Fifth Avenue; and in 1981, to 2 Park Avenue.)

At the time of the move to West 42nd Street, an automatic letter-opening machine (capable of opening 100 letters a minute), an automatic date stamper, and an envelope-sealing machine that could seal 150 letters a minute were installed to handle the increasing load of mail.

Excerpts from the treasurer's reports of 1941 and 1950 appear in Appendices 3-A and 3-B. They attest to the growth and vitality of the Association's first 10 years.

As the Association grew, so did concerns about membership categories. By 1950, the Committee on Membership and the Constitution had been wrestling

Vivisection:
An Issue For More Than Forty Years

Concerns about anti-vivisection were first raised at the sixth ADA Annual Meeting in 1946, which commemorated the discovery of insulin. By then, the anti-vivisectionist movement had become extremely emotional and controversial. ADA leaders felt that a public statement in support of the use of animals in research was both necessary and appropriate at this time. Therefore, the Council passed the following resolution:

"*Whereas*, The ADA at this meeting is commemorating the 25th anniversary of the discovery of insulin; and

"*Whereas*, Insulin has been instrumental in restoring the health and saving the lives of countless human beings suffering from diabetes; and

"*Whereas*, The great work of Banting and Best in discovering insulin, and the subsequent investigations clarifying its actions and uses, would have been impossible without the use of dogs and other domestic animals as experimental subjects; therefore be it,

"*Resolved*, That the American Diabetes Association hereby testifies to the value of the use of dogs and other domestic animals for the purposes of scientific research and urges all enlightened citizens to refrain from supporting the misguided efforts of so-called anti-vivisectionists, who constantly try to hamper the advancement of scientific medicine."

(The anti-vivisectionist movement accelerated again in the 1980s, and in June 1985, the Association issued a Policy Statement, "Responsible Use of Animals in Research" [*Diabetes Care*, Vol. 8:4, 1985] reiterating the position taken in 1946. See Chapter Eleven.)

with membership categories for 10 years, yet there was still a lack of unanimity. In 1940, membership consisted of four categories: active, associate, honorary, and corporate. Only active members were eligible to vote. By 1950, there were six categories: active, fellow, associate, corporate, corresponding, and honorary.

The committee pointed out that the criteria for active membership was so restrictive that it had not led to broad general practitioner membership, which was a necessary part of the Association's general activities, including physician participation in the Diabetes Detection Drive. The committee recommended that active membership be extended to physician members of local affiliates, but the Council took no action. At this time, the committee also raised the question of lay membership. This question was referred to the newly formed Committee on Purposes and Policies.

Pieces Of The Puzzle:
What We Knew About Diabetes

1946

With the introduction of insulin, the risk of pregnancy for women with diabetes diminishes greatly. However, toxemia is still a great danger. Toxemia is a condition in which poisonous substances, especially toxins produced by bacteria, are carried throughout the body by the bloodstream. Some statistics show that toxemia occurs 50 times more often in women with diabetes than in those without diabetes.

1947

As evidence accumulates that diabetes causes complications of the circulatory system, many researchers become convinced that the outstanding unsolved problem in the treatment of people with diabetes is the development of vascular disease.

While it is clear that insulin is of great value in the treatment of diabetes, its structure and precise mode or site of action remains unknown. One theory suggests that insulin is a catalyst that might work on one or two enzyme systems.

1948

The use of insulin and antibiotics results in a decrease in the number of deaths of people with diabetes from diabetic coma and infection. However, this decrease seems to be accompanied by an almost equal increase in the number of deaths caused by complications of arteriosclerosis (thickening and loss of elasticity of the walls of the arteries).

Two Harvard University researchers examine the medical records of 110 people with diabetes who died between 1940 and 1946 and conclude that good control of diabetes seems to postpone severe vascular lesions in people with diabetes.

There are several distinct schools of thought on what the best diet for people with diabetes is and how much the diet should be restricted. For example, some clinicians recommend a high-protein diet, while some recommend an "almost free diet" (with restriction only on sugar and sweets).

1949

Evidence seems to suggest two types of diabetes, one due to lack of insulin and the other due to insensitivity to insulin. Researchers in England devise a test to measure insulin sensitivity in which a standard dose of glucose is given by mouth, followed by an intravenous injection of a standard amount of glucose. Results indicate that people with diabetes fall into two groups according to insulin sensitivity. Those sensitive to insulin tend to be young and thin, with "severe" diabetes of sudden onset. Their diabetes responds readily to insulin. Those insensitive to insulin tend to be older and obese, and often have arteriosclerosis and high blood pressure. Their diabetes is milder and of slower onset; they are often surprisingly insensitive to insulin.

The debate over whether tight control can delay or prevent complications continues. Edward Tolstoi, M.D., one of the founders of the American Diabetes Association, becomes a controversial figure because of his treatment regimen for people with diabetes. He recommends giving only the amount of insulin necessary to keep a person with diabetes feeling well. Dr. Tolstoi does not consider hyperglycemia and glycosuria (sugar in the urine) to be of major concern. His critics insist that people with diabetes who have repeated episodes of uncontrolled hyperglycemia will develop serious complications. However, Tolstoi's experience with 3,000 patients treated over 12 years does not seem to substantiate these criticisms.

Physicians suspect that heredity and infection are prime factors in causing diabetes in children. One survey of 500 cases of "juvenile diabetes" shows that about 30 percent of children had had an infection before being diagnosed with diabetes. In most of these cases, diabetes appears within two months of the infection. As for diabetes in adults, advancing age, obesity, and endocrine disturbances are thought to play important roles in the development of the disease.

Another insulin appears on the market: modified protamine insulin, also called NPH-50 (N = neutral; P = protamine; H = Hagedorn, for Hans C. Hagedorn, M.D., who improved the insulin). It has a relatively quick action, taking effect in about two hours. Its maximum blood-glucose lowering effect occurs 10 to 20 hours after administration, and its effects last about 28 hours. Priscilla White, M.D., reports that 95 percent of 336 people with severe diabetes were able to successfully manage their diabetes with a single daily injection of NPH, as opposed to taking separate injections of crystalline and protamine zinc insulins. NPH insulin was first developed by Nordisk in 1946.

Increasing numbers of clinicians are using mixtures of insulins to help people with diabetes control their disease. A mixture of 2-3 units of regular insulin to 1 unit of protamine zinc insulin (PZI) is typical.

1950

After an 18-month study examining the effect of NPH-50 insulin on 28 people with diabetes for 18 months, Thomas P. Sharkey, M.D., (who would later serve as ADA president) and Harry E. King, M.D., report that 12 of those patients required additional regular insulin. However, they report, while NPH-50 is not the "ideal" insulin, it does give better control than PZI or a combination of PZI and crystalline zinc insulin. They also note that insulin reactions to NPH-50 or mixtures with NPH-50 are not as severe as with other kinds of insulin and that it is easier to make adjustments in dosage using NPH-50.

Several studies on the relationship between degree of control and development of complications in young people with diabetes indicate that a high level of control delays and may prevent the development of degenerative changes (such as retinopathy, nephropathy, and arteriosclerosis).

Chapter Four
Growth and Reorganization 1950-55

ADA PRESIDENTS

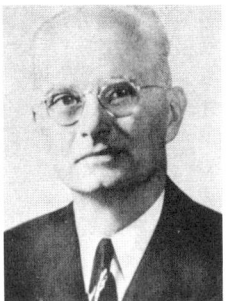
Lester J. Palmer, M.D.
(1950-51)

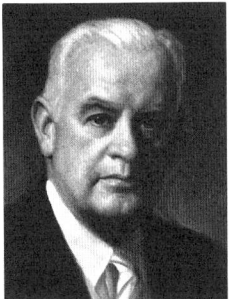
Arthur R. Colwell, M.D.
(1951-52)

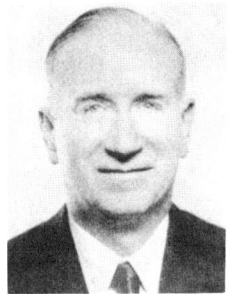
Frank N. Allan, M.D.
(1952-53)

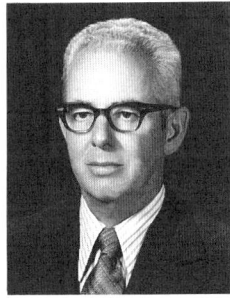
Randall G. Sprague, M.D.
(1953-54)

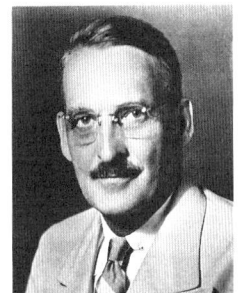
Henry B. Mulholland, M.D.
(1954-55)

In the spring of 1951, there was uncertainty over the Korean conflict and fear of an atomic attack. The United States was once again in a state of war emergency. In January 1952, the maiden issue of the journal *Diabetes* featured an article titled "The Diabetic and Civilian Defense, A Statement by the Committee on Emergency Medical Care of the American Diabetes Association." The purpose of the statement was to help physicians care for people with diabetes in the event of a nuclear attack. Included was information on available insulin supplies, appropriate treatment for casualties and evacuees who had diabetes, and diabetic diets vis-a-vis wartime food restrictions. *ADA Forecast* followed with a similar article for people with diabetes and a dramatic full-page poster, "The Diabetic and the Atom Bomb," for use with the government's civilian defense pamphlet "Survival Under Atomic Attack."

Also of significance was a notice in *Diabetes* later that year announcing that the Department of Defense would accept physicians with diabetes if the disease were under good control. This was an unprecedented departure from custom. Heretofore, people with diabetes had not been permitted to join the armed forces, nor remain in the service after a diagnosis of diabetes. This move was obviously necessitated by a scarcity of military physicians.

In 1953, at the request of U.S. President Dwight D. Eisenhower, Congress created a new department: Health, Education and Welfare. This department was to have a far-reaching influence on the nation and on diabetes research.

In medicine, the U.S. Surgeon General issued the first warning on the causal effect of cigarette smoking and lung cancer. For two consecutive years, the Nobel Prize in Physiology and Medicine was awarded to developers of anti-viral vaccines: to Jonas Salk in 1954 for the polio vaccine and to Max Theiler in 1955 for his work on a yellow fever vaccine.

In 1950, Solomon A. Berson and Rosalyn S. Yalow began their investigation into the application of radioisotopes. These studies, done at the Veterans Administration Hospital in the Bronx, New York, resulted in 1959 in the radioimmunoassay test for measuring the amount of insulin in the blood. This test gave new insights into the nature of diabetes. When insulin levels in the blood could be tested, it became clear that there were two types of diabetes. One of these was caused by the body's ineffective use of insulin, not by the lack of this hormone. With this finding, the riddle of insulin resistance in non-insulin-dependent (NIDDM or type II) diabetes began to unfold.

The early 1950s brought self-examination and change to the American Diabetes Association. ADA President Arthur R. Colwell, M.D., (1951-52) and others agreed that the time had come for an in-depth look at the operations of the American Diabetes Association. To chart the best future course and to better serve Americans with diabetes and the professionals who treated them, the Committee on Purposes and Policies was appointed.

The committee held its first meeting December 2-3, 1950, in Cleveland, Ohio. Present were Drs. Arthur R. Colwell (chairman), Joseph T. Beardwood, Jr., Jerome W. Conn, Francis D.W. Lukens, Howard F. Root, and Randall G. Sprague. Franklin B. Peck, M.D., also a member, was absent. Others who attended were W. W. Bauer, M.D., of the

American Medical Association, ADA President Lester J. Palmer, M.D., Secretary John A. Reed, M.D., and Executive Director J. Richard Connelly (*ex officio*).

At this initial meeting, Dr. Colwell presided over deliberations as to how the Association should support its activities without undertaking general public fund raising. It should be noted that at this time, the American Diabetes Association was the only large medical organization engaged in health education programs (through detection drives, scientific publications, and affiliate associations) comparable with those of voluntary health organizations. Voluntary health agencies were supported by public fund raising, but the American Diabetes Association, at that time, was anxious to avoid falling into that category, at least until it had undergone further maturation.

The committee recognized the following problems in the Association's operations: 1) scanty contributions to research; 2) vague definition of affiliate relationships with each other and the national organization; 3) lack of program development for affiliates, both lay and clinical; 4) disorganized/insufficient publications program, especially at the professional education level; and 5) lack of funds for national health education work.

Addressing these problems would lead to significant changes within the Association.

A New Emphasis On Research

In his presidential address at the 1951 ADA Annual Meeting, Lester J. Palmer, M.D., reminded his colleagues that the original purpose of the Association was to improve the lives of people with diabetes. He warned against overspecialization at the expense of treatment and said that the greatest need and the responsibility of the Association now lay in more energetic research in diabetes and metabolism. It was not until 1953, however, that a Committee on Research was appointed.

At the committee's first meeting, individual members were requested to submit views on the use of research funds if, and when, they became available. The majority favored basic investigation in diabetes through fellowships based in established laboratories. This way, the fellow could be accommodated and guided in his work. A preliminary report signed by Charles H. Best, M.D., chairman of the committee, recommended: 1) that $5,000 be transferred from the General Fund to the Clinical and Research Fund; 2) that two ADA fellowships for the study of fundamental aspects of diabetes be created; and 3) that the successful applicants be paid from $2,000 to $3,000 per year, depending upon their seniority. Alternatively, one senior fellowship at $5,000 a year might be created.

The committee did not meet again until almost two years later, at which time members were informed that the Executive Committee had made $23,000 available to them for research. This amount included $7,500 from the Atlas Powder Company for the study of sorbitol in human diabetes. This gave the committee $15,000 to use for applications in hand.

The grant from Atlas Powder was reviewed. Inasmuch as it was to be used specifically for research on the metabolism of sorbitol in human diabetes and there were no applications that met these criteria, the committee agreed that a notice of the grant should be published in *Diabetes*.

In a discussion of procedures, the committee adopted the following broad principles for the use of research funds: the American Diabetes Association would conform to the salary scale of the USPHS fellowships—$3,000 for an unmarried post-doctoral applicant, and $3,600 for a married post-doctoral applicant. The committee retained full freedom to adjust salaries to each particular situation. Recognizing the desirability of two-year fellowships, for both the fellow and the laboratory where the work was to be done, the committee asked for complete assurance that

THE DIABETIC AND THE ATOMIC BOMB

Read the Government's small pamphlet called SURVIVAL UNDER ATOMIC ATTACK. Get it from your Civil Defense organization. READ IT!

Carry your identification (diabetic) card with you at all times, if you have one. If not, Civil Defense may supply one.

WHERE TO GO In the event of an atomic bomb attack on your city, the chance of you and your home escaping injury is very good. If, however, you are within the destruction range of the bomb, you could either be injured or uninjured, but your home would probably be partially or entirely destroyed. If you are injured, you will be cared for, and your diabetic condition will have attention—rest assured of that. If you are homeless and you have friends who will care for you, you need not worry.

PREPARE TO TAKE CARE OF YOURSELF completely, if you are uninjured. Your family and friends should be taught enough about diabetes to take care of you in an emergency.

EVERY DIABETIC should know how to take insulin. There is plenty of insulin.

INSULIN EVERY DIABETIC TAKING INSULIN should have his usual ONE extra bottle in addition to current needs, and one EXTRA insulin syringe with two needles. This is because insulin is your best friend and with it you have the best insurance there is. ALWAYS USE YOUR OLDEST BOTTLE FIRST. Regular insulin is superior to the other forms for emergency purposes. Carry a little case with your insulin syringe, if you have one. If an emergency arises and you must change from long-acting insulin (protamine zinc insulin, globin insulin, or NPH insulin) to regular insulin, take 2 doses of the regular—the morning dose equalling 3/5 of the number of units of your usual dose of the long-acting insulin, and the evening dose, 2/5 of the units. If you have no food, reduce your dose to 1/2 or 1/3 of these amounts to avoid reactions. TEST YOUR URINE. KEEP TO YOUR DIET AS NEARLY AS POSSIBLE IN ALL CIRCUMSTANCES. It is better to eat too little than too much. Here is a simple emergency diet one can get under most any circumstances:

EMERGENCY DIET

BREAKFAST	NOON & NIGHT
Bread, 2 or 3 slices	Meat or cheese sandwich, or
Butter or margarine	bread and butter, 3 slices, or
Coffee and canned milk, or in place of bread, a cereal and a can of milk	meat and potatoes, with such vegetables as are available

You can get along on this simple fare for several days, if necessary.

future support be guaranteed. Also approved was a supplementary grant, not to exceed $500, to the institution in which the fellow was located, toward the expenses of his work. Fellowships were to be limited to U.S. citizens for work done in American institutions (although occasional exceptions to this rule were granted.) Fellows were to work full time; no grants were to be awarded to committee members; and the committee was to maintain broad authority to act in all matters of research policy.

Thirteen initial fellowship requests were reviewed for the 1955-56 fiscal year. Two applications were unanimously approved and granted in January 1955. John A. Owen, Jr., M.D., of Duke University, was granted $4,800 to work with Frank Engle, M.D., on "The Diabetogenic Action of Pituitary Growth Hormone in Rats." And E.R. Froesch, M.D., was granted $4,000 to work with Albert E. Renold, M.D., at Peter Bent Brigham Hospital in Boston on "The Determination of Glucose by Glucose Oxidase and its Clinical Applications."

Although it was generally agreed that fellowships were to be awarded to United States citizens, an exception was made for Dr. Froesch because, "although not a citizen, he was already working in this country under the best auspices."

To stimulate interest among young medical students and acquaint them with the American Diabetes Association, an essay contest was established in 1951. The contest was open to interns and students within two years of graduation from medical school. Any subject relating to diabetes and basic metabolism was acceptable. A prize of $250 (raised to $500 in the mid-1960s) was offered to the author of the best paper reporting an original work of laboratory investigation or clinical observation. An award of $50 was offered for the best review article or case report. All papers were judged on the value of the material and the method of presentation. The contest was held annually until 1970, when it was discontinued.

Addressing Affiliate Concerns

The affiliate structure established in 1945 provided for an informal confederation of local societies, each a facsimile of the national organization. They were incorporated in the various states as nonprofit organizations. Each society elected officers, and most had a clinical society (physicians and health-care professionals only,) and a parallel lay society. These affiliate societies

Official ADA Emblem Adopted

A Committee on Emblems was appointed in 1950 to design a suitable symbol for the Association. The committee submitted three designs for consideration.

The first design showed a little girl with diabetes. A dog was at her side. She was shown in the act of taking insulin into a syringe. In a circle around the picture appeared the name "American Diabetes Association." Proponents of this design felt it reduced "the idea of diabetes to its simplest form, for no one could mistake the meaning of it for something other than diabetes."

The second proposed design was the ADA logo already in use on the cover of *ADA Forecast*. It had the advantage of recognition, and was widely perceived already as the official ADA emblem.

The third design—which was accepted—consisted of an inverted triangle with a lamp of learning, symbolizing research, upon which was superimposed "1940," the year the Association was founded. Also depicted were a scale, symbolizing balance in diet, and a caduceus, the symbol of the medical profession. The triangle was enclosed in a circle, indicating unity and continuity. Around the circle were the words "American Diabetes Association, Inc."

In the orginal composite, a book (representing the clinical aspects of diabetes) and an hourglass (symbolizing life) were also included, but were later dropped.

The adopted logo was used until 1974, when the present symbol came into being. The current logo shows the three sides of a triangle. The base represents research; the left side, detection; the right side, education. The left side is broken to indicate undetected cases of diabetes. The base is likewise broken to show the gap that yet exists in diabetes knowledge. That gap also represents the anticipated cure that will someday fill the space.

could expect "guidance" from the national organization, but had no voice in planning or policy making. In financial matters, they operated independently.

Under such a loose structure, there was no established formula for sharing dues or contributions with the national organization. Conversely, no provision existed for elected representation of local affiliates on the parent board of directors. Change was needed if orderly growth was to continue on a national scale.

The Association leadership saw the need clearly. At the twelfth Annual Meeting in Chicago, Dr. Arthur Colwell confronted the problem in his presidential address. Speaking on June 7, 1952, he cited organizational structure as the Association's most pressing concern. He acknowledged that future growth would require "constitutional changes of both national and local bylaws." But such changes were necessary to accommodate "dues adjustments, definition of geographical responsibility, arrangement of representation for lay groups on local professional boards and for local professional groups on the national board," he said.

Dr. Colwell concluded by stressing the importance of organizational restructuring. "If we fail to recognize the need or to meet it as we see it," he said, "we shall stop growing stronger and may even relapse."

The Association soon acted. An interim Council meeting was held January 17-18, 1953, in Toronto. There, the Committee on the Constitution submitted a revision of the Constitution and Bylaws. New proposals were offered that would broaden the base of membership and reorganize the affiliate structure and its relationship to the Association.

At the Annual Meeting in May 1953, a new Constitution and Bylaws were adopted. But the membership sidestepped the affiliate issue, and dealt instead with defining future ADA activities and extending membership privileges to more physicians. The affiliate question continued to chafe.

Affiliate associations had already been established under the auspices of the national organization. On June 1, 1953, a Conference of Delegates of the affiliate associations met in New York. Of the 33 affiliate associations then in full existence, 26 were represented by 57 delegates.

The chief topic considered by the conference was the evolving relationship between affiliates and the national organization. The group also discussed the increasing problem of securing adequate financial support for the activities of the national organization, and debated (to no conclusion) the role of laymen in the future of the affiliate association program. In closing, however, the conference unanimously adopted a proposal that governors be appointed representing each state, as affiliate representatives to the national organization. They urged that such appointments be made by the ADA Council as soon as possible.

Real change finally came in June 1954, at the fourteenth Annual Meeting in San Francisco. A Board of Governors was formally created by the Association as liaison between the national organization and the affiliates. Its members were appointed by the Council. On June 18, 1954, the new governors—one from each of the affiliate states—met for the first time with the ADA Council, and then with its first chairman, Louis K. Alpert, M.D., of Washington, D.C.

The governors would come to play a vital role in ADA affairs. They would serve to coordinate all activities pertaining to diabetes in their respective states; they would interpret policies and programs of the national organization for local groups; they would establish liaison between the Association and its affiliates. In turn, local interests and needs would be carried to the national Council by the governors.

In 1955, more change came when the Association established an Assembly of Delegates. The Assembly consisted of one delegate from every clinical and lay society in the organization. These delegates were to consider issues and problems and bring them to the Board of Governors, which would pass them on to the ADA Council.

The revised organizational structure was intended to give each affiliate a place in the national hierarchy. ADA President Henry B. Mulholland, M.D., (1954-55) said: "For this plan to work, there has to be mutual respect on both sides. The ADA expects to be more helpful to its affiliates, standing ready to aid them not only in their financial drives but in any aspect of their activities."

In return, the affiliates would henceforth be expected to assume more financial responsibility for the welfare of the national organization. "The future course of our Association," Dr. Mulholland said, "may well depend on the manner in which our affiliates respond to our request that they organize fund-raising campaigns to provide money not only for their own needs but an additional amount to help support the activities of the National Association."

Dr. Mulholland correctly predicted that it would take several years for the new structure to establish itself. Nevertheless, a significant turning point in ADA history had been reached. A difficult and potentially fractious challenge had been surmounted. The national organization was not only intact, but stronger than ever.

Expanding Publications

In 1950, the Education Committee appointed a subcommittee on Health Information to make recommendations to the Council on the development and dissemination of information to the laity. After a survey of existing materials distributed by insurance companies, the subcommittee recommended that the Association develop an inexpensive, basic information piece for wide distribution to respond to its many public inquiries. "Facts About Diabetes" was published in 1950.

In 1951, *ADA Forecast*, then in its fourth year of publication, was read avidly by 20,000 subscribers. Frederick Williams, M.D., was appointed editor to succeed Elizabeth M. Mullann.

The magazine's message was upbeat: "You can live a normal life with diabetes." Inspirational articles, such as "My Diabetes is an Asset" and "The Miracle of Diabetes," appeared frequently. "Young Folks Corner" became an instant hit with children, and continues to this day as "Kid's Corner." "The Funny Side," which allowed readers to share amusing anecdotes, was never lacking in submissions. Deaconess Maude Behrman, director of Mercer Memorial House in Atlantic City, served as consulting dietitian to *Forecast* and provided a monthly column on food, tips on nutrition, and recipes. Most of the recipes were for single portions, because at that time it was generally accepted that individuals with diabetes required special meals.

One very popular feature in those early years was "Dave's Diary." Dave was a gregarious young man with insulin-dependent (type I) diabetes living an energetic life and meeting big and small challenges with good humor and common sense, in spite of diabetes.

ADA Forecast also served as a vehicle for reporting advances in diabetes treatment and the latest news on issues affecting the lives of people with diabetes, such as employment, insurance, and affiliate and camp activities. In 1950, the magazine reported that the U.S. government had lifted the ban keeping people with diabetes out of civil service jobs. This concession was most likely the result of the strong wartime employment record established by many people with diabetes.

Dave's Diary: A Healthy Dose of Humor

The March 1951 issue of *ADA Forecast* was an important one in the publication's three-year history. For the first time, the

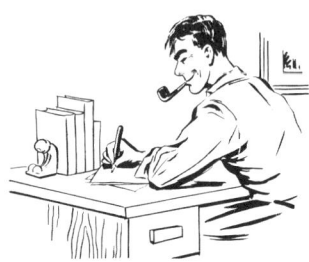

magazine was produced in New York instead of Philadelphia. That issue also marked the debut of Frederick W. Williams, M.D., as editor in chief, in place of Elizabeth Mullann.

For early readers, though, the March 1951 edition is best remembered as the first to carry "Dave's Diary," a popular feature that ran in *ADA Forecast* for nearly 20 years.

The simultaneous appearance of Dr. Williams and Dave was no coincidence, for they were the same person.

When Dave first introduced himself, he was 25 years old. "My name is Dave," he wrote, "and I am a diabetic. Of course, I have a second name or family name, but it isn't important. Ever since I can remember, everybody who knew me has always called me Dave, and that suits me."

Dave had a contagiously positive outlook on life despite his diabetes. He referred to those with diabetes as "Club Members." His observations on life with diabetes (and life in general) were down-to-earth, warm, and devoid of self-pity. "You know," he wrote, "as far as my experience goes, most diabetics who take insulin and keep sugar in their pocket always snitch it. They'll never go out and buy it! I call them 'sugar-snitchers', a 'Chapter' of the 'Club'—and I'm one myself!"

Hidden in Dave's breezy style was sound advice on coping with the everyday experience of having diabetes. There was always a lesson in the "Diary"—on exercise, overindulgence, doctors, or diet. Dave often discussed the social aspects of diabetes with wit and common sense.

Dave eventually was married, and his helpful wife, Marge, became a standing character in the "Diary."

In truth, Dave's creator was somewhat older than 25. Dr. Williams was born in New York City in 1900, 50 years before bringing Dave to life. He was one of the original founders of the American Diabetes Association in 1940 and served for many years on ADA's Council. He later served as Association president (1956-57) and was awarded the Banting Medal in 1957. He was also president of the New York Diabetes Association and president of its Clinical Society. In large measure, Dr. Williams was responsible for the establishment of Camp NYDA, one of the oldest summer camps for children with diabetes.

As editor in chief of *ADA Forecast*, Dr. Williams made many changes. Along with "Dave's Diary," he introduced another department called

Studies on absenteeism showed that employees with diabetes lost less time due to illness than their nondiabetic counterparts; this was generally ascribed to the disciplined life style people with diabetes must follow.

ADA Forecast did not accept advertising. Because the magazine was published by a medical organization for a lay audience, ADA leaders agreed that advertisements could be construed as product endorsement. (This policy was changed in 1974 by the newly created Advertising Committee. Committee members believed that information about products and devices should be made available so that individuals with diabetes could make their own decisions. To this day, all advertisements for use in ADA publications are reviewed by the Advertising Committee, and each publication carries a disclaimer stipulating that advertisements do not constitute endorsement by the American Diabetes Association.)

A journal had been the ardent wish of the members since the founding of the American Diabetes Association. In January 1952, the first issue of *Diabetes*, a bimonthly journal, was published. Addressed to the medical professional, this journal incorporated the two earlier publications, *Diabetes Abstracts* and the *Proceedings*, and included original articles and editorials. Dr. Joslin expressed the hopes of many in his lead article, which appeared in the first issue: "When we were young we were told: Hitch your wagon to a star. The ADA is still young and I think it is hitching its wagon to a very important star with its new journal *Diabetes*." His analysis was correct. The journal was an instant success, has been published continuously since 1952, and graduated to monthly publication in 1965.

Advertising in *Diabetes* in the early years was limited to producers of medical supplies, devices, and a few selected foods. In general, advertising was permitted because the journal was circulated only to physicians.

A Handbook for Physicians, originally published by the American Diabetes Association and subsequently taken over by E.R. Squibb, was advertised on the back cover of the first issue of *Diabetes*. Other ads in that issue included Lilly NPH Insulin, "featuring one daily injection," and Globin Insulin, "for a good night's sleep," from Burroughs Wellcome & Company, Inc. While syringe manufacturers had generally accepted the standard scale and markings advocated by the American Diabetes Association, in 1951 there remained a choice of no less than 13 different types of syringes, according to a Becton, Dickinson and Company (later

"The Funny Side" in May 1951. In July 1951, he added an art editor to the staff, improving the magazine's visual appeal. In January 1952, the first *ADA Forecast* cover appeared in a color other than blue. The blue had symbolized the Benedict urine test, in which a blue color meant sugar-free urine.

In the January-February 1953 issue, *ADA Forecast* used a front-cover photograph for the first time, instead of the table of contents. A year later, a Canadian edition of the magazine was launched.

Dr. Williams remained with *ADA Forecast* until 1966, when he retired. He was named the magazine's editor emeritus—the first person to be so honored. He retired to Vermont, where he died December 24, 1975.

In a lifetime devoted to people with diabetes, Dr. Williams made numerous contributions to research, organization, and communication. Perhaps none was as important—or beloved—as the one he made with his good friend, Dave.

Becton Dickinson Consumer Products) advertisement. Abbott Laboratories invited people with diabetes to use "Sycaryl, the new non-caloric sweetener that stays sweet in cooking and baking."

The Debate Over Fund Raising

Fund raising had become an omnipresent concern in the Association. After the war, the Association had expanded its programs and activities rapidly as needs and demands arose, with little thought as to how these were to be financed. There was the naive assumption by many that dues, subscriptions, the sale of publications, and corporate contributions would take care of these growing activities. By 1953, it became apparent to many that the treasury was being strained. How to find the funds necessary to go forward was a nagging concern, but one the Councilors were slow to explore.

Many felt that the American Diabetes Association had built a prestigious organization, widely recognized and well respected in the medical community. They did not want to abdicate this position of leadership by

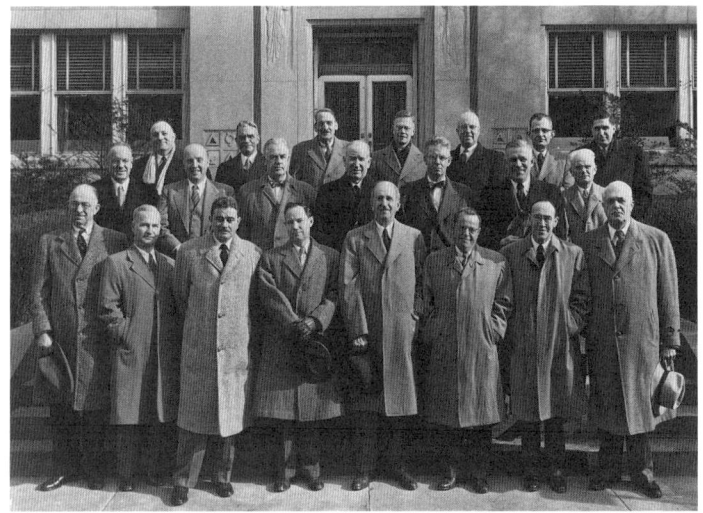

The American Diabetes Association Council, January 18, 1952, at the Lilly Research Laboratories. Front row, left to right, are Drs. Edward S. Dillon; George M. Guest; Edwin L. Rippy; Robert L. Jackson; Joseph H. Barach; John A. Reed; Franklin B. Peck; and Blair Holcomb. Second row, left to right, are Drs. Edward L. Bortz; Charles H. Best; Arthur R. Colwell; Frank N. Allan; Randall G. Sprague; Frederick W. Williams; and Lester J. Palmer. Top row, left to right, are Drs. George E. Anderson; William H. Olmsted; Henry B. Mulholland; Henry T. Ricketts; Howard F. Root; and George C. Thosteson; and Mr. J. Richard Connelly.

seeking public funds; such activity seemed unprofessional to them. Several years earlier, however, the Council had given tacit approval to affiliates to raise funds locally for administrative and program purposes—if the fund raising was done in a "dignified manner." The Council reserved the right to decide what was dignified and appropriate. In the interim, affiliates were left in limbo, unable to go forward or backward.

In his presidential address in 1952, Dr. Arthur Colwell had noted, "It seems obvious that it would not be feasible to create an active national membership of working lay people, no matter how interested they might be. As a homogeneous society they simply could not serve or be served on a country-wide basis because of the distances and mechanical problems involved.

"Therefore it seems rational to continue the formation of local societies, to assist in their work towards a common goal by providing inspiration and strength . . . . As affiliates grow in number and strength, however, they should support the parent which nourished them." (*Diabetes*, Vol. 1:4, 1952)

In 1954, ADA President Randall G. Sprague, M.D., (1953-54) stated frankly, "Our problems are of our own making. By creating greater public awareness of diabetes we have created a demand for services beyond our ability to pay. Now the Association must choose. If we are to make steady progress toward our original goal, namely a better life for the diabetic patient, we should concentrate on the activity that has the most significant impact on this objective, and that is education. It would, of course, be advantageous to have more money for research, but the Council has voted their opposition to that. Logically, the next step is to appeal for funds to diabetics and their families."

Addressing the issue head-on, Dr. Sprague said, "Not all of our activities are self-supporting. We should not try to raise funds as an end unto itself. Rather we should decide what programs we want, how much they will cost, and then plan strategies to pay for them." (*Diabetes*, Vol. 3:4, 1954)

In an editorial in *Diabetes* in 1955, ADA President Henry Ricketts, M.D., (1955-56) pointed out two committee reports with conflicting recommendations (*Diabetes*, Vol. 4:6, 1955). In June 1955, the Committee on Purposes and Policies recommended that the Council reaffirm its opposition to general public fund raising by national and affiliates. On the other hand, the Committee on Finance recommended by a majority vote that a public fund-raising program be developed. The

The Continuing Search For Undiagnosed Diabetes

The introduction of the "Dreypak" for mass screening of diabetes in 1953 revolutionized screening programs. The Dreypak originated in St. Louis and was a kit for the collection of dried urine specimens. Kits consisted of a strip of coarse, treated filter paper sewn to a piece of polyethylene, with a stiff paper sewn to the other side on which the subject was to write such pertinent information as name, age, and medical history.

The kit came with instructions and a return envelope. It had been established in experiments that once dried, sugar was preserved for 90 days. Initially, the Association arranged for the production of one-half million kits, which were offered to local affiliates at cost—one cent per kit. The Dreypak had several advantages over earlier methods of screening. It was just as accurate, but was quicker and easier. And for the first time, detailed studies could be made from the test results.

However, at the eleventh hour, the American Diabetes Association learned that the U.S. Post Office would not permit dried urine specimens to be sent through the mail. It was quickly arranged for the Dreypaks to be distributed by pharmacists, industrial concerns, offices, and stores, which would also handle collections. Specimens were processed, and individuals with a high level of sugar in their urine were advised to see their physicians. The postal regulation was changed some time later, and by the time self-monitoring of blood glucose was introduced in 1981, millions of people had been tested for diabetes using Dreypaks.

basic issue was whether a program of *limited* fund raising among people with diabetes and their families, as approved by the Council in 1954, could provide funds to meet modest financial commitments. If not, a movement toward general public fund raising with its far-reaching implications for the future would doubtless be accelerated.

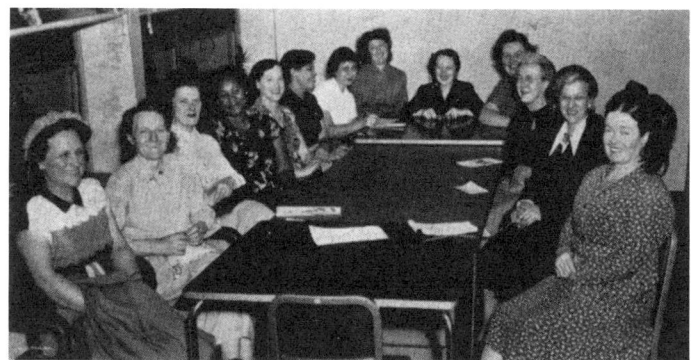

Cleveland's 1950 Diabetes Week was a most successful occasion. Twelve Detection Centers were set up in various parts of the city. Here, Mrs. Rodney C. Sutton (at head of table) tells neighborhood leaders of the importance of the Diabetes Week program.

Changes In Membership

The ADA leadership had long recognized that it needed to broaden the membership base if its message was to reach a nationwide audience. As ADA President Frank N. Allan, M.D., (1952-53) put it in his 1953 president's address: "If we are to grow and reach the general practitioner which has been our goal, we need to actively pursue new professional members."

In 1950, the Committee on Purposes and Policies had been asked to review the membership criteria. In 1953, the committee recommended a modification in membership, reducing the seven existing categories to three: active, associate, and corporate. The Council accepted this recommendation and requirements were modified to include 1) an interest in diabetes; 2) a high standing in the medical profession; 3) certification by two physician members in good standing; and 4) review and approval of each application by the Council.

But as membership grew, demands on the time of the Councilors increased, and the process of review and certification proved impractical. Both procedures were dropped in 1975.

From the beginning, associate members were accepted but never aggressively recruited. But gradually, from 1965 to 1975, the "team approach" to diabetes treatment became increasingly important. This approach delineated the role of the nurse educator and the dietitian. Eventually, associate membership, made up of non-physician health professionals, became an entity unto itself. In 1975, regional health-education programs with continuing education credits were established for associate members. These programs continued until 1977, when the ADA Postgraduate Course was opened to associate members.

The American Diabetes Association started out solely as a professional organization; eventually, the professional section of the Association became part of a larger organization. The evolution of the professional membership in the Association was a long and tedious process, with frequent changes in the Constitution and Bylaws as adjustments were made. In 1987, membership categories were simplified to full, research focus, clinical focus, and associate. (Emeritus status was established in 1970, and is offered to retired physicians 65 years and older who have had continuous membership in the Association for at least 20 years.)

The International Diabetes Federation

The postwar growth of diabetes associations was not limited to the United States. Such groups were sprouting up around the world. In 1949, representatives of offical diabetes organizations in various countries joined forces and established the International Diabetes Federation (IDF). The group held its first IDF Congress July 7-12, 1952, in Leyden, Holland.

Although the American Diabetes Association was not a charter member of IDF, it was well-represented at that first meeting. Elliott P. Joslin, M.D., was the keynote speaker, and Charles H. Best, M.D., was sworn in as the IDF's first president. Dr. Best delivered the first inaugural address. In addition, Howard F. Root, M.D., became IDF vice-president. ADA Executive Director J. Richard Connelly also attended.

In all, 30 American physi-

Nordisk Insulinfond: The Research Program Begins

For the fiscal year ending May 31, 1950, ADA Treasurer Joseph H. Barach, M.D., reported a balance of $305.00 in the Association's Clinical and Research Fund. That was an increase of $5 over the previous year, thanks to an unknown contributor.

Dr. Barach also had news of a more spectacular nature to announce. At the group's annual business meeting in San Francisco that June, he said:

"At this time I wish to call to your attention the deposit, with the Boston Safe Deposit & Trust Company of Boston, Massachusetts, of $100 to establish the Research Fund of the American Diabetes Association, which is a parent fund for the Nordisk Insulinfond Foundation for the Elliott P. Joslin Fellowship. The Foundation is a $50,000 gift from the Nordisk Insulinfond of Copenhagen, Denmark. The income from the Insulinfond Foundation during the lifetime of Elliott P. Joslin is to be applied to the study of diabetes as he shall direct, and thereafter applied to that purpose as may be directed by the Advisory Committee of the Research Fund of the American Diabetes Association, Inc., subject to certain requests of the donor and provisions of the trust agreement."

This $50,000 windfall marked the real start of the

cians were informally present in Leyden along with 241 delegates from 15 countries.

The Association continued to support the activities of the IDF, but did not become an official member of the group until 1955. Early that year, the ADA Executive Committee and Council accepted the IDF's Constitution and Bylaws, which were duly published in the January-February issue of *Diabetes*.

The second IDF Congress was held July 4-8, 1955, in Cambridge, England. ADA President Henry T. Ricketts, M.D., was named medical delegate to the Congress; ADA Executive Director J. Richard Connelly was appointed lay delegate.

Dr. Joslin—an honorary IDF president along with Dr. Best—delivered the Banting Memorial Lecture of the British Diabetic Association on July 4 in Cambridge, to coincide with the opening of the second IDF Congress. His lecture was entitled "Diabetes for Diabetics."

Association's research funding capability. The original fund has continued to benefit the Association over the ensuing 40 years. It came about because of the close contact and professional admiration that existed be-

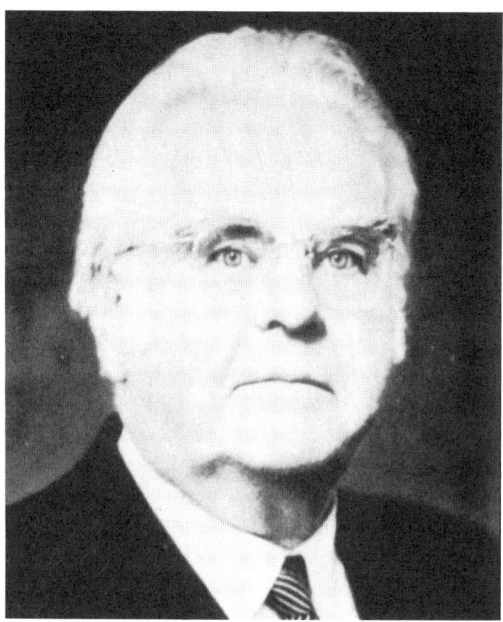

Hans C. Hagedorn, M.D.

tween two pioneers in diabetes treatment and research: Elliott P. Joslin, M.D., of Boston and Hans C. Hagedorn, M.D., of Denmark.

Dr. Hagedorn was the first researcher to develop long-acting—or protamine—insulin in 1936. He was also one of the founders of the Nordisk Insulin Laboratory, and served as its head from 1923 to 1963. With the invention of protamine insulin, Dr. Joslin and others were eager to test the new preparation. Joslin's protege, Howard F. Root, M.D., spent some weeks in 1936 at the Nordisk Laboratory, becoming acquainted with the newest breakthrough.

The success of Dr. Hagedorn's protamine formula was immediate. American insulin manufacturers paid substantial royalties to the Nordisk Institute. During World War II, when Denmark fell to the Germans, these funds were retained in the United States. They were returned to the Institute in 1949.

In friendship and gratitude, Dr. Hagedorn and his associates decided to donate $50,000 of that accumulated wealth to the study of diabetes in America.

The first fellowship was awarded to a young Danish doctor, Niels Ried Keiding. He worked as a research associate at the Joslin Clinic in Boston from 1952 to

1954. There, he initiated his doctoral thesis, which was published in 1957.

In 1962, Dr. Joslin died at the age of 92. Since then, the Nordisk Fund has continued to grow under ADA administration. The market value of the assets of this fund amounted to approximately $251,700 as of June 30, 1989.

New Developments In Treatment

In 1950, the question of "free diet" (a diet for people with diabetes that did not strictly regulate food intake) came under intense scrutiny and was widely debated.

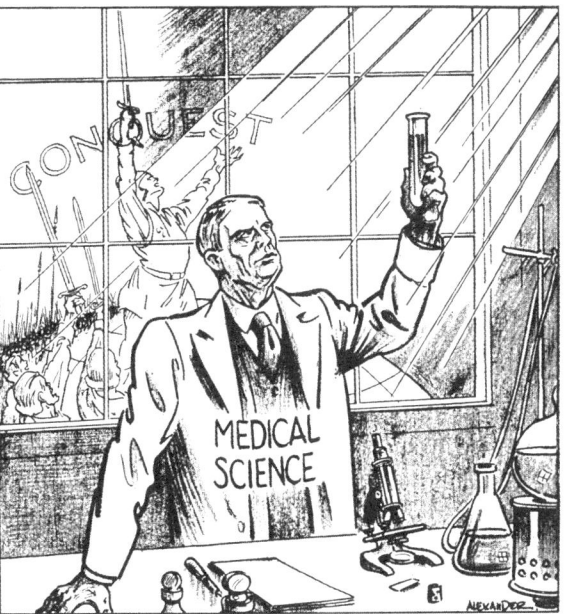

This was the real beginning of the debate on "tight" control. (Keeping diabetes in tight control means keeping blood-glucose levels as close to normal, or nondiabetic, levels as possible.) It was a debate that would continue into the 1980s.

In his president's address, ADA President Howard F. Root, M.D., (1950-51) said, "The problem in treatment is to discover the best way to prevent kidney and eye disease. Since the discovery of insulin, children with diabetes rarely die under the age of 15, and seldom develop serious complications in the first 10 to 15 years of diabetes. This does not mean, however, that treatment pursued in childhood can be carried on throughout a lifetime without serious results. In patients with retinal hemorrhages, improved control has halted progression of the disease."

In the 1950s, many studies were done on people

who had an early onset of the disease and who had had diabetes on a long-term basis. The vast majority of researchers felt that people with good control of their diabetes were less likely to have degenerative complications of the disease, such as retinopathy, arteriosclerosis, and nephropathy, and the results of study after study seemed to support this viewpoint. Two of the pioneers of diabetes care—Frederick Allen, M.D., engineer of the pre-insulin "starvation diet," and Elliott P. Joslin, M.D.—strongly supported good control as a means of preventing or delaying complications.

Yet not everyone agreed that good control of diabetes would have this effect. Some clinicians took the stance that if a person with diabetes felt good, he or she was in good control of the disease; these clinicians considered high blood-glucose levels or sugar in the urine relatively unimportant. Some clinicians, such as Cleveland's Henry J. John, M.D., (one of the first ADA Council members), believed that the diet for people with diabetes should be liberalized, thus doing away with the need for planning, weighing, and estimating food portions as called for by advocates of restricted control. Dr. John thought that people with diabetes should eat in moderation and watch their weight, but need only eliminate sugar from their diet; otherwise, they could eat whatever was served to the rest of the family.

A paper entitled "Degenerative Vascular Complications in Juvenile Diabetes Mellitus," by Drs. Larsson, Lichtenstein, and Ploman of Stockholm, Sweden, appeared in *Diabetes* (Vol. 1:6, 1952). The authors concluded that the use of measured diets do not protect children with diabetes against later vascular complications any more than does treatment with a free and normal diet. Thus the free and normal diet was considered preferable, because, as the authors noted, it has "obvious advantages in offering the diabetic children a chance of a more natural and normal life."

In the same issue, an editorial debated the pros and cons of a free diet. George M. Guest, M.D., pointed out that a "free diet" was not totally free. "Simply speaking, it means a self-selected, unmeasured diet, eaten within reasonable limits of appetite, and in accordance with family habits. Hyperglycemia and glycosuria are not important as long as these do not lead to ketosis." And, Dr. Guest continued, the free diet had the advantage of lessening psychological trauma.

In another editorial, Alexander Marble, M.D., defended a prescribed, disciplined diet. He said that an adequate, nutritious diet that restricted the amount of carbohydrates within the total number of calories allowed was essential to prevent long-term complications. Psychological trauma was minor compared with the deleterious physical effects observed in patients in their thirties and forties after years of poor control, according to Dr. Marble.

The First Postgraduate Course

A milestone in professional education occurred when the first Postgraduate Course (PG) in Diabetes and Metabolic Problems was held January 19-21, 1953, under the direction of Charles H. Best, M.D. The PG Course was held at the University of Toronto, where Dr. Best was director of the Banting and Best Department of Medical Research. Ray F. Farquarson, M.D., professor of medicine, and Dr. Andrew L. Chute, M.D., professor of pediatrics, served as clinical directors of the course. The facilities of the Hospital for Sick Children were placed at the disposal of the participants, and the hospital's lecture theater was used for the presentation of papers and discussions.

The PG Course was designed to be a clinical course for continuing education, primarily for general practitioners. The Course was established to provide clinicians with an opportunity to discuss problems related to clinical practice. It was not meant to examine the most current laboratory research—that was the purpose of the ADA Scientific Sessions, held each year in conjunction with the ADA Annual Meeting.

In attendance at the first Postgraduate Course were physicians from 24 states and the District of Columbia, as well as Canadian physicians from three provinces—a total of 176 registrants. Due to limited facilities, 78 applicants had been turned down, albeit with regret. The Postgraduate Course has been held annually in January since 1953.

At the end of the Course, three-page questionnaires were distributed to registrants. These yielded high praise for the Course. As a result of the Course, the American Diabetes Association received many applications for membership, as well as a substantial number of new subscriptions to *Diabetes*.

Recognizing Progress

On October 4, 1954, the Association was invited to participate in public hearings before a House Committee on Interstate and Foreign Commerce in Washington, D.C. The subject of the hearing was "The Causes, Control and Remedies of the Principal Dis-

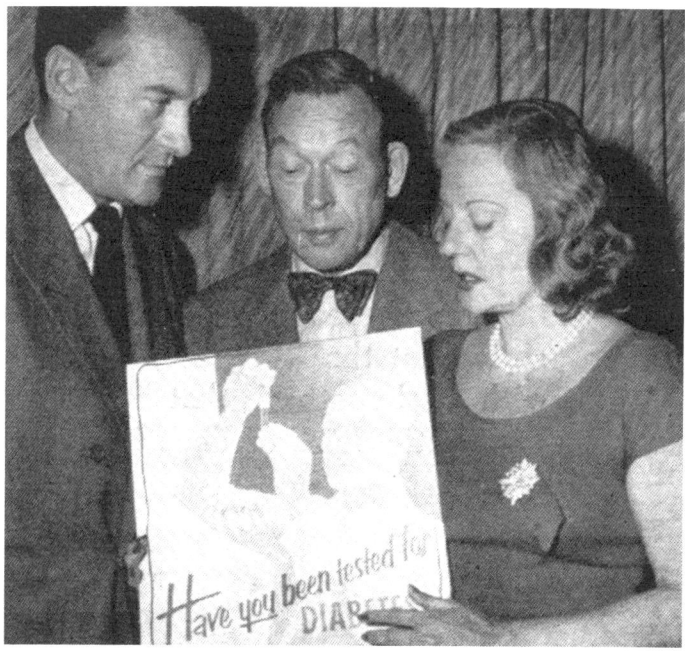
Fred Allen, center, helps promote 1951 Diabetes Week with a half-hour radio show.

eases of Mankind." This was the first time the Association had been invited to make a presentation at a hearing before Congress, and there was very little time to prepare for it—the hearing on diabetes was held October 7. The Association was represented by ADA President Randall G. Sprague, M.D., Secretary John A. Reed, M.D., and Executive Director J. Richard Connelly. Each delivered a statement, but since there had not been sufficient time to clear the statements with the Council, the statements were presented as purely personal observations. Comments dealt with diabetes, its general importance as a cause of illness and death, the methods of control, research activities, and major problems.

At the conclusion of the hearing, Representative John Heselton, of Massachusetts, asked why the Association had not devoted more funds to the support of research. Mr. Connelly read a prepared statement describing the activities and programs of the Association. In response, Charles A. Wolverton, chairman of the House Committee on Interstate and Foreign Commerce, said, "Mr. Connelly, I think the Association for whom you have spoken is entitled to a great deal of credit. Your program is one of the most comprehensive that has been presented to us by any organization. When I realize what you are doing as a private organization, with no public appeal for funds, I am astounded that you could have such expansive and expanding programs. I think you are to be highly commended for the evident worthwhile work that is being done by your Association."

Less than a year later, assessing the status of the American Diabetes Association on its fifteenth anniversary, ADA President Henry B. Mulholland, M.D., (1954-55) said that the Association had passed from a period of adolescence to maturity. "Since 1941 our operating budget has increased 133 percent; our membership 8.4 percent; and our corporate contributions some 67 percent. Our publications have expanded to two bimonthly magazines and a number of other publications. Our annual detection drive has screened over one million people. Now it is time to look forward. The Association is not in dire straits financially, but if we want to continue our programs in education and establish a research program, much more money will be needed."

For the Association, the early 1950s was a time of great growth and change. In 1949, the organization had six paid employees. There were 18 in 1955. The 16 committees that existed in 1949 had grown to 22 by 1955. In 1949, income amounted to $48,024 against expenses of $49,130. By 1955, income had reached $210,033 against expenses of $206,311.

There were 67 county and state Committees on Diabetes nationwide in 1949. In 1955, such groups numbered 905. Affiliates grew from 20 to 38 during the same period. Subscriptions to *Forecast*, which num-

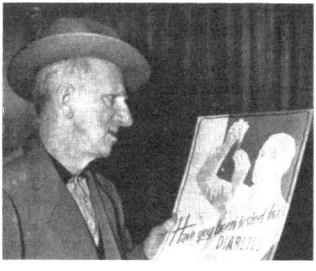

Jimmy Durante, the "Schnozzola," looks at the 1951 Diabetes Week poster.

bered 8,000 in mid-1949, reached 31,352 by 1955. Total ADA membership stood at 1,239 in 1949; it was 2,100 in 1955.

By every yardstick, the Association was thriving. It was ready to face new and bigger challenges as the second half of the decade began.

Pieces Of The Puzzle:
What We Knew About Diabetes

1950

At the 1950 Annual Meeting, E. T. Bell, M.D., reports the results of a long-term study made of 1,214 people with diabetes. The study was conducted at the University of Minnesota from 1910 to 1948. The 1,214 people with diabetes were among 49,922 postmortems done at the University during those years. Among the findings:

- For those with diabetes, coma was responsible for 10 percent of the deaths from 1936 through 1948.

- Among those with diabetes, deaths from vascular disease increased from 12 percent in the third decade of life to 58.7 percent in the eighth decade.

- Fatal coronary disease was about twice as frequent in men with diabetes than in men without diabetes, and three times as frequent in women with diabetes.

- The duration of the diabetic state has a definite influence in accelerating vascular disease in those who die before the age of 60 years, but little or no effect on those who die after that period.

1951

Many people with diabetes are able to control their diabetes with a single daily injection of NPH insulin. If Regular insulin is needed, too, it is combined with the NPH in the syringe. However, NPH apparently has no advantage over other insulins in the treatment of children with diabetes, who often experienced tremendous variation from day to day while following the same diet, exercise, and insulin regimen.

In addition to NPH insulin, other preparations on the market include Regular (or amorphous) insulin—the original form; crystalline insulin; protamine zinc insulin; and globin insulin.

Good medical and obstetric care result in the lowest fetal mortality rate ever recorded for pregnant women with diabetes.

Better recognition of the imbalance of electrolytes and the need for the prompt replacement of fluids and electrolytes results in improvements in the treatment of diabetic coma.

1952

It is thought that environmental stresses can affect diabetes. After examining the life circumstances of 64 people with diabetes, researchers from the New York Hospital/Cornell University Medical Center conclude that there is a causal relationship between stresses and fluctuations in diabetes control.

The role of cholesterol levels and their possible relationship to vascular complications becomes a topic of research.

1953

Lilly Research Labs prepares a highly purified form of glucagon, extracted in crystalline form. Researchers at the University of Chicago Medical School show that glucagon causes hyperglycemia in a nondiabetic dog. Research elsewhere on humans shows that an injection of glucagon causes an abnormal elevation of blood glucose.

In addition to the Benedict's test for glucose in the urine, tablets are now routinely available for urine testing. The tablet method is simple and convenient, but because the tablets may lose their potency (and thus give false negative results), they are greeted with skepticism by some.

In Europe, new preparations of insulin—Lente, Ultralente, and Semilente—are introduced by Novo. Lente corresponds to a mixture of soluble insulin and protamine zinc insulin; Ultralente, to a longer-acting protamine zinc insulin without any action on the morning of administration; and Semilente to Regular insulin. Clinical trials in Denmark show that most people with diabetes can control their disease with a single daily injection of Lente (a mixture of three parts amorphous insulin to seven parts crystalline insulin).

In Vienna, researchers attempt percutaneous administration of insulin: people with "mild" diabetes rubbed 40 Units to 100 Units of standard insulin into the skin on their chests for 10 to 15 minutes. But because of its uncertainties and tediousness, this method of insulin administration is considered impractical.

1954

Research on glucagon indicates that it increases utilization of glucose in the body tissues, and thus can be considered a true hormone. Previous theories had considered glucagon to be a breakdown product of insulin or a "contaminant." It is postulated that glucagon and insulin work together to enhance the use of glucose in the body and to maintain relatively constant blood-glucose and liver glycogen levels. And because glucagon acts rapidly, it is thought to serve an emergency function.

1955

The first heart-lung machine is developed for use in heart surgery. This machine is now used routinely during surgery and other stress situations. Its technology paves the way for later development of the kidney dialysis machine, used for the treatment of diabetic renal disease.

Chapter Five
Expanding Our Reach
1955-60

ADA PRESIDENTS

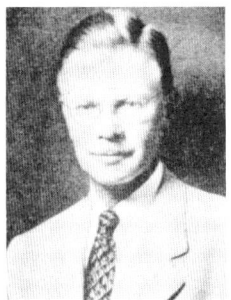

Henry T. Ricketts, M.D.
(1955-56)

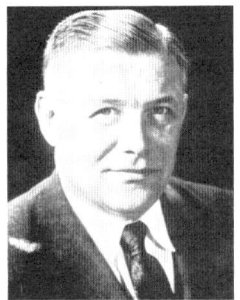

Frederick W. Williams, M.D.
(1956-57)

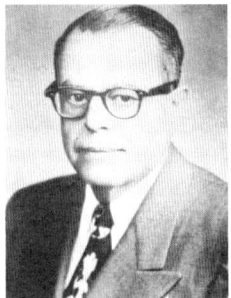

John A. Reed, M.D.
(1957-58)

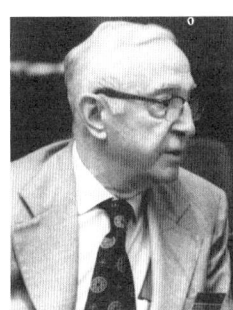

Alexander Marble, M.D.
(1958-59)

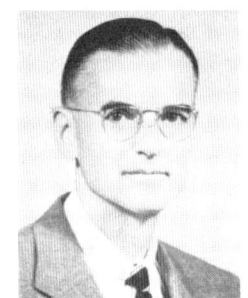

Francis D.W. Lukens, M.D.
(1959-60)

In the years 1955 to 1960, the world was changing rapidly. With the Korean armistice, the nation was technically at peace. Yet the tensions of the Cold War mounted. In 1957, Russia successfully launched two satellites into orbit around the earth and the race for space began.

In the United States, Supreme Court rulings on the desegregation of schools led to racial friction and unrest. The first U.S. space efforts failed, and when the Soviets shot down an American U2 spy plane over Russia in 1960, a major confrontation nearly resulted.

In medicine, Albert Sabin, M.D., produced the first oral vaccine for polio, a discovery that ultimately saved millions from life in a wheelchair. Scientists developed the laser, which would have many uses, not the least of which would be the successful treatment of diabetic retinopathy. The American Heart Association published statistics showing higher death rates among middle-aged men due to smoking, introducing a health issue that was to affect the lives of many, including those with diabetes.

The big news in diabetes treatment was the introduction of oral drugs that lowered blood-glucose levels. However, these oral antidiabetic sulfonamide compounds and sulfonylureas received early and overly optimistic publicity as "a pill instead of insulin." In a report on the new drugs in *ADA Forecast*, ADA President Henry T. Ricketts, M.D., (1955-56) said that studies of these compounds in Germany and the United States showed that when taken by mouth, the drugs did lower blood and urine sugars in *certain* patients. However, predictions as to the future role of the drugs in the treatment of diabetes were premature.

The late 1950s was a time of expansion for the American Diabetes Association. By 1960—the twentieth anniversary of its founding—the Association had 2,575 professional members. Growth was largely attributed to greater awareness of diabetes fostered by the Association, and not to any particular drive for new members.

In addition to increased membership, there was also a steady stream of money coming for research by 1960. Contributions came from wills, bequests, corporations, and individuals. In 1960, the Association received $392,000 in bequests, of which $260,000 came from a single source. Of the total figure, $360,000 was earmarked for research. Had research contributions been less generous during these years, there may have been more urgency for public fund raising. As it was, that issue continued to be debated during the late 1950s.

In his 1960 president's address, ADA President Francis D. W. Lukens, M.D., (1959-60) spoke to the present and future progress of the Association: "In the welter of your various opinions and in the proper search for organizational growth and improvement, let us not forget the ABCs of our own history. We have come to this point because for twenty years many devoted people have worked for the cause of the diabetic, albeit in their varied, individual fashions.

"Let us not forget as we talk of organization and policy, that not too long ago Dr. Ricketts asked, 'Where, oh where will the money come from?' Remember that administration, government, organization, and even money, accomplish nothing of themselves. At best they smooth the path for people, and as long as we have an interest in diabetes we will be, in Biblical words, seeking 'laborers for the vineyard.' We have had loyal and active workers in these first twenty years. I pay them all my personal tribute on this twentieth anniversary, and I remind you never to cease asking this paraphrase of Dr. Ricketts' question: Where oh where will the labor come from? If our present enthusiasm matches that of our charter members, the future course of the American Diabetes Association will be one of continuing progress,'' said Dr. Lukens.

**Elliott P. Joslin, M.D.
1869-1962
The Sage Of
Diabetes Departs**

The following text is reprinted in its entirety as it appeared in the March-April 1962 issue of *ADA Forecast*.

As this issue of *Forecast* goes to press, word has been received of the death in his ninety-third year of Dr. Elliott P. Joslin. Blair Holcomb, M.D., of

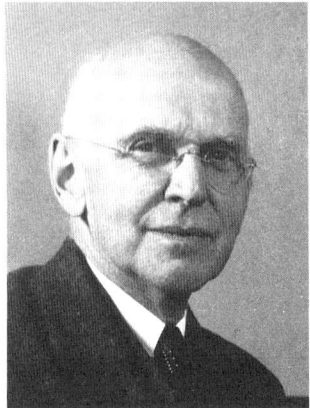

Elliott P. Joslin, M.D.

Portland, Oregon, President of our Association, issued the following statement on behalf of the Officers, Councilors and Members, on learning of the death of their beloved and esteemed colleague:

"In the passing of Dr. Joslin, the world has lost one of the great physicians of our times, a man whose creative clinical advances over half a century have made life easier and longer for millions of people with diabetes.

"Dr. Joslin's passing leaves an unappeasable feeling of personal loss in the hearts of the many physicians who trained at the renowned clinic in Boston which bears his name, and the tens of thousands of diabetics who have received individual care and meticulous instruction from Dr. Joslin and his associates, thus enabling them to lead active

Oral Drugs for Diabetes Introduced

In 1956, American, Canadian, and German researchers, as well as representatives from a number of laboratories and clinics, determined that oral antidiabetic sulfonamide compounds and sulfonylureas were not a substitute for insulin, nor did they imitate the action of insulin. Their major effect was to diminish destruction of insulin in the body, thus making any available insulin more effective.

Studies in all three countries showed that the drugs reduced high blood and urine sugars in people whose diabetes had been diagnosed in adulthood. However, the drugs did not lower blood sugar in the majority of children with diabetes or in adults who had had the disease since childhood. (Some studies showed that in children who had diabetes only a short while, the compounds did have a hypoglycemic effect—but only for a brief time. This was consistent with the theory that during the first months after onset, many children with diabetes were able to produce some insulin—but only for a while.) Such observations indicated that the age of onset and the duration of diabetes determined the effectiveness of the drugs. In general, older patients with diabetes of relatively short duration seemed to respond best—usually those whose diabetes was easiest to control with diet. (It was stressed, however, that dietary restrictions must continue to be observed when using the sulfonamides.) The implication was that some pancreatic insulin must be present for these compounds to work, and therefore, that a functioning, presumably insulin-producing pancreas must be present.

At this time, assessment of the long-term effects of oral sulfonamides was not possible. But studies indicated that the toxic effects were negligible; liver tests revealed no evidence of deterioration, and there was no apparent kidney damage.

However, Dr. Ricketts spoke words of caution. "There are risks in using these new drugs. (Injected) insulin is a specific hormone, and replaces or makes up for a relative or absolute insulin deficiency. Indiscriminate replacement of insulin with sulfonamides could result in loss of (blood-sugar) control, ketosis, or even coma. When complications of infection, surgery, or acidosis exist, insulin is indispensable, and these drugs should not be used.

"The well-being, comfort, and convenience of the patient is our continuing concern, but further evidence is needed before the ultimate usefulness of the sulfonamides can be determined. Until we have more definitive information on the mechanism of their action, and

and productive lives.

"I know that I express the feelings of sorrow felt by every member of the American Diabetes Association, of which Dr. Joslin has been Honorary President since its founding in 1940, when I say that we have lost an irreplaceable physician and human being, a man whose life and achievements as a scholar, teacher, author, and scientist have been an inspiration to us all. His guidance and positive, vital approach to the control of diabetes and to life in general will be truly missed.

"Elliott Proctor Joslin was born June 6, 1869, in Oxford, Massachusetts, and died in Boston, January 28, 1962. The world's foremost authority on the care and treatment of people with diabetes, he was active in his clinic until the day before his death.

"In addition to his work as a practicing physician, Dr. Joslin was an outstanding medical educator, having been Clinical Professor of Medicine at the Harvard Medical School from 1922 to 1937, and Emeritus Professor thereafter. His reputation and influence were both worldwide, as is indicated by the fact that he had been Honorary President of the International Diabetes Federation since it was founded over ten years ago. Dr. Joslin, who was a skilled and inspirational speaker, presented the first Banting Memorial Lecture for the American Diabetes Association in 1941. This honorary lecture, given annually, is a memorial to the co-discoverer of insulin, Sir Frederick G. Banting.

"As author, Dr. Joslin wrote the standard textbook on the treatment of diabetes, which he first published in 1916. He and his associates revised this landmark in publishing for the

the long-term observation for possible chronic harmful effects, the drugs will not be available for sale," Dr. Ricketts said.

Studies on another sulfonylurea, known as Compound 860, showed that it was useful in lowering blood sugar. Compound 860 was given the generic name of tolbutamide and licensed in the United States under the name of Orinase in 1957. Chlorpropamide, a compound with the trade name of Diabinese, was tested and then released by the Federal Drug Administration in 1958. Precautions for physicians prescribing these new drugs stipulated: They are not beneficial for "juvenile" or "brittle" diabetics, and are suitable only in middle-aged and elderly patients taking 40 units or less of insulin daily.

In 1958, an addendum to the *Diabetic Guidebook for Physicians* was revised to include information on the new oral hypoglycemic drugs. At that time, the guidebook was the definitive reference book on diabetes for physicians.

Research that began in 1954 on a different family of chemicals, the biguanides, produced phenformin in 1959. Phenformin was of sufficient importance and interest to warrant a symposium by the American Diabetes Association in 1960, "A New Oral Hypoglycemic Agent." ADA President Alexander Marble, M.D., (1958-59) summarized the conclusions of the symposium with the following statement: "Phenformin is a biguanide which, when taken by mouth, has a blood-sugar lowering effect in certain diabetic patients of all ages . . . . Phenformin is a compound of great interest. Further studies are needed to clarify its mechanism of action and define its place in the management of diabetes."

(Phenformin was eventually withdrawn from the market by the FDA in 1977, when it was found to cause lactic acidosis. In July 1977, the American Diabetes Association and the Committee on Materials and Therapeutic Agents issued a "Statement on Phenformin," supporting the FDA decision to withdraw the drug from the market. "Mounting scientific data from the United States and other countries indicated that phenformin may constitute a significant health risk in that lactic acidosis may develop and death may even result in some diabetic patients using this drug," the statement said [*Diabetes*, Vol. 26:8, 1977].)

The Lilly Award

In 1956, the Lilly Award was established to recognize demonstrated research in the field of diabetes, taking

tenth edition as recently as 1959. Dr. Joslin was at work on an eleventh edition at the time of his death. He also published a manual for diabetic patients in 1918, and a tenth revised edition in 1959. In addition, he was the author or coauthor of many basic scientific and clinical papers on diabetes. He was the recipient of such honorary awards as the Distinguished Service Medal of the American Medical Association, which he received in 1943, and the Honorary Diploma of the Swiss Academy of Medical Sciences, which was awarded him on his visit to Geneva, Switzerland, only last July, to attend the Fourth Congress of the International Diabetes Federation.

"A story about Dr. Joslin and the Fourth Congress, and also a vital and informative article by Dr. Joslin himself called 'Diabetes in the Future,' appeared the November-December 1961 issue of the *ADA Forecast*, and his photograph was featured on the cover.

"Dr. Joslin, to the very last, was active, alert, and interested in life. The Friday before his death he kept regular office hours, seeing several patients with diabetes; and on Sunday he attended church as was his usual custom. His death that same evening was sudden and without any illness or pain.

"He will truly be missed by those who were privileged to know him and to benefit from the blessings of his work."

into consideration originality and independence of thought. Any investigator who is in an appropriate field of work closely related to diabetes, is less than 40 years of age on January 1 of the year in which the award is presented, and is a resident of either the United States or Canada is eligible to receive this award. Today, the Outstanding Investigator Award, sponsored by Eli Lilly and Company, continues to be bestowed. The winner is announced at the Annual Meeting and receives a cash award and a gold medal. Travel expenses are also covered for the recipient so that he or she may receive the award in person.

The recipient of the first Lilly Award, in 1957, was Solomon A. Berson, chief of Radioisotope Service at

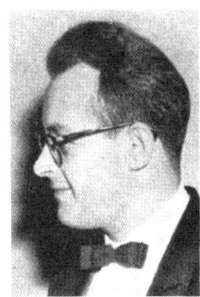

Solomon A. Berson, M.D., the first Lilly Award recipient

the Veterans Administration Hospital, Bronx, New York. Dr. Berson subsequently collaborated with Nobel Laureate Rosalyn S. Yalow on the radioimmunoassay test for determining the exact amount of insulin in the blood. (A list of Lilly Award recipients can be found in Appendix 7-C.)

More Debate Over Fund Raising

In no matter, great or small, can it be said that the American Diabetes Association ever acted recklessly. The monumental struggle over whether to engage in public fund raising was debated by ADA leaders over several years, and even after a general vote was taken, action was slow to follow. In June 1956, the Council accepted the following recommendations:

1) That the American Diabetes Association continue its policy of not engaging in general public fund raising at the national level.

2) That the Association withdraw its opposition to general public fund raising by an affiliate, provided its clinical society or medical advisory group considered it essential in the local situation, and approved the methods employed, and provided that such activities be restricted to the geographical area as defined in the terms of its affiliates. Further, the advice and counsel of the

A New Marketing Strategy

In 1959, the Association published *A Cookbook for Diabetics* by Deaconness Maude Behrman, author of the popular food and recipe section of *ADA Forecast*. The *Cookbook* was the first of its kind written especially for people with diabetes. It became an instant bestseller. Published in paperback, spirally bound, the book included 176 recipes based on the *Exchange Lists* and sold for $1. The original printing of 50,000 sold out quickly. The book was reprinted, selling over one million copies between 1959 and 1976.

One reason for the wide popularity of the *Cookbook* was a simple, inexpensive promotional idea, whereby printed postcards describing the publication, its modest price, and availability were distributed to physicians by salesmen from pharmaceutical firms. Physicians then gave the cards to their patients with diabetes, who could order the *Cookbook* directly from the American Diabetes Association. Thanks to this promotional technique, sales of the book remained high for years. In 1970, when the price was raised to $2 because of rising costs, five to ten postcard orders per week were still being received.

national Association would be available and the affiliate would be expected to act in accordance with the objectives, principles and policies of the American Diabetes Association.

3) That the American Diabetes Association would welcome appropriate contributions from the affiliates to further the objectives of the Association.

4) That the American Diabetes Association reserve the right to terminate affiliation of any affiliate employing fund-raising techniques that are unethical, undignified, or otherwise unacceptable to the national Association.

5) That a committee be appointed to draw up means of giving advice and counsel to affiliates employing, among other means, a revision of the *Fund Raising Manual for Affiliate Diabetes Associations of the American Diabetes Association*.

6) That the implementation date of supplying advice and counsel, as provided above, be January 1957.

In the subsequent *Fund Raising Manual*, published in 1957, there was a section on "undesirable practices," which listed campaigns with other agencies, appeals during detection drives, use of fear techniques, and appeals for camps that make reference to "crippled" or "handicapped" children as unacceptable.

Another section outlined "unacceptable solicitation techniques," such as telethons; paid newspaper advertising; buying radio or television time; collection cans or containers; bingo, raffles, or other games of chance; general door-to-door canvassing; general mail appeals; general telephone appeals; mailing of unordered tickets, merchandise, or stamps; high-pressure methods using intimidation or coercion; and payment in any form of commissions for fund raising. According to the guidelines, use of any of these techniques placed the affiliate in jeopardy.

In his presidential message in 1957, ADA President John A. Reed, M.D., (1957-58) said, "Perhaps the most important development that occurred within the past week is the modification of the fund-raising policy of the Association, permitting general public fund raising on the part of affiliate organizations. This action puts a different complexion on the organization from that which it has worn since its founding. I should like to admonish the members that this move, possibly, could lead to a decidedly different kind of control in the local affiliates, unless physician members are determined to retain that control in their own hands. This may take some watchdog activity. I hope it will be exercised."

Diabetes, Pregnancy, and Priscilla White: Progress by the 1950s

Before the advent of insulin, most women with diabetes were sterile and could not bear children at all. Of those who could, few were able to go through a normal pregnancy and bear a healthy child. Thus, the problem of pregnancy was one physicians rarely encountered. Even when they did, they could do nothing.

For several years after the discovery of insulin, successful pregnancies were still relatively rare among women with diabetes. Young women with insulin-dependent (type I) diabetes found that they could indeed become pregnant; but for some reason their babies were born dead or died soon after birth.

Thanks to insulin, many young girls with diabetes had grown to marriageable age by 1930, and refused to be denied the rights of motherhood. The results were not encouraging. Over the first post-insulin years, records showed that even in cases where women with long-duration diabetes had successful pregnancies, only half of the infants survived. It was a difficult and discouraging time. But a considerable amount of highly valuable information was being discovered by several exceptional physi-

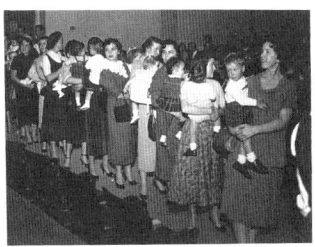

These mothers with diabetes line up for a meeting of the Greater Boston Diabetes Society. Photo courtesy of the Joslin Diabetes Center.

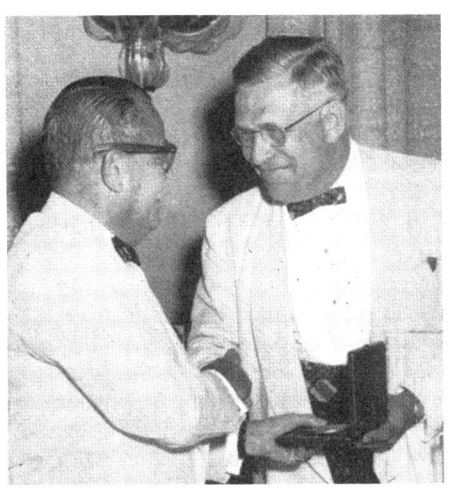

In June 1958, John A. Reed, M.D., left, retiring ADA president, receives the Banting Medal from immediate past President Frederick W. Williams, M.D.

The comments of J. Richard Connelly, executive director, at the Council meeting that followed reflect the concern felt by many in the organization. "The recent change in policy adopted by the Council, for affiliates to engage in general public fund raising, I am sure will present many problems. To those of you who are members of affiliates, I would personally like to urge conservative campaigns if your affiliate decides to enter into this kind of activity. We urge you to wait until the national organization has had an opportunity to set forth certain principles and guides. Although the Council did not intend for the parent organization to become engaged in various campaigns themselves, we will try to provide whatever counsel is necessary."

Over time, the fund-raising issue evolved into today's formula. Local affiliates and chapters perform their fund-raising functions with planning, coordination, and assistance from the national Association.

Pregnancy and Diabetes

A panel discussion, "Pregnancy and Diabetes," was convened at the Annual Meeting in 1957. Moderator and former ADA President Lester J. Palmer, M.D., said in his introductory remarks that despite numerous studies, methods of treatment and other aspects of diabetes management during pregnancy remain controversial and unresolved.

Noted physician Priscilla White, M.D., said, "Only one in 1,000 diabetic women conceived in the pre-insulin era, but fertility in the post-insulin period has

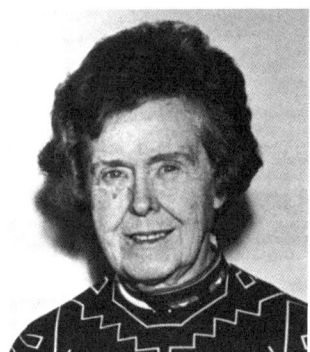

Priscilla White, M.D.

cians who entered the unknown field of diabetes and pregnancy. Foremost among them was Priscilla White, M.D.—a pioneer in many ways.

Priscilla White was born in Boston in 1900. She attended Radcliffe College and graduated third in her class at Tufts University Medical School, which she attended after Harvard Medical School refused her admission on grounds of gender.

Dr. White met Elliott P. Joslin, M.D., in 1924 and joined his staff by invitation. It was one of the great collaborations in diabetes history. She remained at the Joslin Clinic through her entire career—over 50 years. During that time, she became one of the world's foremost authorities on pregnancy and diabetes, as well as in the field of juvenile diabetes.

Her remarkable achievements earned her countless honors, including the Banting Medal (1960). She spoke and taught all over the world, and had the ultimate satisfaction of living to teach classes at Harvard. She wrote hundreds of medical articles and texts, many of which were published in various Association periodicals. She was an active ADA member, and served on numerous committees.

been unimpaired, resulting in more diabetic pregnancies. However, the statistics on successful deliveries and healthy babies are discouraging. With increasing fertility there has been increased fetal wastage. A pregnancy in the pre-insulin era could be summarized as destructive, because most women died undelivered. Today, with insulin, diabetic women survive, but without intervention only one woman out of three delivers a living infant. Perinatal loss is 45 percent; previable loss 20 percent, and toxemia 33 percent. Therefore, the causes of abnormalities must be found and modes of prevention discovered in three areas, maternal, placental and fetal. Chemical, functional, and structural abnormalities occur in all three areas and may be related to fetal fatalities."

Speaking on "The Significance of Glycosuria and the Abnormal Glucose Tolerance Curve During Pregnancy," Edmund L. Shelvin, M.D., of New York City, said, "There is abundant evidence that diabetes may start long before clinical recognition, and fetal mortality in the unrecognized diabetic may be as great, if not greater than, in the known diabetic. Retrospective studies indicate that unexplained intra-uterine deaths, large-sized babies, episodes of pre-eclampsia, and even habitual abortions, may be due to diabetes lurking in the background." His remarks are among the earliest to recognize the seriousness and extent of "gestational diabetes."

(Gestational diabetes was officially identified by the National Diabetes Data Group in 1979 as one of four types of diabetes. That same year—along with the American College of Obstetricians and Gynecologists, the National Institutes of Health, the Centers for Disease Control, the U.S. Public Health Service, and McNeil Laboratories—the American Diabetes Association sponsored the first International Workshop on Gestational Diabetes [*Diabetes Care*, Symposium on Gestational Diabetes, Vol. 3:3, 1980]. The American Diabetes Association has devoted considerable attention and study to pregnancy and diabetes over the years, with particular emphasis on gestational diabetes, which is often unrecognized and left untreated.)

Employment And Insurance

In 1957, the Committee on Employment mailed questionnaires to 434 business and industrial concerns throughout the country to ascertain the attitude of employers toward people with diabetes.

The survey was a prodigious accomplishment in the pre-computer age. The entire job was handled by a na-

Soon after joining Dr. Joslin in 1924, Dr. White started the Joslin Pregnancy Clinic. At the time, only 56 percent of babies born to women with diabetes survived. Fifty years later, Dr. White had achieved a 90 percent survival rate among her patients.

How did she do it? M. Donna Younger, M.D., who heads the Joslin Clinic's Pregnancy Center today, was a long-time protegee of Dr. White, and has a keen insight into her methods and techniques.

"Through meticulous, pioneering research," wrote Dr. Younger, "Dr. White learned that insulin and blood sugars had to be carefully controlled to reduce greatly the risks of birth defects and maternal and infant death. She emphasized the importance of strict blood-sugar control before and during pregnancy, and showed that stillbirths in the last few weeks prior to term could be avoided by early (Caesarean section) delivery."

By 1952, Dr. White was able to write in *ADA Forecast*: "Today no diabetic woman should hesitate to try having a child if she wants one, if her physician approves, and if the father is nondiabetic."

Dr. White stressed five rules of treatment to be followed "if pregnancy in a diabetic is to have a chance of success." First was *diet*, with weight kept down but strength and blood supply increased. Dr. White believed in a diet high in protein and fairly liberal in carbohydrate. Second was *insulin therapy*, often meaning an increase in dosage during pregnancy. Third "for certain diabetic women" was the administration of *female hormones*, preferably by injection. Dr. White's fourth rule stressed the desirability of *early delivery*

tional office staff of 20. "Analysis of a Survey Concerning Employment of Diabetics in Some Major Industries" (*Diabetes*, Vol. 6:6, 1957) reached these conclusions:

- An enlightened attitude on the employment of diabetics existed to an encouraging extent in the country's leading businesses and industrial concerns.

- A corollary of this conclusion was that the larger the company, the more enlightened the attitude.

- Most companies, small and large, employed known diabetics, though companies who did not, did continue employment when diabetes developed.

- In general, the picture was not good. Some companies, even larger ones, did not employ known diabetics; most did not make any concessions as to rotation of shifts for diabetics they did employ.

That same year, the U.S. Civil Service Commission distributed the leaflet "Employment of Diabetics in the Federal Service." The commission stated that "persons with controlled diabetes may be good employees and it is good business to hire them."

In 1957, an article in *ADA Forecast*, "The Truth About Life Insurance for Diabetics," challenged readers to learn whether they could obtain life insurance. Until 1940, people with diabetes were denied insurance because mortality statistics were unavailable and insurance companies could not decide how much more to charge for premiums. Subsequently, it became customary to add an arbitrary amount, originally $10, to the annual premium (more or less, depending on age) for people with diabetes. In general, the applicant had to:
1) be between the ages of 20 and 70;
2) be able to carry on normal activities;
3) be able to lead a stable, well-regulated existence, as to rest, work habits, and exercise;
4) have no abnormality or complications likely to decrease life expectancy;
5) be under adequate medical supervision; and
6) control diabetes with no more than 75 units of insulin daily.

As reasonable as the criteria seemed, many people with diabetes just could not qualify. Common reasons for rejection were:
1) lack of control;
2) abnormal condition of the blood vessels and heart;
3) kidney disorders;
4) too high an insulin dose;
5) alcoholic habits;

in many cases. "Some patients appear to do well if their babies are delivered two to three weeks early; others sometimes have to be delivered as much as five to six weeks early," Dr. White wrote. Her fifth rule stressed the health of the newborn infant itself by insisting upon *special care at birth*. Dr. White saw this extra care as the surest means to avoid difficulties for the infant: breathing problems, low blood sugar, and other diabetes-connected malfunctions.

Dr. White assured prospective mothers with diabetes that pregnancy did not increase the severity of their disease. She told them that diabetes usually did not develop in a child if only one parent inherited a tendency toward it. She emphasized close and constant cooperation between patient and physician during the term of pregnancy.

Throughout her career, Dr. White followed her own precepts. She attended mothers-to-be with skill and understanding, and went personally with them to the delivery room. She felt it was her place to care for and support the mother, and to direct survival procedures for the newborn infant. Over time, she became an "associate mother" to more than 2,500 children—by far the largest group of its kind in the world.

In 1974, Dr. White retired. She still came to the Clinic, although she conceded slightly to age by cutting her workday to 10 hours. She remained active and alert while pursuing a new interest: the emotional problems of youngsters with diabetes.

Dr. White died December 16, 1989, in Boston. She was 90. Her immense contributions to diabetes medicine have secured her place in history.

6) too recent a diagnosis;
7) excessive weight;
8) visual disturbance; and
9) age.

A typical life insurance premium in 1957 for a person with diabetes 45 years of age was about $48 per thousand for a 20-year basic endowment policy—a high price for that time.

It is easier today for people with diabetes to obtain life insurance, due to a better understanding of the nature of the disease and new technology that has improved management of diabetes. With the growth of group insurance policies, many people with diabetes are covered through their employer. However, individual policies for people with diabetes usually require a higher premium.

Providing Information to Professionals

Recognizing the need for greater access to information on diabetes, a *Diabetes Related Literature Index*, which listed appropriate articles by author, title, and key words, was established in 1960. It incorporated 2,500 diabetes-related articles from the cumulative 1960 *Index Medicus* and was published as *Diabetes Supplement* 1, Vol. 14:, 1962. It was distributed to all members. This first attempt to systemize information retrieval later evolved into a specialized computer service similar to the National Library of Medicine's Literature Analysis Project. A second and a third index were also published in *Diabetes, Supplement* 1, Vols. 15 and 16, 1963 and 1964.

About the same time, the Cleveland Diabetes Association, which was not affiliated with the American Diabetes Association, began a similar endeavor. It gathered and evaluated patient and professional diabetes education materials. The resulting bibliography was known as *The Cleveland Book*, or the *DAC Index*, and was widely used from 1965 to 1975. Mary Ann Keller, R.N., M.S., C.D.E., who would later serve as the Executive Director of the ADA North Dakota Affiliate, was the nurse educator who compiled the bibliography.

(With the passage of the National Diabetes Research and Education Act of 1974, and the establishment of the National Diabetes Advisory Board, funds were allocated for a National Diabetes Information Clearinghouse. Charged to gather, analyze, and evaluate information and publish bibliographies on all diabetes literature, the clearinghouse accomplished this in a mere three years. Since then, the information has become part of the Combined Health Information Data-

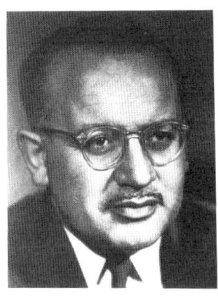

**Rachmiel Levine
And The Key To Insulin**

With their discovery of insulin in 1921, Frederick Banting and Charles Best revolutionized the world of diabetes treatment. It was not until the late 1950s, however, that another man discovered how insulin actually works. His name is Rachmiel Levine, and many consider him the father of modern diabetes research.

Rachmiel Levine was born in Poland and orphaned at an early age. Looking to the new world, he tried to get a United States visa but failed. He went instead to Canada, where a Canadian physician adopted him, and, at age 16, he entered Montreal's McGill University. In the early 1930s, at McGill, he studied with James Collip, the biochemist who first purified insulin extract with Banting and Best. After taking his medical degree, Dr. Levine went to Michael Reese Hospital in Chicago to work in diabetes research with Samuel Soskin, M.D.

The two formed a great research team. Together, they published Levine's first paper, "The Effects of Blood-Sugar Level on Sugar Utilization." It showed that the greater the amount of sugar in the blood, the greater the amount of blood sugar used. Even in those early years, Levine was thinking along the lines that would later result in his solution of the insulin mystery. He was already intrigued by the idea that substances can work

bank. Today, the National Diabetes Information Clearinghouse is the authoritative source of all diabetes literature.)

The first National Conference on Teaching and Research in Diabetes, sponsored by the American Diabetes Association and the National Institutes of Arthritis, Metabolic and Digestive Diseases (NIAMDD), the Public Health Service, and the U.S. Department of Health, Education and Welfare, was held May 1958. Proceedings of the conference were edited, published, and distributed by the American Diabetes Association. They went to all participants; ADA members; deans of medical schools; professors of medicine, diabetes, and metabolism; program directors; and International Diabetes Federation members.

In January 1960, the American Diabetes Association cosponsored a "Diabetes Program Directors Workshop" with NIAMDD. Immediately following the Postgraduate Course, the workshop provided an opportunity for program directors to exchange information and experiences.

Product Endorsement Policy

A Policy Statement prohibiting the use of photographs or citations of individual physician members in the endorsement of pharmaceutical products was passed by the Council in 1959. Members were apprised of the possible misinterpretation by persons with diabetes. The policy strictly prohibited the endorsement of any product by a member of the American Diabetes Association.

Reaching The Public

Celebrities with diabetes have always been in demand for fund raising. Public acknowledgement of diabetes by a prominent person dispels fears about the disease and gives encouragement to those who have it. In 1959, the Association was fortunate to have Carol Haney, dancer, choreographer, director, singer, and actress, serving as national chairman. She was appearing in "Pajama Game" on Broadway, and the image of a young, energetic, hardworking, successful actress was a good role model for young people with diabetes. Some years later, Mary Tyler Moore, actress and television star, was featured in a cover story in *Diabetes Forecast*. The reaction to this story was phenomenal—hundreds of letters were received at the national office. People had no difficulty relating to her as a real person with real problems, one of which was diabetes.

through mechanical as well as chemical means.

The Levine/Soskin research team continued and captured the attention of researchers around the world. Albert Renold (who became a Levine associate) first read their 1946 book, "Carbohydrate Metabolism," in Switzerland. He called it "the first orderly and comprehensible summary of the basic sciences. (It) laid the groundwork for a greater knowledge and better treatment of diabetes."

Levine then began researching the question of how insulin works. By the 1950s, other researchers were uncovering details of how a cell uses a glucose molecule. They were figuring out the complex biochemistry of the breakdown of sugar. "We found that a molecule of glucose goes through many, many steps before its energy can be used," Levine recalled. Everybody knew that insulin speeded up these processes. What nobody knew was how.

Levine found out. His idea was deceptively simple but radically different. What if insulin had nothing to do with the individual actions of breaking down sugar inside the cell? What if, instead, insulin simply helped glucose to get inside the cell?

"Everyone thought insulin caused a chemical change like an enzyme," said Levine. But couldn't insulin have a mechanical rather than a chemical effect? Couldn't it work by *transporting* glucose into the cell rather than by *transforming* it, once inside?

This theory—now called the Levine Effect or the transport theory—holds that insulin permits glucose to be moved into cells. Like a key, insulin opens a gate into the cell, allowing glucose to get inside.

National Diabetes Week, which began in 1948, continued to be a success. Each year, thousands more people were screened for diabetes. Physicians were asked to play a bigger role in these drives and they willingly did. In a fortuitous merger of professional

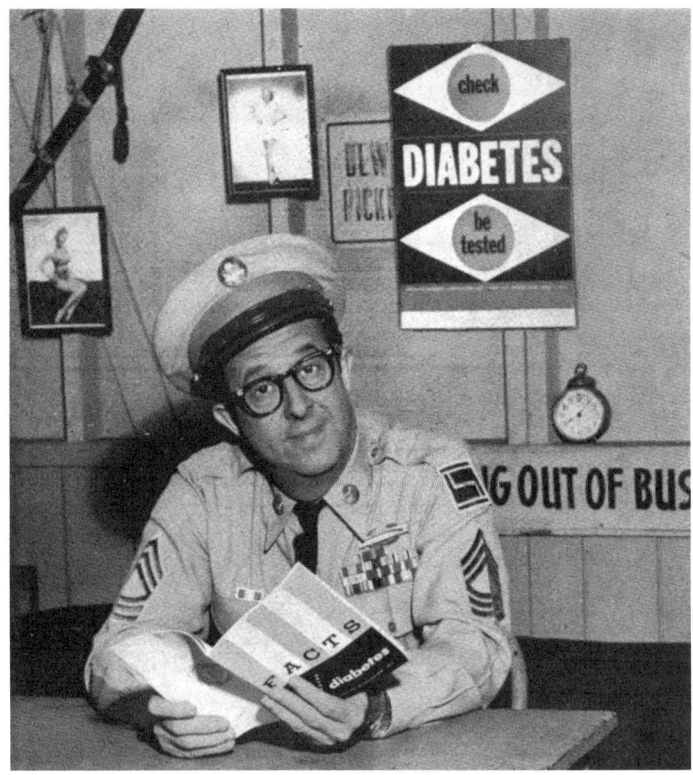

In March 1957, Phil Silvers, better known as the popular Master Sergeant Ernie Bilko, requests that all members of his audience join in the national Detection Drive by taking a test for diabetes.

with public education, a new scientific exhibit was added annually. By 1960, three exhibits were displayed at large medical meetings by affiliate clinical societies. Intended primarily to educate and interest the physician in diabetes, displays at the exhibits consisted of "The Management of Diabetes Mellitus," "Vascular Complications of Diabetes Mellitus," "Diabetes Detection by the Physician," and "Diabetes Today and Tomorrow: The Expanding Role of the Doctor." The exhibits were available without cost and were widely used.

In collaboration with the American Foundation for the Blind (AFB), the "talking book" *Encore* was developed in 1958. It contained a transcription of selected articles from *Forecast*. *Encore* was a series of records, available on loan to anyone registered as le-

It took many years for Levine and his associates to prove their theory. By the 1960s, though, the scientific community was convinced. The Levine concept put medical science on the road to today's quest for the specific cell receptors for the insulin molecule. It ushered in a whole new era in which investigators began to ask how hormones, such as insulin, modify fundamental functions of the cell.

In 1960, Levine became professor and chairman of the Department of Medicine at the New York College of Medicine. A diabetes center there was later dedicated in his name. In 1964-65, he served as twenty-third president of the American Diabetes Association.

He moved across country in 1971 to become director of the City of Hope Medical Center in Duarte, California. His first act there was to establish a department for diabetes clinical care and research. Under Levine's direction, the City of Hope helped produce human insulin from recombinant DNA.

Fakers, Quacks, and Diabetes

Quacks and charlatans have flourished for decades on the fringes of diabetes medicine.

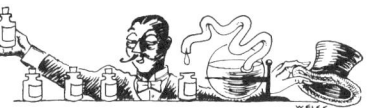

Long after the discovery of insulin, many people with diabetes fell easy prey to newspaper ads like the following, which appeared around the country in the mid-1950s: "DIABETICS. Modern Medicine will take you off the needle and reduce your diabetes to a point where you can control it. Control costs you less than 10 cents per day . . . ."

gally blind. At that time, the records could be borrowed from regional libraries or purchased from AFB. In the early 1980s, with the advent of new recording techniques and the floppy disk, the records were given out free. This service is still available. Registration is through the Regional Libraries for the Blind or through the Library of Congress. The American Diabetes Association is justly proud of its role in this unique service, which has been provided to the blind without interruption since its inception.

Reaching The Volunteers

The *Affiliate Builder*, forerunner of today's *Management Letter*, served as chronicle of the era when the Association was gradually changing over to a voluntary health agency. It was launched in 1959 as a bimonthly newsletter to keep the burgeoning affiliates and chapters informed about Association programs and activities. It was published continuously until 1974. Today's *Management Letter* is issued from the office of the national executive vice president every Friday and sent to each affiliate.

Growth And Activity

In 1958, the American Diabetes Association was listed for the first time as one of 59 health and voluntary organizations in the *Givers Guide to National Philanthropies*. The *Guide* was published by the National Information Bureau, a nonprofit organization founded in 1918 for the purpose of advising and protecting contributors.

At the Annual Meeting banquet in June 1960, ADA President Francis D. W. Lukens, M.D., (1959-60) described the physical condition of the Association: "Every member of this Association knows that we are suffering from growing pains. The syndrome, not yet in the text books, consists of Councilors' headaches, spastic stasis of committees, laudable restlessness of many individual members, and miscellaneous forms of affiliate itching. The treatment consists of decalcification, reorganization, representation, and mental catharsis all directed to achieve a clear definition of the purposes and directions of our future activities. It is a gladsome fact that on our twentieth anniversary, I should mention growth as our principal problem. Would any of you wish it otherwise?"

To treat these "ills" and solve the problems confronting the Association, the Council needed information about the needs and wishes of the professional

It sounded inviting to a young salesman named John R. Fredericks. He answered the ad and stopped taking his insulin. Fredericks died suddenly May 12, 1954—one day before the Federal Drug Administration launched an investigation that closed down the fraudulent operation.

From its inception, the American Diabetes Association was aware that such pseudo-medical chicanery existed. ADA members were physicians, and knew first-hand that some of their diabetes patients were particularly vulnerable to the pie-in-the-sky promises of quacks.

There were two important reasons why people with diabetes were so susceptible to phony treatments, despite the serious consequences. One was the necessity for injections. Many people with diabetes intensely disliked them, which gave the quack his opportunity. By offering a treatment that did not involve injections, the charlatan found

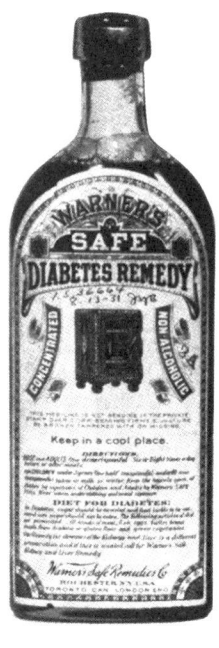

membership. The Council approved sending a questionnaire to that membership. About 2,500 questionnaires were mailed and 850 answers were received. "This 34-percent reply affords a useful sampling of your various opinions, and provides an index of interest in the ADA which is most encouraging," said Dr. Lukens.

Dr. Lukens went on to summarize the responses to the questionnaire sent to members by reading some of the questions and answers.

" 'Are you in accord with the present programs of ADA?' This question turned out to be an ambiguous one. A 'Yes' answer might mean agreement with stated purposes of the program, but reservations about fulfillment of objectives. A 'No' might mean disenchantment with progress, but approval of goals. There were 76 'No' answers, and these were qualified by expressions of a desire for a change in emphasis in the Association's four-fold programs (patient education, professional education, public education and detection, and research.) Some answered 'Yes,' and others qualified their answer by saying 'Yes,' but not with the manner in which programs are carried out," said Dr. Lukens.

In response to the question, "Are you in accord with the present organizational structure of ADA?," 55 percent voted that the Association should become a solely professional organization, while 34 percent voted against the idea.

In answer to the question, "Do you favor public fund raising?" Dr. Lukens noted that there were 495 "No" votes and 260 "Yes" votes.

The last item, which asked for other comments, drew suggestions from 394 respondents (46 percent) for improving the professional education program, the journal *Diabetes*, and the organizational structure.

Dr. Lukens offered the following summary of the survey:

"One, we can become a solely medical organization, terminate the affiliate system as legal units of our Association . . . assuming that members of the ADA would support their local independent units, aid in local fund raising, detection, public education, etc. Under such a plan, the local groups would have complete autonomy, which many comments requested.

"Two, we can become a full-scale national voluntary health agency, with the hazards of this venture. The majority, if not all, of our professional activities, could probably be retained under this structure.

"Three, we can deliberately foster the development

a receptive segment of the diabetes population that wanted to believe him. Second was the nature of diabetes itself, which helped the faker trap his victims. Most people with diabetes have mild or moderately severe cases. Most have non-insulin-dependent (type II) diabetes. With exercise and diet control, they can actually get better, or appear to be getting better. This was a fertile field for exploitation, since a quack could claim that his "treatment" was responsible for the patient's improvement. Often, the victim would seem to be doing well while actually developing the complications of uncontrolled diabetes.

Knowing this, the Association established a Committee on Nostrums at its founding meeting in 1940. The committee's job was to police the marketplace and protect those with diabetes from useless or harmful treatments. In 1950, the Committee on Nostrums was absorbed into the Committee on Scientific Evaluation (now the Committee on Scientific and Medical Programs).

One of the committee's most famous victories came in the late 1940s, when it investigated the Kaadt Diabetic Institute of South Whitley, Indiana. In reality, the "Institute" was a vicious swindle operated by two brothers. Patients stayed three days at $10 per day, then left with a gallon jug of "medicine" consisting of saltpeter and digestive tablets dissolved in vinegar. (This cost an additional $30.) Patients were advised to take two spoonfuls daily, stop insulin, and eat anything they liked—the most deadly advice that could be given.

The results were inevitable. Some Kaadt patients went into comas; some developed gangrene and had to have ampu-

of two national organizations, one for professional activities and another for voluntary health functions, fund raising, etc.

"My own thoughts are, that a Council is probably the best form of government for a group which is small, professional and held together by a common intellectual interest. For this group, money, power, and controversy about policy are essentially unimportant. This was the case when ADA was founded. With an enlarged membership, and with the growth of widespread and varied local interest in diabetes, this may no longer be the case," said Dr. Lukens.

After discussions with the Council, it was agreed that a broader base of representation on the Council

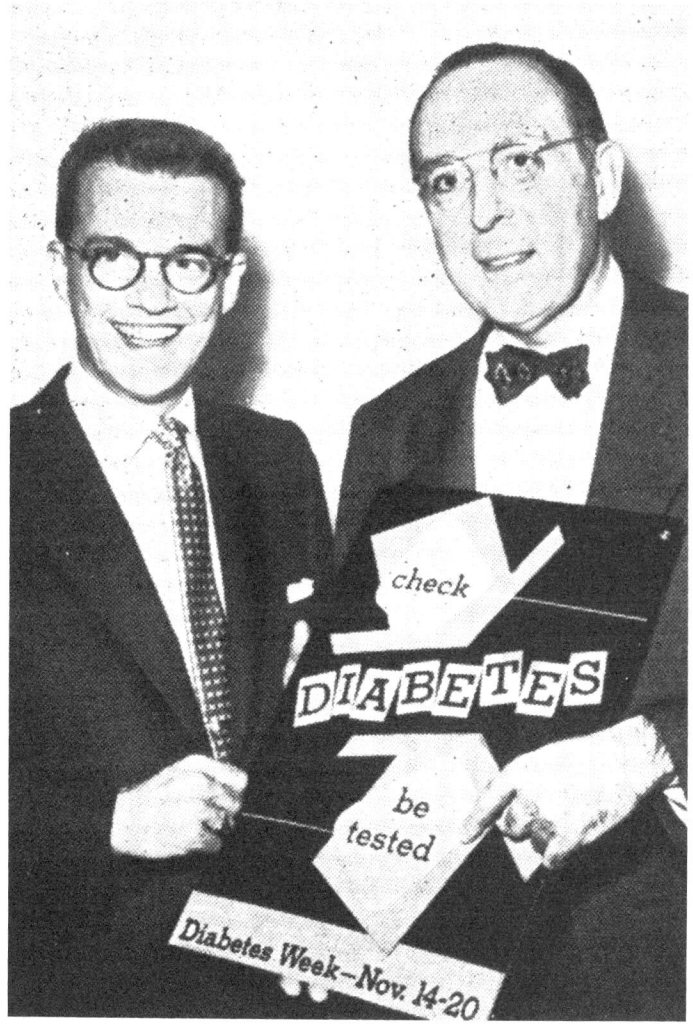

Bill Cullen, television and radio performer, poses with Louis K. Alpert, M.D., right, chairman of the Committee on Detection and Education.

tations; some died.

The Committee on Nostrums began an investigation of the Kaadt brothers in 1946. It contacted the Federal Drug Administration, the Federal Trade Commission, the American Medical Association, the Better Business Bureau, Inc., of Indianapolis, and the Indiana State Board of Registration and Examination "for the purpose of discovering whether more active steps could be taken toward curtailing or abolishing the work of that Institute." ADA members were asked to write letters to the Indiana State Board and Medical Association, urging that "all possible means be taken to eliminate the activities of Dr. Kaadt and his institute."

The Association's efforts resulted in federal investigation of the Kaadt Institute. The brothers were arrested, tried, and convicted of fraud in 1948. They were sentenced to three years in prison and fined $7,000 each.

Over the years, the Association has exposed many such operations. The "Vrilium Catalytic Barium Chloride Tube" was a scam that flourished in the 1950s. The tube was best known as the "magic spike," and consisted of a small brass cartridge containing 1/2000 of a cent's worth of barium chloride. A safety pin was provided for attaching it to clothing, and was included in the cost of $306.

The "magic spike" supposedly gave off emanations that would be effective in treating various disease, including diabetes. Thousands were sold before justice caught up with the manufacturers.

Witch doctors still exist in the age of computers. Until a cure for diabetes is found, an unfortunate part of the old days remains with us.

was needed. It was recommended that the Nominating Committee be enlarged, that affiliates be recognized in the Bylaws, that there be a class of affiliate membership, and that the Council be enlarged by five additional members nominated and elected by the Assembly of Delegates. The Council approved these recommendations and the Bylaws were changed accordingly.

Onward And Upward

As the fifties became the sixties, change was in the air. Man was about to take his first short trip into space. America elected its youngest President ever, to replace its oldest.

Profound change was coming to the American Diabetes Association, too. The signs were there to see as the decade drew to a close. The organization had outgrown its small, club-like atmosphere and was starting to take on aspects of a fair-sized business. Total income for 1959 was $389,000; for 1960, $465,000. But net for the two years amounted to just $17,000 and $24,000 respectively.

Clearly, inflation was hurting the Association at a time of expansion. Expenses rose from $58,000 in 1949 to $175,000 in 1954, and to $372,000 in fiscal 1959. In 1960, they reached $441,000.

Thus far, the Association had been able to keep pace with its ever-growing financial obligations the way it always had: through bequests, grants, donations, and earned income (dues and publications profits).

But funding was becoming increasingly difficult. As ADA activities expanded, as costs spiralled, larger sums were needed. Additional money-raising methods had to be considered. Such realities would change the very structure of the Association in the years just ahead.

Pieces Of The Puzzle:
What We Knew About Diabetes

1955

The British Conference on Diabetes and Pregnancy presents a report to the British Medical Research Council on the use of hormone therapy in pregnant women with diabetes. The conference concludes that the hormones, at least in the doses studied, do not reduce fetal mortality and have little, if any, beneficial effect on maternal health and pregnancy. These data are comparable to those obtained by most investigators and do not support earlier, more optimistic studies on the effects of hormone therapy in pregnant women with diabetes.

1956

Lente, the only one of the three "new" insulin preparations available in the United States (the others being Semilente and Ultralente), continues to receive favorable reports from clinicians.

1957

Studies on the action of glucagon show that it increases the utilization of sugar beyond the effect of hyperglycemia alone.

Glucagon is proven effective in terminating induced insulin coma.

1958

Jerome W. Conn, M.D., delivers the Banting Memorial Lecture at the eighteenth Annual Meeting in San Francisco. His topic is "The Prediabetic State of Man: Definition, Interpretation, and Implications." Dr. Conn describes his methods for predicting the development of diabetes.

For years, Dr. Conn had been conducting experiments designed to uncover individuals with "potential" or "latent" diabetes. He studied two large groups: apparently normal relatives of people known to have diabetes and apparently normal people who knew of no diabetes in their families.

Dr. Conn found that 20 percent of the relatives of those with diabetes had also developed diabetes themselves, while less than 2 percent of people without a family history of diabetes had the disease. His figures projected that 25 percent of those related to people with diabetes would eventually develop it also.

1959

Researchers are in general agreement that insulin works by facilitating the transfer of simple sugars across the cell membrane.

F. Sanger, M.D., of Cambridge University, describes the chemical structure of insulin (thus laying the groundwork for the manufacture of insulin by means of genetic engineering).

At the nineteenth Annual Meeting in 1959, Elliott P. Joslin, M.D., is honored on the occasion of his ninetieth birthday. Charles H. Best, M.D., presented Dr. Joslin with a citation "for distinguished contributions to the medical profession through his work as an investigator, practitioner and educator in the field of diabetes." The award was particularly appropriate, as Dr. Joslin had served as an honorary president of the American Diabetes Association since 1940.

1960

A survey published by the U.S. Public Health Service indicates that there are at least 1.5 million known cases of diabetes nationwide. The survey was conducted by the U.S. National Health Survey through the facilities of the Bureau of the Census. Findings were derived from household interviews. (No interviews were conducted in homes for the aged.) Compared with 1935-36 statistics, when figures showed 660,000 known cases of diabetes in the country, there are now 9 people per 1,000 known have diabetes instead of 5 per 1,000. The increase is explained by population growth, longevity, improved laboratory and diagnostic techniques, and greater awareness of the disease.

Two-thirds of the people interviewed were aged 55 or older; in the 45 and over category, the majority were women. Eighty-five percent interviewed reported no interference with activity and no lost work days in the past twelve months due to diabetes; 75 percent suffered no chronic limitations due to diabetes and could move about freely at home or outside. All reported having seen a physician some time in the past year, and the majority were under a physician's care. The survey showed that among those interviewed, control appeared good, but it was noted that this was no cause for complacency. The survey did not reveal unknown cases or how many were diagnosed annually.

The findings of the ADA Committee on Statistics in 1960 show 1,250,000 known cases of diabetes, with 72,000 cases diagnosed that year. The committee estimated that approximately 5.1 million people could expect to develop diabetes during their lifetime. Every fourth person is a "carrier," free of the disease but able to pass on the tendency to offspring, the report said. The combination of the National Health Survey and the report of the Committee on Statistics presented new and greater challenges to the Association in both treatment and detection.

At the Annual Meeting in June 1960, Dr. Priscilla White delivers the Banting Lecture, "Childhood Diabetes." She was the first woman to receive the Banting Medal, the Association's highest honor.

Chapter Six
Identity Crisis
1960-65

ADA PRESIDENTS

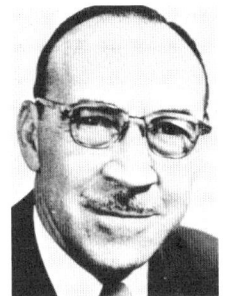
Franklin B. Peck, Sr., M.D.
(1960-61)

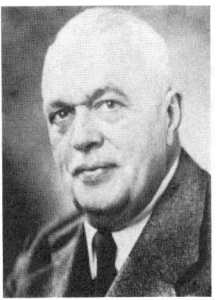
Blair Holcomb, M.D.
(1961-62)

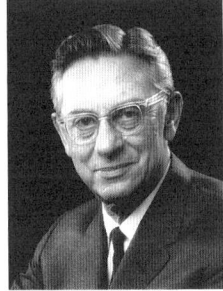
Jerome W. Conn, M.D.
(1962-63)

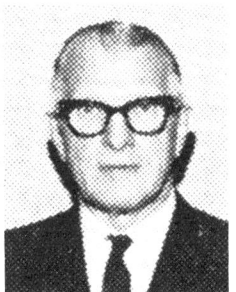
Thomas P. Sharkey, M.D.
(1963-64)

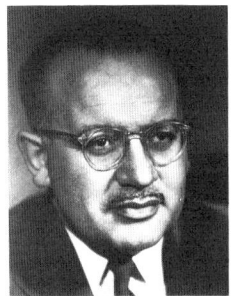
Rachmiel Levine, M.D.
(1964-65)

The 1960s began on a note of high hope as the youthful John F. Kennedy was elected thirty-fifth president of the United States. But his assassination three years later, violence over racial issues, and the nation's progressive involvement in Vietnam would contribute to the unrest that marked this decade as one of the most turbulent in modern history.

The ill-fated Bay of Pigs invasion in 1961 was followed hard by the Soviet Union's construction of the Berlin Wall. With the Cuban Missile Crisis of October 1962, the threat of a nuclear incident again became all too real. A "Statement on Emergency Medical Care," to meet conditions that might result from a nuclear attack, was prepared by the ADA Committee on Emergency Medical Care in late 1962. The statement discussed reserve supplies of insulin and oral drugs, storage, refrigeration, and stockpiling. Testing materials, syringes, needles, and information on appropriate food for people with diabetes were also covered. The statement was cleared with the heads of several U.S. agencies concerned with civilian defense and circulated to all members of the American Diabetes Association. The *Journal of the American Medical Association* (*JAMA*) gave the statement a full-page review. It was discussed December 13, 1962, on NBC's "Today" show, and reprinted by a "considerable number of medical and nonmedical publications," according to the Executive Director's Report to the Board, June 1963.

The Nobel Prize for Medicine and Physiology was awarded in 1962 to F. H. C. Crick and M. H. F. Wilkins, both of Great Britain, and J. D. Watson, of the United States, for determining the molecular structure of DNA. (DNA—deoxyribonucleic acid—is an essential component of all living matter. A basic material in the chromosomes of the cell nucleus, DNA contains the genetic code and transmits hereditary information.) This research would eventually open the door to genetic exploration and the production of human insulin.

What would prove to be the single most revolutionary breakthrough in the management of diabetes since the discovery of insulin was introduced quite inauspiciously in the 1960s. In a two-page advertisement in the journal *Diabetes* (Vol. 31:5, 1964), the Ames Company introduced test strips for blood-glucose monitoring. Dramatic in its simplicity, the ad pictured a finger from which a drop of blood is suspended over a *Dextrostix*. The caption proclaimed, "A One-Minute Test for Blood Glucose."

The next page, addressed to the physician, described the procedure: "With *Dextrostix* quantitative blood glucose estimations are possible in one minute." (The full impact of this test on the daily lives of people with diabetes was not realized until 17 years later, in 1981, when self-monitoring of blood glucose was introduced. A blood test that could be done at home, was more accurate than a urine test, and provided greater control was quickly adopted by many at this time. Why it took so long for this test to be made available to people with diabetes is uncertain. One theory is that there was no easy, painless way for drawing blood until the lancet was invented in England around 1979.)

In 1964, Dorothy C. Hodgkin, Ph.D., received the Nobel Prize in Chemistry for determining the structure of biochemical compounds.

The Association itself changed in the early 1960s. A milestone was reached in 1961 when the Bylaws were changed to give affiliate members a vote in the selection of Council members. A "Statement of

Operation," designed to provide uniform financial reporting by affiliates to the national office, was published that same year. (Complete implementation, however, did not occur until 1984, 23 years later.) In 1963, the name of the Council was changed to the Board of Directors, and the State Governors became the Committee of State Coordinators.

While administrative changes came somewhat smoothly, decisions over the direction the American Diabetes Association should take did not. There was tension and concern among members. Should the Association continue solely as a professional society or should it become a voluntary health organization and actively seek funds from the public? That was the major question the Association had to address in the early 1960s.

Architects of the Modern American Diabetes Association

As medical director of Eli Lilly and Company, Franklin B. Peck, Sr., M.D., was the only pharmaceutical representative ever to head the Association. He assumed the presidency in 1960 at a crucial juncture in ADA history, when fundamental questions of membership and funding had reached critical mass.

Dr. Peck recalled his 1960-61 term of office. Then, as ever, he was not a man to mince words about the turbulent days over which he presided.

"On assuming the presidency of the Association," he recalled, "after having served for many years on its Council, as secretary, and on the Executive Committee, my major concern was focused on the recurrent problem common to each president: the relationship of a growing number of loosely affiliated societies with the parent body, the ever-expanding budget required to support our rapidly-developing fourfold program, and our inability to properly render services so necessary to the broad base of diabetic patients nationwide. . . . I had for some years been inclining toward the view that our function and program was actually that of a voluntary health agency, and I resolved to visit and discuss our situation with as many of our component affiliates as possible during this year in order to obtain their views first hand."

Dr. Peck did just that, making several long trips to visit affiliates in different regions. What he saw reinforced his already-strong views. "I finished my year as president," he wrote, "with the conviction that the only solution to the dilemma was for our Association to become a voluntary health organization in name as it was already in fact. I knew, too, that our Council was still not ready to face this issue and take such a step. Furthermore, we were having acute organizational pains with the Board of Governors which had to be resolved, and required a great deal of attention."

As outgoing ADA president in 1961, Dr. Peck knew he would get to make the president's address—as tradition dictated—at the twenty-first Annual Meeting in New York City. He seized the opportunity and decided to give a rousing valedictory speech. He succeeded.

While short, the speech was memorable and far-reaching. Its most famous line warned the Association that without public fund raising, the dream of a truly national organization was "impossible, irrational, schizophrenic, and obviously doomed to failure."

There were other telling points. Dr. Peck told the

IDF Comes to North America

In 1964, the American Diabetes Association and the Canadian Diabetes Association cosponsored the fifth International Diabetes Federation (IDF) Congress at the Royal York Hotel in Toronto, Canada, July 20-24. This was the first time that an IDF Congress had been held on the North American continent.

In his welcoming remarks, ADA President Thomas P. Sharkey, M.D., (1963-64) paid

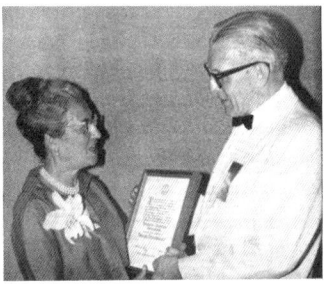

ADA President Thomas P. Sharkey, M.D., presents the ADA's Outstanding Laymen of the Year award to Mrs. Abraham Steigerwald in June 1964 at gala Fifth International Congress banquet.

tribute to the IDF, saying, "It is fitting that this meeting take place in the city where insulin was first discovered. An estimated 10 million lives have been saved by insulin, the discovery of which is an example of the force for good that medical research can exert. Such research will provide the salvation of the human race—if its destruction by atomic holocaust can be prevented. It is indeed an example of the schizoid nature of mankind, that this great international meeting dedicated to the prolongation of human life takes place at the same time that other meetings are being held, where other men devise ingenious ways to destroy life. IDF is an outstanding example of the ways that will lead to a peaceful, healthful world."

In a departure from precedent and in honor of the occasion, Banting Medals were presented to six outstanding physicians and scientists from Belgium, Canada, and the United States (see Appendix 7-A). Other honors conferred at the Toronto meeting included honorary membership to Dr. Striker, scholar, teacher, lecturer, author, philosopher, founder and first president of the American Diabetes Association. Tribute was paid to Dr. Best, in absentia, for his work as a scientist, teacher, scholar, and co-discoverer of insulin, his dedication to the cause of diabetes, and for having served as the ninth president of the American Diabetes Association and having supported the Association from the beginning.

group that it could choose to remain in splendid isolation as a purely professional society. But he also warned that "you, the members of the American Diabetes Association, must determine, and soon, whether uniqueness is a virtue, and your will must determine where we are going." He closed by noting that the most vexing problem of leadership—and its greatest responsibility— was coping with change.

It was not a speech that the majority of members was yet ready to accept.

To address concerns raised by Dr. Peck and decide the future role of the national Association as either a professional organization or a voluntary health agency, the Committee to Study Functions and Structure (F&S) was appointed by the Executive Committee in March 1963. F&S was established at the recommendation of the Committee on Purposes and Policies. Dr. Peck became chairman of the F&S Committee.

Dr. Cecil Striker, first president of the Association, remembered the F&S Committee as "one of the most significant special committees in our history." The committee's sole purpose was "to resolve the torment over the future purpose of the Association," wrote Dr. Striker. "Should it remain a professional organization of doctors and scientists, or should it enlarge its function and become a voluntary health agency with the obligation to conduct a national annual fund raising drive to support its enlarged program? It was a crucial issue fraught with difficult questions within the context of the larger issue."

The committee was charged with examining the structure of the American Diabetes Association and suggesting any changes that would enable the Association to meet its objectives more fully. Specifically, F&S was asked to consider: 1) continuance of the present structure; 2) the formation of a purely professional organization; or 3) the formation of a voluntary health agency.

This important committee was to meet frequently over the next eight years, and its members were the architects of the new voluntary health agency that the American Diabetes Association became. The committee was composed of Drs. Franklin B. Peck, Sr., chairman; Harvey C. Knowles, Jr.; Randall G. Sprague; Thomas P. Sharkey; L.O. Underdahl; and J. Richard Connelly, *ex officio*. Drs. William M. Kirtley and Alexander Marble served as consultants. This original committee was expanded from 1964-67 to include Drs. Addison B. Scoville, Donnell D. Etzwiler, John Bryan, Max Ellenberg, Henry Ricketts, and Robert

Tranquada. All had extensive experience with ADA affiliates.

The committee met for two days in June 1963. Members agreed that the objectives of the Association should be to further increase the dissemination of knowledge and information regarding diabetes. Members believed that this broad statement covered the intent of the Constitution—to promote the well-being of the patient with diabetes. The committee met in August with the American Medical Association's Committee on Voluntary Health Agencies, which offered its cooperation in future ADA efforts.

Finally, at a meeting in September 1963, it was agreed that the American Diabetes Association should *not* remain an entirely professional organization. It was noted that the Association had by that time all the characteristics of a voluntary health agency, except that it was not an "association of citizens," in the broad sense, and not "supported by voluntary contributions primarily from the general public."

Whether the Association was, in fact, already a voluntary health agency and was willing to acknowledge this status and take steps to implement it became the obvious question. Certainly, in terms of program and structure it was. Except for the fact that membership for laypersons had not yet been implemented, it was conceded that the American Diabetes Association was already performing most of the functions of a voluntary health agency.

The committee next met in October, with Sidney J. Shipman, M.D., and Barbara Farley, both of the American Medical Association's Committee on Voluntary Health Agencies. Several hours of questions and answers yielded the recommendation from Dr. Shipman that the American Diabetes Association should form a voluntary health agency. However, no action was taken. The question of a merger with another agency was rejected as neither feasible nor desirable.

In Chicago, in December 1963, the committee "agreed that if the Association is to alter its functions and structure, the change should not be precipitous, but should be carefully and cautiously developed. Time must be taken to develop constructive lay leadership which will be essential."

A second decision by the committee members was the irrevocable step that had been deliberated for so long: They agreed that the structure of the American Diabetes Association be changed to conform to that of a voluntary health agency.

The committee met in January 1964 and agreed that

a letter be sent to all active members of the Association and to affiliates, apprising them of the actions taken and the recommendations made. The letter also solicited their opinions. But the record shows that from nearly 2,600 active members and 50 affiliate associations, a total of 28 and 6 replies, respectively, were received. This meager response was disappointing, and as in President Lukens's survey of 1960, the response failed to show a consensus.

At this meeting, Dr. Wakerlin, medical director of the American Heart Association, reassured ADA members on a point of leadership about which there was general uneasiness, saying, "Medical guidance can be established and resolved as long as lay and medical components are approximately equal, and ADA should have no difficulty maintaining medical guidance of a voluntary health agency since physicians would be starting it."

At the Executive Committee meeting in April 1964, it was agreed to submit to the Board of Directors a set of principles "which would not be unduly affected by future operational changes." These basic guidelines were approved:

- Continue and expand the Association's four-point program of professional education, patient education, public education and detection, and research;

- Maintain guidance of the national Association by physicians and scientists, with a substantial majority of physicians on a single governing board (approximately 60 percent);

- Develop a single type of voting membership in the Association, with board and committee participation and voting rights extended to lay, medical, and scientific persons;

- Align the objectives, policies, and programs of affiliate associations with those of the national Association;

- Sponsor fund raising by both the national Association and affiliate associations, with the national governing board being responsible for definition of the goals, as well as the policies and techniques employed;

- Adopt uniform accounting principles of the National Health Council for the national Association and its affiliates; and

- Require an annual remittance of a specified sum to the national Association by affiliate associations, calculated as a percentage of the gross income, to be determined.

At the ADA's twenty-fourth Annual Meeting, held in Toronto in July 1964, the ADA Board of Directors agreed to accept the report of the Committee to Study Functions and Structure with its recommendation that the Association be restructured to become a voluntary health association.

The course of the Association was forever changed from that day forward. Growth and progress became inexorable and irreversible. To many within the organization, the advance from tacit agreement to reality was tediously slow, requiring many committee meetings and much debate before full agreement on structure was achieved. But all voices were heard during that debate, and all schools of thought considered before final action was taken. Once again, cautious change proved best in serving the cause of unity.

Education And Awareness Programs Expand

ADA President Blair Holcomb, M.D., (1961-62) succeeded Dr. Peck and presided quietly amidst the changes around him. During his tenure, a number of the Association's founding figures passed from the scene. Dr. Holcomb paid tribute to Dr. Elliott P. Joslin, honorary ADA and IDF president; Dr. John A. Reed, past president and secretary; Dr. Christopher J. McLoughlin, Council member and ADA governor for Georgia; and Dr. William Muhlberg, the Association's first treasurer. (It was Dr. Muhlberg who, as medical director of the Union Central Life Insurance Company, obtained the first ADA grant of $500 from that firm.)

By 1961, National Diabetes Detection Week was an established tradition, but the Committee on Public Education wanted to do more. Recognizing that diabetes is a year-round problem—not a seasonal one—the committee developed press kits for affiliates to distribute. The kits contained basic facts about diabetes and printed guidelines to help affiliates interest local media stations in using the "spots" on a year-round basis. In addition, postage meter indicia were made available to affiliates. (A meter indica is a slogan or symbol used in combination with a postal permit as part of the postmark.) The slogan that year, "Be Alert - Be Tested - Be Sure - Check Diabetes," appeared on thousands of letters making their way across the country, and helped inform local industries, utility companies, banks, insurance companies, and department stores about Diabetes Detection Week.

In 1963, a 15-minute public education film, "How Sure Are You?" was an instant hit with affiliates, and many requests were received for copies, including some from other countries.

Two states decided to bring diabetes screening programs to their rural areas via traveling trailers. The

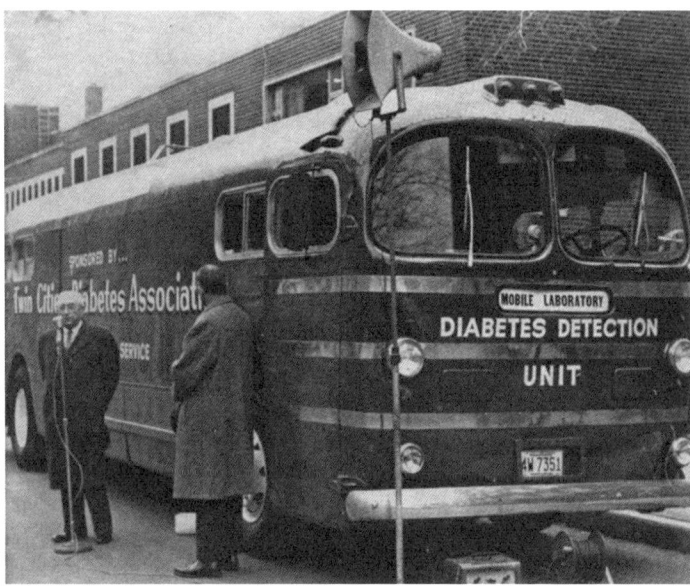

The Twin Cities Diabetes Association's Mobile Diabetes Detection Laboratory is dedicated Wednesday, November 28, 1963, on the University of Minnesota Medical School campus. Pictured at the left is diabetes researcher Moses Barron, M.D.

first year that a trailer was used in Michigan, 151,821 people were tested for diabetes during Diabetes Detection Week. A prevalence of 6 persons with diabetes per 1,000 tested was found. In Minnesota, a city bus was converted into a mobile laboratory. The bus was dedicated in 1963 on the campus of the University of Minnesota Medical School and was used for screening throughout the year.

In 1962, President John F. Kennedy sent the following message to the American Diabetes Association: "The annual Diabetes Detection Drive sponsored nationally by ADA performs a valuable public service by informing the American People of the need for early detection, thus helping to find the hidden cases of diabetes. It is a great misfortune that there are still so many people in America who have diabetes without being aware of it."

Celebrities who helped in the national diabetes awareness campaign included comedian Bob Hope, singer/movie star Bing Crosby, Senator Gale McGee, Jackie Robinson, and TV weatherman Tex Antoine. All were heard on radio or appeared on television or other media during the early 1960s.

Educating the public about diabetes included informing correctional institution personnel about the disease. One in 140 prisoners incarcerated in U.S. penal institutions had diabetes. In the early 1960s, two individuals with diabetes, one in New York and one in New Jersey, died while in custody, due to alleged misunderstanding of proper diabetes treatment.

In 1961, the article "Facts About Diabetes, Insulin Reaction, and Police Protection" was published in *Police Chief*. Written by William Grishaw, M.D., chairman of the ADA Committee on Information for Diabetics, the article was reprinted and widely distributed among law enforcement officers and prison personnel. That same year, ADA President Franklin Peck, M.D., spoke before the County Jail Warden's Association to explain the various aspects of diabetes and the need for prompt treatment in emergencies.

(Between the years 1971 and 1985, the national office received numerous letters from prisoners with dia-

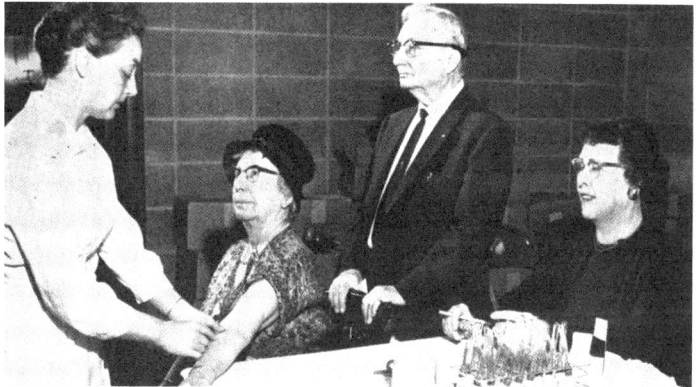

Blood testing at a two-day Diabetes Fair held by the Reading Diabetes Association and the Berks County Medical Society during Diabetes Week 1962.

betes, whose problems ranged from inadequate meals and inappropriate treatment to a lack of emergency care. For the most part, the letters revealed a basic misunderstanding of the facts about diabetes on the part of both inmates and prison personnel. By 1986, the prison population had tripled that of 1961, and 30,000 of the 600,000 confined had diabetes. Because of the letters that had accumulated, indicating the need for education, the American Diabetes Association joined the National Commission on Correctional Health

One Father's Recollections

In 1964, Ed and Gloria Hirsch's son Irl was diagnosed as having insulin-dependent (type I) diabetes. Irl was six years old. Ed Hirsch recalls what it was like to raise a child with diabetes in the 1960s—before there were disposable needles and syringes, diet soda, and home blood-glucose monitoring devices.

Irl was diagnosed at St. Louis Children's Hospital. There, a nurse taught the Hirschs how to give an insulin shot by injecting distilled water into an orange and how to sterilize steel needles and glass syringes in a strainer over boiling water.

To test the amount of sugar in the urine, a tablet was dropped into a test tube of urine and color changes were noted. Blue was "negative"—no sugar. A blue-green color indicated a trace amount of sugar in the urine; this, Mr. Hirsch noted, was considered ideal. Orange was "positive" for sugar. "The readings were duly noted in a diary, which accompanied us to the doctor on our regular visits," Mr. Hirsch said.

"The most difficult part of living with a child with diabetes in those days was meal planning," he continued.

When Irl was eight years old, the Hirschs' received special permission for him to attend the St. Louis summer camp for children with diabetes (children were supposed to be at least ten years

---

Care [NCCHC]. The purpose in joining NCCHC was to extend the many ADA patient and professional education programs to prisons, in an effort to ensure better care and treatment for inmates with diabetes. As of 1986, the Association had the distinction of being the only voluntary health agency represented on the NCCHC Board.)

A Boost for Diabetes Research

In response to requests from many professional members, an Annual Research Symposium was established in 1962. The subject of the first symposium was "Cellular Metabolism in Relation to Cell Structure." (A chronological list of subsequent symposia appears in Appendix 8 and provides insight into the trends in research from 1962 to the present.)

By 1962, many members realized the urgent need for greater funding for diabetes research. ADA President Jerome W. Conn, M.D., (1962-63) proposed that a research foundation be established, saying, "Encouragement of research in diabetes is an active function of the ADA, and like all other areas of research, it must expand if problems are to be solved with reasonable speed. Creation of a research foundation will facilitate receipts and disbursements of funds and expedite the growth of diabetes research."

He went on to explain that "the sole assets of the foundation will be funds contributed by those with a real desire to help. The foundation will be financed only as well as its donors make possible. The larger the gifts, the more research programs can be accelerated. Presently, the Association awards a number of Research Fellowships each year, and plans and supports annual research symposiums. Other activities will be added as donations make possible." The Council accepted his recommendation, and subsequently, discreet advertisements began to appear in *ADA Forecast* reminding readers that donations or bequests to research were tax exempt and that more information could be obtained by contacting the national office.

Insurance and Employment: New Hope

In the early 1960s a hands-off attitude still prevailed among insurance companies when it came to insuring people with diabetes. For many years, the industry had considered a higher premium paid for a higher risk to be impractical, comparing the policy with insuring the burning house. However, with improved methods of diabetes control and resultant delays in the onset of

old to attend the camp in those days). "At the camp, our son learned to give his own shots, which gave us (and him) a new sense of freedom," Mr. Hirsch said. For one thing, this meant that Irl could now stay overnight at a friend's house. This new independence, plus the introduction of disposable needles and syringes, "truly changed our lives," Mr. Hirsch said.

complications, insurers began to take a new look at coverage for diabetes. In 1964, insurance companies were writing at least 15 percent of the health insurance issued each year on the basis of equalized risk, according to Groff Conklin in the article "Facts About Health Insurance for Diabetics," published in *ADA Forecast* (Vol. 17:6, 1964). Pioneer plans to make health insurance available to some if not all people with diabetes, through equalization of risks were under consideration by several companies, Conklin wrote.

(With the advent of employee group health insurance plans, the picture for people with diabetes brightened, particularly for those employed by a large company. Still, even today, individual health insurance plans for people with diabetes are considered "high risk," expensive, difficult to obtain, and may even be unavailable if complications exist. There is no doubt that the relaxation of restrictions starting in 1964 contributed to a more liberal attitude on the part of underwriters, but progress has been slow.)

Along with the desire for fair insurance coverage for people with diabetes came concerns for full and equal employment. In 1961, the American Diabetes Association published its own pamphlet, "Diabetics are Desirable Workers," stating that people with diabetes are an asset to employers, because they usually have good attendance records, are often superior or outstanding workers, and present no special problems. The pamphlet also provided standards for employers to use in hiring people with diabetes. The purpose of the pamphlet was to dispel the myth that diabetes was a physical handicap. This pamphlet was one of the most popular ever published by the Association and was distributed until 1973.

A survey conducted by the ADA Committee on Employment showed that by the mid-1960s, more than two-thirds of the responding companies employed people with diabetes. The figure was somewhat misleading, however. It included those companies that continued to employ people who developed or discovered their diabetes after being hired. Many of those same firms simultaneously maintained a strict no-hire policy toward the job-seeker with diabetes. Moreover, most companies made no distinction among those with diabetes. Corporate policies—whatever they were—lumped everyone together, whether the individual was under diet control alone, diet and insulin control, or diet and oral compound control.

Employment prejudice against those with diabetes was not confined to the United States. In 1964, exten-

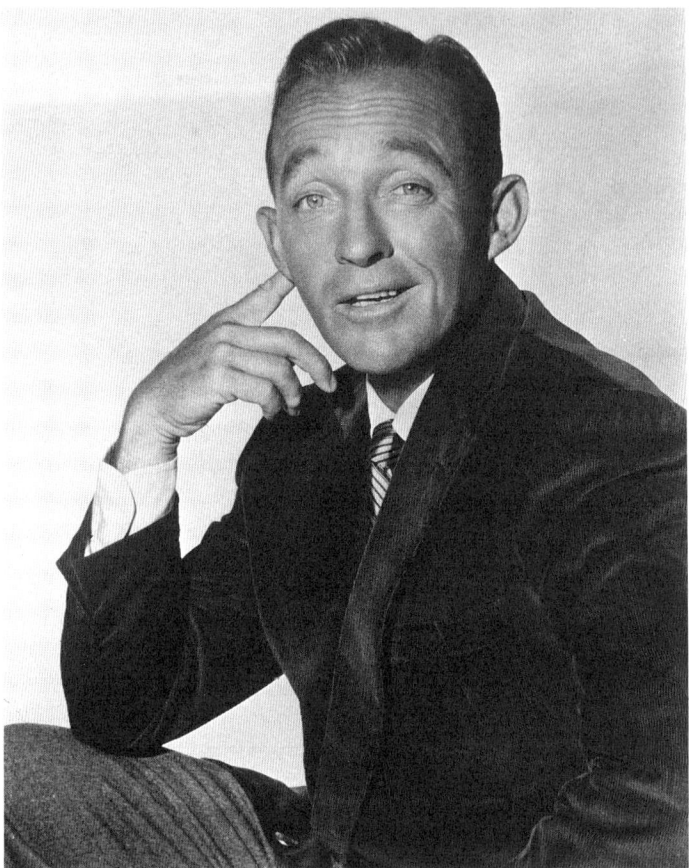

Bing Crosby, one of America's best-loved movie and television personalities, supports the 1964 Diabetes Week campaign with a persuasive television announcement alerting people to the dangers of undetected diabetes.

sive attention was given to the subject at the fifth International Diabetes Federation meeting in Toronto. In 1965, the World Health Organization issued the following statement which not only illustrated the scope of the problem but summarized it:

"The Organization views with dismay the restrictions in many countries hindering the employment of diabetics. All too often these restrictions are purely negative and are based on prejudice or ill-formed opinion about the effect of diabetes on a person's working ability or capacity. This injustice is perpetuated and even increased by the tendency to regard all diabetics as a group of patients with identical characteristics. This is bound up with the failure to distinguish between mild cases and cases under proper medical control on the one hand and uncooperative, uncontrolled cases on the other. The Organization urges strongly

Twenty-Five Years of Growth

The Annual Meeting in 1965 marked the twenty-fifth anniversary of the American Diabetes Association's founding. Attendance at the Scientific Sessions and at the banquet was among the highest in the Association's history. In addition to the awards for scientific achievement, special tribute was paid to the founders. Twelve of the founders were present; the thirteenth was represented by his widow.

Personal citations signed by ADA President Rachmiel Levine, M.D., (1964-65) and Secretary Joseph H. Crampton, M.D., were given to each of the founders present: Drs. George C. Anderson, Joseph T. Beardwood, C.B.F. Gibbs, J. West Mitchell, Paul F. Polentz, William S. Reveno, Beverly Chew Smith, Cecil Striker, George C. Thosteson, Edward Tolstoi, and Frederick W. Williams. Mrs. Charles Bolduan, representing her husband, was also presented with a citation (*Diabetes*, Vol. 14:8, 1965).

In conferring citations on the founders, Dr. Levine said, "Twenty-five years ago, because the problems arising from diabetes were so unusual, so complex, and growing so rapidly that only organized action could have enabled the medical profession to cope effectively with them, the founders had the courage, vision, and conviction to recognize the needs, and designed programs to educate, to alleviate suffering, and to create a greater public awareness of diabetes."

that a much more liberal attitude of mind be adopted which would aim at the elimination of discrimination against diabetics that has arisen simply on diagnostic grounds. In short, a diabetic should have the same chances as any other person at obtaining and performing work for which he is medically and vocationally suitable."

Slowly but steadily, the employment picture improved. Small signposts indicated major changes to come. In Minnesota, for example, citizens with diabetes were severely restricted in their right to drive a car, which in turn limited their employment opportunities. Minnesotans with diabetes who had accidents came under the provisions of a statute dealing with "unpredictable loss of consciousness, such as occurs in epilepsy." They were subject to automatic two-year license suspensions.

In 1963, the Minnesota Highway Department adopted new guidelines, as suggested by the Advisory Committee on Diabetes of the State Medical Association. These provided for a six-month suspension, but only if poor diabetes control caused the accident. The new policy benefited both the public and most drivers with diabetes. It was also a relief to the State Highway Department, which had been plagued by lawsuits filed by drivers with diabetes who felt they had been treated unfairly.

In such small ways were equal rights gradually extended.

A Time To Look Back; A Time To Look Ahead

At the silver anniversary Annual Meeting held at the Hotel Roosevelt in New York City, June 19-20, 1965, ADA President Rachmiel Levine, M.D., summarized the Association's many achievements of the past 25 years. "The first treasurer's report showed an income of slightly over $2,000 and expenditures of around $860. The latest reported annual income is $617,000, with expenditures of $604,000. These figures are the numerical reflections of the variety and intensity of the work, which is aimed to fulfill the objectives enumerated in the Constitution." All the labor and achievement of the past 25 years were "impressive," said Dr. Levine.

He concluded his president's address with a look to the changing future of the Association. "The Committee to Study the Functions and Structure of the Association has worked out a proposed transformation of the

Association into a national health agency with broad scopes and objectives—one designed to serve the broadest interests of the public and profession, with the widest possible participation and activity.'' That change would still be years in coming.

Pieces Of The Puzzle:
What We Knew About Diabetes

1960

A study by Dr. Sven Johnsson, of Malmo, Sweden (*Diabetes*, Vol. 9:1, 1960), shows that careful control of diabetes delays the development of nephropathy (kidney disease) and retinopathy (eye disease). The study included people with diabetes from Malmo who were under 40 years of age. These patients were divided into two groups. Series I included those whose diabetes was diagnosed between 1922 and 1925, and who had carefully controlled diets for an average of 10 years prior to the liberalization of diets in the 1930s, or 18 percent of their total course. Series II included those diagnosed between 1936 and 1945 who had a controlled diet for only two and a half years before liberalization, or 85 percent of their total course. Those in Series I had had diabetes longer than those in Series II. Despite this, nephropathy, severe retinopathy, and visual impairment were all greater among people in Series II, who had been on a liberal diet. This suggests that careful control of the diet may delay development of these complications.

1961

A new injectable emergency drug for those with diabetes appears on the market. Called "glucagon," the substance helps people with diabetes recover from insulin shock (hypoglycemia). *ADA Forecast* readers learn that glucagon "is a white powder which comes in a vial similar to that in which insulin is bottled." The magazine recommends that everyone with insulin-dependent diabetes "have at least one injection of glucagon on hand all the time—especially those who take a large amount of insulin and are subject to variations in meals and exercise."

1962

"Current Concepts in Diabetes Mellitus," by Max Ellenberg, M.D., and Harold Rifkin, M.D., is published in the *New York State Journal of Medicine*, June 1, 1962. The article covers the future in the field of diabetes, the role of genetics, beta cell lesions, glands, and the value of knowledge through teaching and testing. Reprints of the article are distributed by the American Diabetes Association.

"Treatment of Diabetes," by George J. Hamwi, M.D., is published in *JAMA* (Vol. 181, Sept. 1962). A guide for physicians and patients in the initial education of diabetes mellitus, it is widely distributed.

"The Diabetic Child" by William H. Grishaw, M.D., is published in the *National Education Association Journal* (Vol. 41:1, January 1962). It is addressed to teachers and educators to help them in understanding children with diabetes in the classroom.

1963

Panayotis G. Katsoyannis, M.D., associate research professor of biochemistry at the University of Pittsburgh School of Medicine, produces the first synthetic insulin. Dr. Katsoyannis and his collaborators achieve a partial synthesis of human insulin and develop the first completely synthetic "A" chain of the insulin molecule. It proves effective in tests conducted by Dr. G.H. Dixon of the University of Toronto.

"Diabetes Suspect," by Thomas P. Sharkey, M.D., published in the *Ohio State Medical Journal* (Vol. 59:12, 1963), reveals updated statistics on diabetes: 3 million in the United States—1.6 million known and 1.4 million unknown.

1964

World Statistics on Diabetes: "Diabetes in a World Survey," published in *Diabetes* (Vol. 4:4, 1964) by Paul S. Entmacher, M.D., and Herbert H. Marks, M.D., reports mortality rates from diabetes in 41 countries. It is the first such study and becomes one of the most widely circulated journal reprints of all time. The report, presented at the fifth Congress of the International Diabetes Federation, held in Toronto, Canada, on July 20, 1964, states that diabetes is a universal disease. It presents incidence, prevalence, and mortality figures. The authors point out how these figures are influenced by genetic and environmental factors. The report confirms the belief that obesity, as it relates to abundance of food, daily physical labor, and pace of technology in a given society, is a prime factor in the increasing prevalence of diabetes. The survey concludes that quantity and quality of medical care, public health programs, and cultural mores all have an influence on the quality of life and life expectancy of people with diabetes. However, increasing longevity brings new challenges, primarily vascular complications and their control, and nephropathy (kidney disease), a special problem for which there is no effective therapy at this time. Tabulation of the data of this comprehensive study is accomplished with funds from the U.S. Public Health Service.

"Known diabetics in the United States number about 2 million or 11 per 1,000 population. The proportion increases with age from about 1 in 900 for persons under 25 years of age to 1 in 20 for those 65 and over,'' according to the authors.

"Characteristics of Persons With Diabetes," published by the National Center for Health Statistics in October 1967, shows the number of people with diabetes reported for the period July 1964-June 1965 is 12.2 per 1,000 population. The prevalence of diabetes is essentially the same in all regions and residential areas. Of the 2.3 million Americans with diabetes, 58 percent are women.

1965

The ADA Research Committee establishes the Association's first Research and Development Awards Program. The first recipient of this program's highest award—the Elliott P. Joslin Research and Development Award—is Ronald A. Arky, M.D., then associate director of Boston City Hospital's Diabetes Clinic, who went on to serve as ADA's president (1979-80).

Chapter Seven
Years of Transition 1965-70

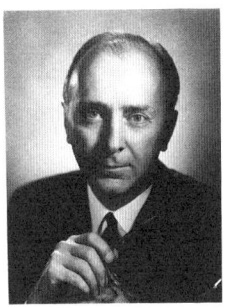
Thaddeus S. Danowski, M.D.
(1965-66)

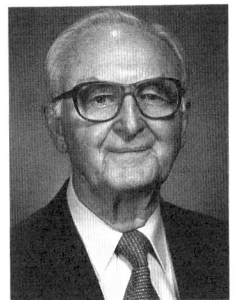
Laurentius O. Underdahl, M.D.
(1966-67)

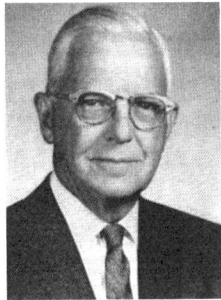
Edwin W. Gates, M.D.
(1967-68)

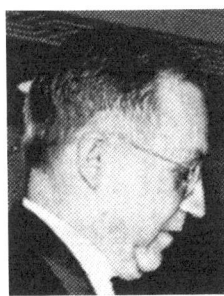
Harvey C. Knowles, Jr., M.D.
(1968-69)

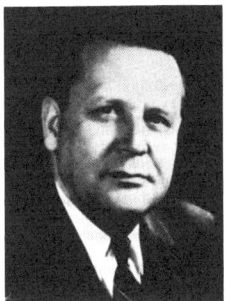
Robert C. Hardin, M.D.
(1969-70)

In 1965, newly elected President Lyndon B. Johnson announced plans for the "Great Society," a program of sweeping domestic reforms that would affect the young, the old, the poor, the sick, and the disenfranchised. A year later, the Social Security Act was amended to include Medicare, which provided for low-cost health insurance for people 65 and older, and Medicaid, which guaranteed subsidized health insurance for families with low incomes. The next year, disability insurance was added to this package. This had a profound effect upon people with chronic diseases, such as diabetes, and ultimately upon the American Diabetes Association.

Dramatic, turbulent events marked the later 1960s. Yet against a backdrop that included an unpopular war in Vietnam, rioting in American cities, and the assassinations of Robert Kennedy and Martin Luther King, Jr., science and technology forged ahead. Christiaan Barnard, M.D., performed the first successful human heart transplant, United States astronauts walked in space and later on the moon, and scientists developed synthetic DNA. Work with synthetic DNA opened the door to genetic exploration and led to the production of human insulin in the laboratory.

In 1968, Arthur R. Colwell, M.D., gave the ADA Banting Lecture, "Fifty Years of Perspective in Diabetes," in which he provided a glimpse of what he expected from future research. "A prophet is one regarded or inspired by divine guidance," Dr. Colwell said. "My inspiration is certainly not divine, but to extrapolate from the past about the clinical future in diabetes the following developments may well be revealed . . . genetic mechanisms may soon be understood and perhaps manipulated, and the metabolic basis for diabetic microangiopathy [small blood-vessel disease] and neuropathy made clear and prevention become possible."

The American Diabetes Association faced its biggest challenge: conversion from a professional society to a voluntary health agency. The decision to take this step had been slow in coming, and the vote by the Board of Directors in 1964 had not been unanimous. But the conversion coincided with a notable trend in American society, which was to have both a stormy and a beneficial effect upon the Association: People, particularly the young, were breaking with traditions of the past. They wanted—and were demanding—more control over their lives and environment. This sentiment spilled over into the realm of diabetes. No longer willing to assume a passive role in their care, people with diabetes began to question their doctors, seek more knowledge, and assume greater responsibility for their own well-being.

Physicians suddenly found the old ways of providing health care challenged by both patients and allied health professionals. Formerly looked upon by physicians as purely supportive, non-physician health professionals began to change their role, seeking more direct responsibility for the delivery of health care. This ultimately resulted in the "health-care team" approach to diabetes management. The team concept, initially strongly opposed by many physicians, was an idea whose time had come. As health professionals—nurses, dietitians, social workers and others—pushed for more recognition and began providing both health care and patient education, the idea caught on. Physicians began to see the positive effects of this approach to health care. And for the person with diabetes, the beneficial effect of this trend was better treatment.

The Charles H. Best Birthplace

Charles H. Best, M.D., co-discoverer of insulin, enjoyed the distinction of being appointed ADA honorary president, and was later elected as the ninth president of the Association.

In 1959, a group of ADA members and people interested in diabetes formed The Charles H. Best Birthplace Trust under the leadership of

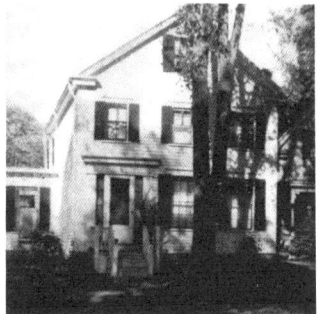

Birthplace of Charles H. Best, M.D.

Edwin Gates, M.D., (ADA president in 1967-68) to raise money to buy the house where Dr. Best was born. This, they said, "will be a fitting tribute to Dr. Best's high achievements and noteworthy contributions to diabetes, and his devotion and unceasing efforts on behalf of the well-being of diabetics throughout the world." By acquiring and maintaining the Best birthplace, the group felt the Association could make certain that its public importance and historical value would be preserved.

The trustees raised the money, bought the property, and did some minor restoration. In June 1968, the deed was turned over to the Association at the Annual Meeting in San Francisco. In his presentation, Dr. Gates said, "In tribute to Dr. Charles H. Best, B.E., M.D., F.R.S., Honorary President, the American Diabetes

Reorganization: Why It Took So Long

The Committee to Study Functions and Structure (F&S), appointed in 1963, continued to meet regularly until 1970. Continuity was assured by the fact that the original members continued to serve, with only the officers changing from year to year.

On March 19, 1966, F&S presented its plan for a national structure to representatives of affiliate associations gathered in Chicago. The 35 who attended studied 1) the structure of affiliates, 2) interrelationships of affiliate associations, 3) proportionate representation and the development and implementation of programs, and 4) the role of the Central Council.

A complete revision of the Bylaws was presented by F&S at the Fourteenth Assembly of Delegates in Atlantic City, June 1966, where Chairman Thomas P. Sharkey, M.D., reported on the reorganization. Panel discussions on *Model Bylaws for Affiliates*, the *Annual Affiliate Agreement*, and the *Statement of Purposes, Principles, and Policies* followed Dr. Sharkey's report. The Bylaws revisions were not adopted at this time.

In addressing the Delegate Assembly, outgoing ADA President Thaddeus S. Danowski, M.D., (1965-66) said, "The magnitude of diabetes warrants ADA becoming among the top voluntary health agencies. We cannot shift overnight. Transition must be phased and programmed. Even at this moment our planning is ahead of our resources. There is great need to support

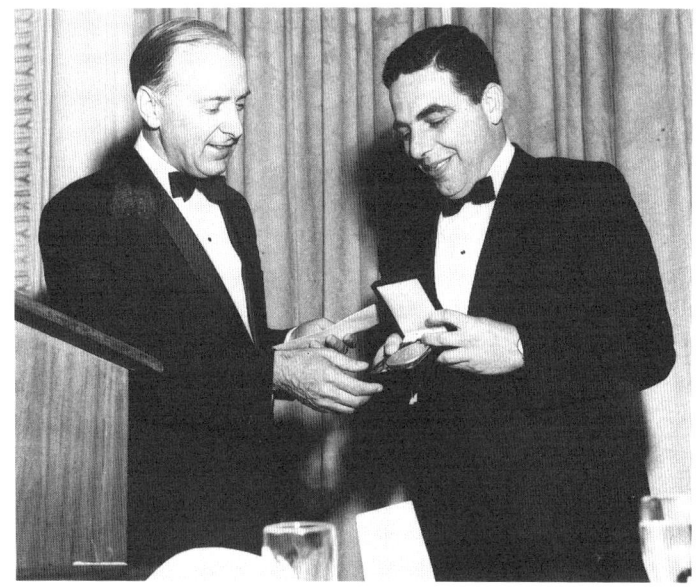

Norbert Freinkel, M.D., right, receives the Lilly Medal from ADA President Thaddeus S. Danowski, M.D., June 1966 (LaSalle Hotel, Chicago, Illinois).

Association is proud to announce its acceptance from the trustees of the Charles H. Best Birthplace Trust, full ownership of title to the residence and property on Old State Highway One, Town of West Pembroke, County of Washington, State of Maine, where he was born February 27, 1899. The residence and site will be maintained as a symbol of gratitude, from all those who owe their lives and their well-being to the historic discovery of insulin in which he shared, and to the subsequent research performed by him and those under his direction." The document was signed on June 15, 1968, by ADA President Edwin M. Gates, M.D., and ADA Secretary James B. Hurd, M.D.

Noble as the idea was, there were problems almost immediately with maintaining the property. During the Association's period of transition, when every dollar was counted carefully, it became apparent that the Association could not afford to maintain the Best Birthplace, which by this time needed considerable restoration. Executive Vice President John L. Dugan, Jr., initiated discussions with the National Trust for Historic Preservation. In 1978, the Board voted to give the property to the National Trust.

The Trust found an interested buyer—a medical doctor familiar with the work of Dr. Best—who was eager to renovate and restore the property. Since he planned to use the house as his office, this seemed the ideal solution. The American Diabetes Association assumed ownership of Dr. Best's surgical instruments and these now are on display at the ADA National Service Center in Alexandria, Virginia. The consulting room furniture and original operating table have

training, research, epidemiological studies, and other activities." These remarks were addressed to those individuals in the organization who felt that the conversion process was going much too slowly.

At the same Annual Meeting, ADA President Laurentius Underdahl, M.D., (1966-67) announced detailed plans for the first national fund-raising campaign. He reported that the executive director had been authorized by the Executive Committee to engage fund-raising counsel to make a feasibility study in connection with the first campaign. F&S met with the fund-raising counsel during the summer of 1966, and a committee was appointed to consider the divisibility of funds between the national organization and the affiliates, and related matters.

In the summer of 1967, *A Guide to Accounting and Financial Reporting for Affiliates* was distributed to all affiliates. The guide had been prepared by the accounting firm of Peat, Marwick, Mitchell and Company. Designed to provide the basics of financial reporting in compliance with the requirements of the National Health Council, the guide fulfilled one of the original recommendations of F&S, namely that when the American Diabetes Association became a full-fledged voluntary health agency it would conform to uniform accounting principles.

At the Board meeting in June 1967, these recommendations pertaining to affiliates were adopted:

- The principle of proportionate representation on the Central Council be based on the voting membership of each affiliate.

- Upon implementation and execution of the *Annual Affiliate Agreement* by affiliates, under conditions of special need, the ADA national office would advance funds on a loan basis without interest, to an organization that showed promise of achieving its goals.

- All affiliates, chapters, and branches would use the official emblem of the American Diabetes Association.

- Affiliates would be encouraged to establish professional education/training programs in teaching institutions.

- Affiliates would support new and existing research projects in their respective geographic areas. If no research projects exist in local areas, affiliates would obtain from the national Association a list of possible projects.

been restored by the owner of the house, and the remainder of the property was completely renovated. Today, a bronze plaque attests to the authenticity of the birthplace and the Association's role in helping to preserve the site.

On March 16, 1968, F&S met with 43 representatives from 26 affiliates to review the *Statement of Purposes, Principles, and Policies of ADA*, the *Annual Affiliate Agreement*, *Proposed Model Bylaws of Affiliates and Chapters*, and *Regulations for Branches and Units*. All these documents had previously been approved in principle by the Board of Directors and ultimately became the Magna Carta of the new organization. Workshops at this meeting covered fund raising and interorganizational division of funds.

In late 1968, the fund-raising firm of Bowen, Gurin, Barnes, and Roche was hired to do a feasibility study to help determine the future of the Association. Representatives traveled across the United States, questioning physicians, lay persons, affiliate and chapter members, and community leaders. The results of their study were circulated to affiliate delegates prior to the 1969 Annual Meeting. In addressing that meeting, team leader Mr. Gurin said, "We found the Association a sleeping giant in terms of its potential. Six things are necessary if you want to become a viable voluntary health agency: 1) build a strong case for diabetes, one that will provide greater financial support; 2) enlist qualified leaders; 3) enlist as many workers as possible; 4) line up prospective contributors; 5) plan effective fund-raising campaigns; and 6) build a stronger organization."

Mr. Gurin went on to say that, interestingly enough, while the Association thought the reason for converting to a voluntary health agency was to raise more money for research, answers to the study questionnaires placed patient education and detection as top priorities. Several physicians questioned why research was given a lower priority. Some felt that it belied their own experience. However, as the survey indicated, there were some doctors who did not place research first. To this Mr. Gurin said, "The low rating on research was affected perhaps, by the feeling that the government is doing a lot, and 'How can a small organization contribute very much?' Secondly, patient education and detection are visible things in the community, whereas research going on in some laboratory somewhere is intangible. People can't see where their money is going."

Some affiliates were dependent on monies from the United Fund for their existence. The study's architects, therefore, encouraged affiliates to mount independent campaigns outside of the United Fund. They emphasized that affiliate campaigns should be conducted simultaneously all across the country—a consolidated effort would attract more visibility and attention. Suggestions for campaigns included membership promotion, special gifts solicitation, bequests, memorials, special events, benefits, and community and industry appeals, all of which have been incorporated into ADA's fund-raising programs.

F&S outlined the areas of responsibility for a national and an affiliate fund-raising program as follows: 1) the national organization will establish an ad hoc committee to cover areas where no affiliates exist; 2) a national campaign committee will be appointed to develop fund-raising programs; 3) the national organization will solicit funds from sources beyond the reach of affiliates, such as national corporations, foundations, wealthy individuals, etc.; and 4) the national organization will apply for entrance into the Combined Federal Campaigns, whereby federal government workers would more easily be able to donate charitable funds to the Association. It was also suggested that the Fund Raising Committee should establish a timetable for preparations and build a field service, public information, and fund-raising staff. In addition, a director of fund raising should be hired to explore sources of immediate funds, plan a full-scale campaign for the Association and affiliates, and arrange for additional office space to accommodate this activity. In order to retain the general focus, program ideas and projects should be referred to the Executive Committee for feasibility determination and prioritizing.

In accordance with the recommendation of F&S, in early 1969 William Ferguson was named director of affiliate development and service, to work closely with the Committee on Affiliates on the development of fund-raising programs. Mr. Ferguson had formerly been field director for the National Council on Alcoholism. In his first interview with ADA Executive Director J. Richard Connelly, he was given a copy of *Diabetes Mellitus: Diagnosis and Treatment.* "Up to that time," Mr. Ferguson said, "I had known several people with diabetes, but was totally ignorant of the potentially devastating consequences of the disease. The book convinced me of the seriousness of diabetes, and the need for research, and I assumed that everyone in ADA shared this opinion. It came as a great shock to me that this was not so."

At the national office, Mr. Ferguson found a small group of dedicated workers, led by Mr. Connelly, who had grown up with the Association, and contributed greatly to its impressive growth. A no-nonsense executive, Mr. Connelly was highly capable, totally dedi-

Living With Diabetes in the 1960s

Jean Betschart was a student at the University of Pittsburgh when, in 1966, she was diagnosed as having insulin-dependent (type I) diabetes. She recounts what her diagnosis and treatment were like.

"Between September 1965 and February 1966, I made numerous trips to the Student Health Service at the University of Pittsburgh. I had palpitations, leg cramps, blurred vision, thirst, weight loss, fatigue, and infections of my fingers. The staff there would briefly examine me and send me back to class feeling somewhat neurotic. Then, on a routine physical, diabetes was diagnosed.

"I was not admitted to the hospital because I was in the middle of finals . . . . I was sent to my physician's office for follow-up care. He told me I would need to take insulin and showed me how to give the injection." Her doctor also gave her a copy of the ADA *Exchange Lists* and told her to read it and follow the 1,500-calorie diet listed.

"I was to take 5 units of NPH U-80 insulin and was to go to the University Health Service to take it. The next morning, therefore, I came to the surprised nurse with my insulin but no syringe. She had no insulin syringe, either, so we ended up using a tuberculin syringe and calculating the dosage in cubic centimeters. I was clumsy with the injection and the nurse was angry."

Ms. Betschart bought a glass insulin syringe and 10 stainless steel needles. They had to be boiled for 20 minutes, then cooled and dried before use. "The needles were sharpened on a stone but they clanked around while boiling and became dull again," Ms. Bet-

cated, formal, and courteous. He gave of himself tirelessly, and he expected—and received—the same dedication from his staff.

In a second interview, Mr. Ferguson was asked by the office manager, "Can you type?" He couldn't, and thought this a strange question to ask of someone who was being hired for an executive position. He soon found out, however, just how understaffed the national office was, and that everyone at the American Diabetes Association was expected to perform any task that needed to be done. This delayed his plans for setting up his new department. The biggest surprise of all, however, was that the 50 affiliates, which were to be the foundation of the new organization, were not all "chomping at the bit" to reorganize and raise funds for research. Some affiliates were completely inactive, many had only marginal bank accounts, and at least one had not held a meeting in more than a year.

It should be noted here that of the active affiliates at that time, most were counterparts of the national office, with physician members who held local professional meetings to pass along the latest information on treatment methods to colleagues. These were known as clinical societies. In addition, some affiliates had lay societies; the primary purpose of the lay societies was to sponsor patient education programs.

In 1969, three affiliates—Los Angeles, Michigan, and New York City—each had an income of just under $100,000 a year. All of the other affiliates had a combined income of $200,000 and were sending a total contribution to the national office of $15,000 a year. There was open hostility between some affiliates and the national organization and, as in any merger, there was some resistance and tension. To understand this, two things should be remembered: some local lay societies predated the national organization; and, lay membership in many affiliates was made up of a majority of people with non-insulin-dependent (type II) diabetes. These latter affiliates were more concerned with immediate management problems and were unaware of how research into the seriousness of diabetes or its long-term complications would improve their lives—and the lives of countless others. These affiliates were receiving modest amounts of money from the United Fund and were content with the status quo.

Both groups felt threatened: the professionals, by a loss of autonomy; the lay members, by the new emphasis on fund raising for research. As time went on, however, the need to fund more research took precedence. Typical of this new trend in thinking was the

schart recalled. "You couldn't sharpen them after boiling because you'd contaminate the needle. What an effort to get up in the morning, boil, drain, and cool my syringe, and find the key to the dormitory refrigerator to get my insulin before breakfast and make an eight o'clock class."

In the meantime, her doctor increased her insulin dose, based on urine Tes-Tape readings. "At 13 units, I got dizzy before supper, and when I reported this he cut the dose to 11 units," she said. This was her first experience with hypoglycemia. Her doctor told her that if it ever happened again she should eat some Life-Savers. "But," Ms. Betschart said, "I was afraid to eat sugar because I thought it was really dangerous for a diabetic to eat sugar."

In addition to daily insulin injections, Ms. Betschart said her diet presented a struggle as well. "At that time," she noted, "it was fairly restrictive for carbohydrates. Trying to eat measured portions of proper foods was tough in the cafeteria . . . . Most of the time, I was hungry." She said that the sugar substitute cyclamate was helpful and was a real improvement over saccharin.

plea of one mother whose daughter had recently lost her vision due to diabetes. She wrote, "When are you going to start telling the truth about diabetes? When will you embark on a national campaign similar to other health organizations?"

Reorganization: Approaching The Change

ADA Presidents Edwin W. Gates, M.D., (1967-68) and Harvey C. Knowles, Jr., M.D., (1968-69) served the Association well during this turbulent time of transition to a voluntary health agency. "There can be no other way," said Dr. Gates about the change.

Dr. Gates, a four-time ADA treasurer and a Board member since 1955, presided over the first gathering of the ADA Central Council during the 1968 Annual Meeting in San Francisco. Convened on June 13, 1968, the Council meeting included 47 delegates representing 32 of 53 affiliates. After a welcome address by Dr. Gates, President-Elect Knowles presided. According to the record, the composition of delegates selected by affiliates was 28 physicians and 19 nonprofessional members, in addition to local board members, committee chairmen, and state coordinators. A major organizational policy change should be noted here. Traditionally, the majority of affiliate, chapter, and branch board members had to be physicians, but under the new rules, the number had been reduced to half.

The national Nominating Committee presented a slate of officers, and, for the first time, officers and board members were elected by the Central Council. This election was particularly significant because, for the first time, five lay persons were elected to the Board. They were Dorothy Child, of California; Robert Curran, of Washington, D.C.; Sara Hunt, of Tennessee; Walter Morris, of New Jersey; and William Talbert, of New York City. "Transition to a voluntary health agency is in the final stages," said James Hurd, M.D., chairman of the Committee On Affiliate Associations. "Full acceptance of the proposed Bylaws will be voted upon tomorrow, and implementation by all affiliates will take place within the next two years."

Dr. Knowles, who had been appointed editor of the Association journal, *Diabetes*, in 1967, declared a year later in his own president's address that he had never been through a year like the one he had just experienced. He clearly saw the Association at a crucial point in time. "There is no doubt," he said, "that we have produced some significant advances, but honest evaluation forces us to admit it is not enough. We do have a Fellowship Program of merit, a good Small

Grants Program, a fine Detection Drive, and excellent Postgraduate Programs, as well as many other commendable projects. But there is much more to learn.

"We need to know at least four more factors about diabetes: how to put the facets of the disease together; the influence of environment; the need for predictors of the disease; and how to attend to heredity of diabetes. We need funds and manpower to undertake these tasks. It is no longer sufficient just to control diabetes; we must overcome it," Dr. Knowles concluded. But as the 1960s closed, it was organizational change that dominated the scene.

The conference, "Building an Organization to Advance the Cause of Diabetes," held in Chicago on March 21, 1970, saw another significant turning point. After five years of planning, a consensus was close about the new partnership of professional and lay members and the plan for increasing fund-raising strength.

The agenda of the meeting covered:

1) The need for commitment by the national organization and all affiliates to respond to diabetes as a national health problem;

2) The nature and intent of fund-raising efforts of national and affiliates;

3) The disposition of the 75-25 percent local/national division-of-income provision in the *Annual Affiliate Agreement*, which was being held in abeyance;

4) The need for a temporary fund-raising arrangement until a national campaign could be launched; and

5) The need for affiliates and the national organization to implement an organizational approach and structure as set forth in the *Statement of Purposes, Principles and Policies*.

By the close of the meeting, the national Association's plans to organize as a voluntary health agency were reaffirmed. For the first time since 1964, disparate ideas began to coalesce into consensus. It was a mandate to move forward.

Reorganization: The All-Important Vote

At the Annual Meeting in June 1970, ADA President Robert C. Hardin, M.D., (1969-70) said in his opening remarks, "Today is the day when we must come to a final decision. We need a strong organization to advance the cause of diabetes, and no other organization is doing this. We ask you now to cover all points of the previous discussions and come to a consensus."

Before the vote, Max Ellenberg, M.D., a member of the Board of both the national organization and the

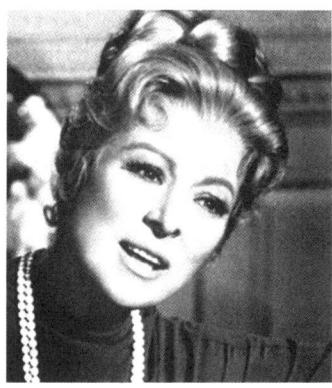 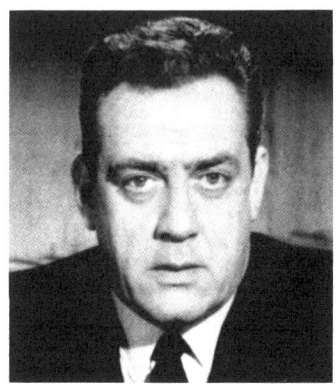

Greer Garson and Raymond Burr made special films for the 1966 Diabetes Week of November 1966.

New York Diabetes Affiliate, had emphasized the rising incidence of diabetes, increasing physician competence, and socioeconomic implications. "The American Diabetes Association is in a position to meet these changing problems with educational programs," said Dr. Ellenberg.

United States Senator Gale McGee of Wyoming, who himself had diabetes, sent a letter endorsing the need for an organization committed to the growing needs of people with diabetes. He promised to work to ensure adequate support for medical research, a promise he later kept by sponsoring a bill in the Senate that resulted in the passage of the National Diabetes Research and Education Act of 1974.

Almost six years had gone into planning for an organizational structure that would be workable and acceptable to all levels of the Association. The long preparation paid off. The vote by the Central Council in favor of the new Constitution and Bylaws passed triumphantly.

Lewis E. January, M.D., past president of the American Heart Association, congratulated members of the American Diabetes Association on the momentous step they had taken and extended an invitation to members of the Central Council, saying, "Please do join the voluntary health agencies at the top. It is not enough to band together in a good cause. ADA has a long and successful record as a professional society, and this identity should not be lost. A strong scientific society can exist within a voluntary health agency. And, a final word of caution to preserve your identity, have well defined goals, exert influence by playing an important role in funding research, which is how tuber-

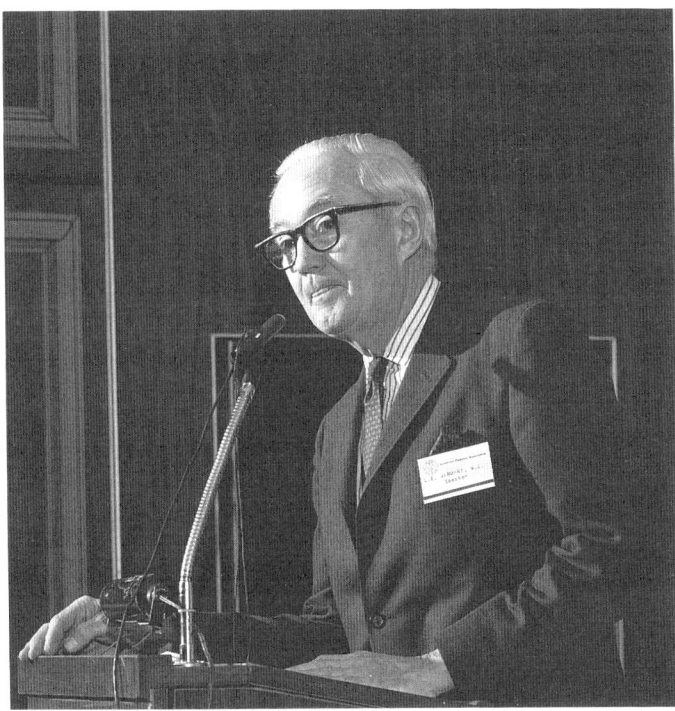
Lewis E. January, M.D.

culosis and polio were finally conquered.''

Richard M. Stephenson, M.D., of the office of the director of the National Institutes of Health, in addressing the group said, "Information, liaison, and lobbying are the three broad categories by which relationships must be maintained. Lobbying is not necessarily a bad word. Political pressure, and activities essential to informing Congress are thoroughly legitimate and to a large extent rest on the shoulders of the voluntary health agency."

To illustrate the need for a greater voice for people with diabetes in the federal government, Dr. Stephenson pointed to a pile of computer printouts of diabetes research programs. Then he pointed to a second pile of research programs funded by the Heart Institute, demonstrating—in inches—how much more was being done in heart research than in diabetes.

Speaking of volunteer involvement, Francis P. Wilcox, past chairman of the board of the American Cancer Society, noted that the cancer control programs in France, Italy, India, Japan, and the U.S.S.R. lagged behind programs in the United States, even though those countries had no shortage of government funds. He attributed this lag to a lack of a broad-based volunteer involvement. "Remember," Mr. Wilcox said,

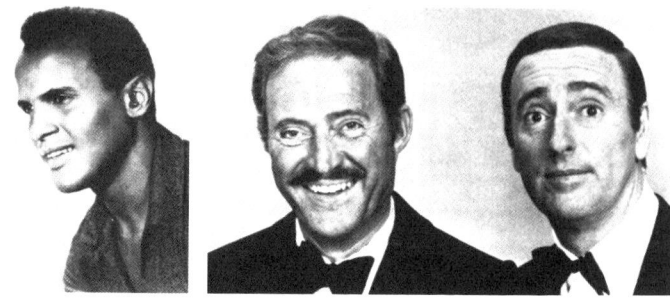

Diabetes Week 1967 featured singer Harry Belafonte, at left, who explained to TV viewers that "even though diabetes sounds dangerous, it need not be if we learn of the condition in time." Diabetes Week 1969 featured comedians Rowan and Martin. The duo did spot announcements shown on TV and movie screens throughout the country.

"people can educate and motivate other people. People listen to people. There is a need for a strong volunteer base for a national fund-raising campaign, and these projects are best done by volunteers."

The Bylaws that the Association passed at the June 1970 Annual Meeting consisted of 16 articles excerpted below:

I. *Membership*, heretofore limited to physicians, health professionals, and corporations, was expanded to include general members of affiliates and direct members, persons who resided in areas not served by an affiliate.

II. *Affiliate Associations* were created, subject to minimal requirements: serve a specific geographic area; be incorporated in state where located; have a commitment to diabetes as a national health problem; and be in compliance with the Association's bylaws.

III. *The Central Council* was designated as the general voting body of the Association.

IV. *Board of Directors*, its general powers, number of members, qualifications, and tenure were delineated. (There were to be 50 people on the Board: 6 principal officers; 1 most recent living past-president of the Association; 15 members of the professional section of the Association; 21 from the past or present membership of the Central Council; and 6 directors-at-large. The executive director was to be a nonvoting member of the Board. The chairman of the Board was to be nominated by the Executive Committee and elected by the Board of Directors from among its members at its first meeting each year.)

V. *Officers*, were identified as president, president-elect, vice president professional, vice president Central Council, secretary, and treasurer.

VI. *Executive Director*, appointment, duties, and responsibilities were described.

VII. *Committees*, including composition of the Executive Committee and provisions for standing and appointment of special committees were described.

VIII. *Contracts, Checks, Deposits, and Gifts*, provided guidelines for handling finances.

IX. *Membership Cards*, were to be provided by the Board.

X. *Books and Records*, the Association was to keep correct and accurate records of meetings and transactions.

XI. *Fiscal Year*, January 1 through December 31.

XII. *Organizational Year*, was to begin immediately following Annual Meeting and conclude with end of next Annual Meeting.

XIII. *Dues*, amounts, payments, defaults, and waivers were described.

XIV. *Seal of the Association*, was to be adopted by all affiliates.

XV. *Waiver of Notice*, described provisions for nonprofit organizations.

XVI. *Amendments*, procedures for amending the Bylaws were described.

The Cyclamate Debate

On October 18, 1969, Robert Finch, secretary of the U.S. Department of Health, Education, and Welfare, announced that all food products containing cyclamates would be withdrawn from the market. Cyclamates were used as artificial sweeteners. Laboratory studies had shown that cyclamates produced cancer in rats, although there were no reported cases in humans. The withdrawal of cyclamates was a great blow to people with diabetes. Cyclamates added a pleasant dimension to the diabetic diet: they were more palatable than saccharin and did not break down in cooking.

In the wake of this announcement, the U.S. Food and Drug Administration (FDA) took another look at several additives to foods and beverages, including saccharin. On November 20, the FDA revised its original order and said that after January 20, 1970, beverages and most drugs containing cyclamates would be banned. However, foods and liquid or tablet sweeteners containing cyclamates would continue to be available on a nonprescription basis, with clear labeling showing the cyclamate content in an average serving.

The American Diabetes Association took the position that since the available information was incomplete, and interpretation of the studies was conflicting, the best approach was caution. The Association advised, "Ask your doctor." The Association took this position to buy time until the FDA had developed guidelines for physicians in prescribing cyclamates. By the end of the year, cyclamates were officially withdrawn from the market. Cyclamates were gone but not forgotten. People with diabetes, as well as Abbott Laboratories, the manufacturer, are still trying to have the ban lifted.

(In 1984, FDA's Cancer Assessment Committee, after an extensive review of the studies, found that "There is very little credible data to implicate cyclamates as a carcinogen at any organ tissue site . . . no newly discovered toxic effects are likely to be revealed by further studies." However, the Committee of the National Research Council of the National Academy of Sciences subsequently reviewed all the available data and concluded that "cyclamates or cyclohexylamine (CHA) are probably not carcinogens by themselves, but there is evidence suggesting that these substances may promote the effects of other cancer-causing substances or cause mutations." This committee concluded that "more investigation is required before cyclamates can again be added to the nation's food supply," *Consumer Reports*, November 1985.)

The University Group Diabetes Program

The University Group Diabetes Program (UGDP) study started in 1961 and was conducted at 12 university medical schools in the United States and Puerto Rico. It was the largest prospective study of its kind—823 subjects—and compared the results of various diabetes treatment regimens using oral drugs, insulin, and diet, against a placebo.

A report of the study's findings—which raised serious questions about the oral antidiabetes compound tolbutamide—was scheduled for presentation and discussion at the ADA Scientific Sessions in June 1970. However, the findings were leaked to the press in the spring. The FDA responded on May 11, 1970, stating, "The FDA agrees with the recent study by the UGDP, that in the treatment of mild, adult-onset diabetes mellitus, use of tolbutamide is no more effective than diet alone."

Commenting upon the UGDP study about to be released, the FDA said, ". . . in the types of patients studied, long-term, a regimen of tolbutamide is no more effective than diet alone, and as far as death from heart disease and related conditions . . . may be less effective than diet or diet and insulin."

The FDA recommended that tolbutamide and other sulfonylurea type agents should be used only in patients with symptomatic adult-onset diabetes who cannot be controlled adequately with diet. This announcement triggered a medical/scientific controversy that lasted for a decade.

Max Miller, M.D., professor of medicine at Case Western Reserve School of Medicine and chairman of the UGDP Study, responded: "Premature release of some of the information from reports which are to be presented to the American Diabetes Association in St. Louis, June 14th is most unfortunate, not only from a scientific standpoint but for the thousands of diabetics in this country who are vitally concerned about the value of various forms of therapy now in use. It subjects to debate in newspapers and other media, very serious questions which have been under study for many years, which must be discussed and evaluated first, by impartial investigators in the field. Naturally, we have been concerned by our findings regarding efficacy of certain hypoglycemic drugs. Final judgment of the relevancy and significance of the UGDP findings will rest on the detailed analyses by our peers and by comparison with other studies. Prior to complete review at the ADA meeting June 14, 1970, it is inappropriate to discuss." (*Diabetes*, Vol. 17 *Supplement* 2, 1970)

The confusion among physicians and patients and a plethora of articles in the lay press made it imperative that the American Diabetes Association state its position. Opinions within the Association were divided. Many physicians were prescribing the drug with good results, and the study findings caused them anguish and concern. Other physicians felt that the drugs should be banned immediately. The issue caused heated debate within the American Diabetes Association.

An ad hoc committee was appointed to draft a response, which was reviewed by the Executive Committee and read at the conclusion of the Annual Meeting in 1970. In a prudent statement, ADA President Robert C. Hardin, M.D., (1969-70) said, "The American Diabetes Association commends those persons who have reported studies concerning the effects of therapy on the course of diabetes and its complications at this Annual Meeting.

"New data have been presented, some of which raise questions about the efficacy and safety of oral therapy. However, it is difficult to generalize from these unpublished data. Careful evaluation of the com-

Mr. Hamster: ADA Symbol?

As part of its ongoing effort to devise new and more effective methods of presenting Patient Education guides for living with diabetes, the Association and the Editorial Board of *ADA Forecast* announced a contest in the spring of 1967.

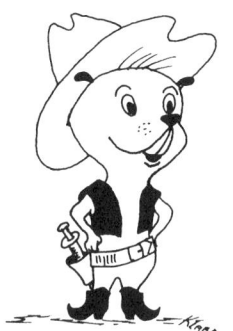

MEET MR. HAMSTER

A cash prize was offered to the individual submitting the best cartoon character that could be used as a symbol in future ADA educational series.

It was believed that an appealing cartoon character would give added impact to almost any message directed toward the fundamental principles of good diabetes control. There were high hopes that such a symbol might catch the public fancy and identify a diabetes message instantly, in the same way Smokey the Bear came to mean "forest fires."

There were hundreds of contest entries. In the November/December 1967 issue of *ADA Forecast*, the winner appeared dramatically on the cover. He was none other than "Mr. Hamster," later known as "Hiram Hamster."

An accompanying press release enthused: "The captivating figure, jaunty in his wide-brimmed sombrero and his loosely-slung hypo-holster, seems to borrow something of

plete data and further study will be necessary to reach final conclusions."

The Association's ad hoc Editorial and Advisory Committee and the Executive Committee agreed with the conclusion that death rates from cardiovascular disease in the UGDP subjects receiving tolbutamide were significantly higher than in study subjects receiving other treatments.

The committees recommended that when dietary treatment failed to control type II diabetes (of mild to moderate severity), insulin should be used in preference to oral agents. Insulin is essential in severe diabetes regardless of age of onset, according to the committees.

Public controversy raged over the study as the debate continued in the media and in prestigious medical journals, such as the *Journal of the American Medical Association* and the *New England Journal of Medicine*. To fulfill a responsibility to patients, physicians, and the cause of research—all of which were primary concerns of the American Diabetes Association—the UGDP data were carefully reviewed and monitored by various committees of the Association. Published statements on these findings appeared in the journal *Diabetes* and in press releases from 1970 through 1984.

Throughout this period, many concerned patients and physicians called the national office. The Association consistently held the position that the study was flawed and that oral hypoglycemic agents have a place in the treatment of adult-onset diabetes. However, a regimen of diet and exercise in the management and control of adult-onset diabetes is the treatment of choice. When such treatment does not achieve normal or near-to-normal blood-glucose levels, physicians need to consider other treatments (i.e., insulin or oral hypoglycemic agents) on an individual basis.

In July 1972, the Association published a statement in support of labeling oral hypoglycemic drugs in accordance with the FDA Drug Bulletin of May 1972, which said, "This labeling and therapeutic regimen for diabetes mellitus are consistent with the therapeutic recommendations of the American Diabetes Association and the Council on Drugs of the American Medical Association with which FDA consulted on the evaluation of the University Group Diabetes Program Study." (*Diabetes*, Vol. 21:833, 1972)

In 1974, Alexander Marble, M.D., then president of the Joslin Diabetes Foundation, wrote in the November/December issue of *Diabetes Forecast*: [Oral agents] are safe for short-term therapy, as safe as al-

the nonchalance and amusing honesty of other renowned cartoon personalities such as Pogo, Smokey the Bear, and similar members of America's menagerie of beloved animal friends . . . *Viva* Mister Hamster!"

For whatever reason, the character never caught on. Adults with diabetes never fully accepted "Hiram," and children refused to adopt him. He made a few desultory appearances in 1968 issues of *Forecast*, and fewer yet in 1969. He lived fitfully into the early 1970s before fading into total eclipse.

Some said he perished of neglect; others thought it was a broken heart. In either case, Hiram's demise served to show that life can be cruel—even in cartoons.

most any drug in common use. As for use over many years, I have seen no consistent evidence that they are not safe if used properly."

Five Years of Progress

The year 1970 was a turning point in ADA history. After years of preparation, the Association had established itself as a voluntary health agency for the pur-

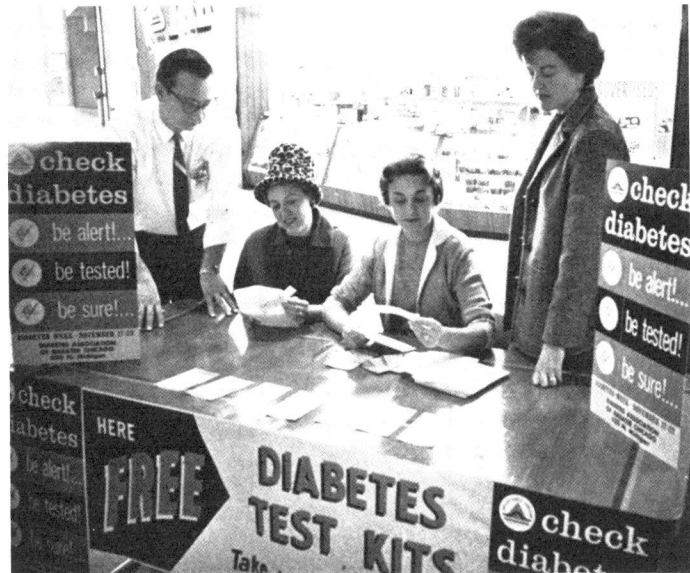

Volunteers in the Diabetes Association of Greater Chicago help distribute Dreypaks, diabetes test kits, during Diabetes Week, November 13-19, 1966.

pose of general public fund raising to continue its programs of patient, professional, and public education, and to pursue more vigorously its funding of research. Administratively, the Association had revised the Constitution and Bylaws to embrace the new organization. For the first time, lay people were granted full and equal membership opportunities.

The six-year period—1965-1970—had seen a long list of accomplishments:

- In 1965, Jerome Conn, M.D., chairman of the Association's Research Committee, proposed the establishment of a research and development awards program to assist exceptionally promising young physicians and other life scientists in the study and investigation of diabetes and related metabolic problems. The top-rated award recipient named would receive the Elliott P. Joslin Research and Development Award for that year. Candidates were required to be members of a university-affiliated institution and to devote 90 percent of their activities to research. The first recipients of these awards were Drs. Ronald A. Arky, of Boston; Michael F. Ball, of Washington, D.C.; Richard J. Mahler, of New York; and Thomas J. Merimee, of Baltimore.

- Under a policy established in 1967 by the National Health Council (NHC), the American Diabetes Association was approved as one of twenty major national voluntary health agencies that met the NHC's standards and ethical guidelines. This assured the public that the Association conformed to a high standard of accounting and financial reporting for voluntary health agencies and welfare organizations.

- The first Postgraduate Syllabus was published in 1965.

- A "Symposium on the Education of the Patient with Diabetes," cosponsored by the American Diabetes Association, The American Dietetic Association, and the U.S. Public Health Service, was held in 1967.

- The Outstanding Layman Award was established in 1969. The first award was given to Mrs. Robert E. Childs, a volunteer with the Michigan Diabetes Association. Mrs. Childs was editor of *News and*

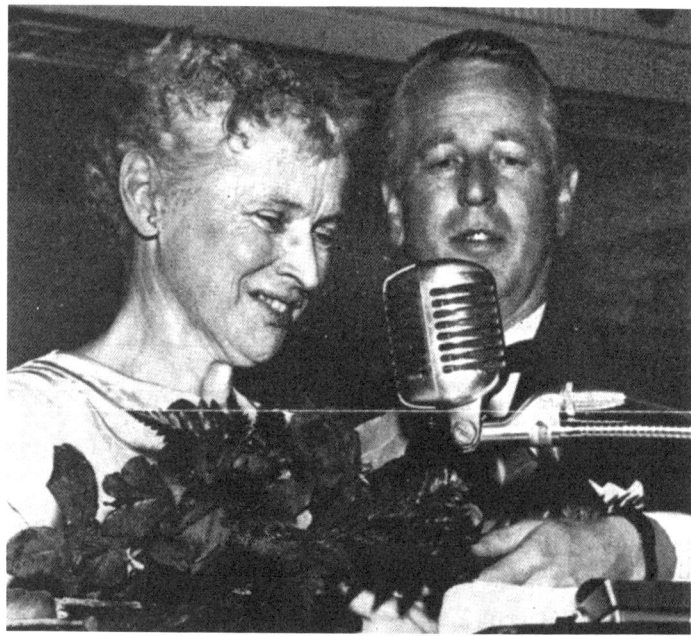

Mrs. Robert E. Childs receives her Outstanding Layman of the Year award from James B. Hurd, M.D., then vice president, Central Council.

Views, a quarterly report published by the Michigan Affiliate. She held the post from 1962 to 1967, when progressive loss of vision forced her to step down. Mrs. Childs turned *News and Views* into a first-rate publication by attending numerous scientific sessions and interviewing physicians for the latest diabetes information.

- The first Postgraduate Course for health-care professionals, cosponsored by the Association's Committee on Professional Education and the Joslin Diabetes Foundation, was held in 1969, and was oversubscribed. (The meeting was originally called the First Paramedical Postgraduate Course. Subsequently, the name was changed to the Postgraduate Course for Allied Health Professionals.) The purpose of the course was to convey current knowledge and teaching techniques about diabetes to non-physician health professionals. The Board had mistakenly held the view that health professionals would not be interested in such a course. However, the success of this course convinced the Board and the Professional Education Committee that they had underestimated the interest. For health professionals, attendance at this course was a quantum leap toward recognition—both in the Association, and as a vital part of the health-care team in diabetes treatment. (In 1974, a third track was added to the annual Scientific Sessions of the Annual Meeting to benefit this fast-growing segment of the membership.)

Echoing ADA President Danowski's comment in 1966—that the Association's planning was ahead of its resources—the Treasurer's Report in 1970 showed an excess of expense over income of $131,997. In giving his report, the treasurer said that in spite of excellent growth, increases in membership, subscriptions, and sales of materials, the treasury was beginning to show the strains of the burgeoning organization. It would take 10 to 12 years before this situation would improve.

Pieces Of The Puzzle:
What We Knew About Diabetes

1965

As part of the Scientific Sessions held during the twenty-fifth Annual Meeting in New York, Benjamin Pansky, M.D., of New York Medical College describes a continuing research program he is pursuing in collaboration with Drs. Lawrence House and Lawrence Cone, in consultation with Dr. Rachmiel Levine, chairman of the school's Department of Medicine. The three doctors found certain cells in the thymus gland that produce an insulin-like substance. The substance—then unnamed—seems to exhibit test reactions similar to pancreatic insulin.

Donald F. Steiner, M.D., of the University of Chicago discovers how insulin is created in the beta cells of the pancreas. He reveals that the hormone begins as a long single-chain molecule, which he calls "proinsulin." This precursor is converted to insulin, a double-chain molecule with a connecting protein bridge, within the beta cell.

1967

Scientists at the Jackson Laboratory of Bar Harbor, Maine, study the people of nearby Vinalhaven Island, 40 miles to the southwest. The island has a very stable population of 1,400, of whom half have abnormally high blood-sugar levels. Only one person in 20, however, has diabetes to a degree that requires treatment. The evidence for heredity in diabetes proves strong. Among those whose ancestors on both sides resided on the island for three or more generations, 60 percent have diabetes. When one side of the family had been there that long, the diabetes rate drops to 30 percent. Among the entire population, there has never been a single reported case of insulin-dependent (type I) diabetes.

1968

Roger Unger, M.D., of the University of Texas at Dallas presents evidence of newly discovered substances on the walls of intestines. These substances are shown to play a part in triggering the release of insulin by the pancreas when food is eaten. One of them appears similar to glucagon, a hormone formed in the alpha cells of the pancreas. Dr. Unger presents the findings at the ADA Postgraduate Course in Cleveland.

The effect of oral contraceptives, or birth control pills, on blood-sugar levels is the subject of several investigations. It had been reported that 80 percent of women receiving oral contraceptive agents developed "subclinical diabetes": diabetes without symptoms. Research confirms that some oral contraceptives do convert normal women into women with subclinical diabetes, although the situation appears reversible when the pills are discontinued. In one study of pregnant women diagnosed with gestational diabetes, the mothers' diabetes does not appear to intensify after delivery, even if the women resume taking oral contraceptives.

1969

A report in the journal *Diabetes* reveals a shocking diabetes incidence rate among certain North American Indian tribes. Whereas the incidence of diabetes among Caucasian populations is 2 percent, it is 35 to 40 percent among the Pima Indians of southern Arizona. The figure is 17 percent among the Cocopahs of southwestern Arizona, 17 percent for the North Carolina Cherokees, and 34 percent for the Senecas of western New York. Generally, the diabetes found is quite mild and usually associated with obesity. An extremely low rate of diabetes is found among the Eskimos and the Athabaskan Indians of Alaska. Both are found to be physically active peoples who consume similarly high protein diets, moderate in fats and carbohydrates.

The exact three-dimensional structure of the insulin molecule is finally discovered. In England, a team headed by Dorothy C. Hodgkin, Ph.D., of Oxford University succeeds in mapping the configuration of the large, complex molecule. The key to success is use of X-ray crystallography. For many years, researchers have known that insulin is a protein containing 51 amino acids. They also knew that each insulin molecule contains 777 atoms arranged in two connected chains or strands. How the chains bonded and what the molecule looked like, however, was previously unknown.

1970

Proinsulin, the protein molecule from which the insulin molecule is derived, is the subject of a paper presented by Albert I. Winegrad, M.D., at the Association's seventeenth Postgraduate Course in Pittsburgh. The 1965 discovery of proinsulin by Donald F. Steiner, M.D., raises the possibility that diabetes may result from proinsulin with an abnormal structure, or from an impairment of the mechanism that converts proinsulin into insulin. Dr. Winegrad reports that early evidence showed some proinsulin is not broken down into insulin and other byproducts, but goes directly into the bloodstream. Most proinsulin, however, is converted into insulin by the beta cells in the pancreas, and released into the circulation as needed. Clifford F. Gastineau, M.D., editor in chief of *ADA Forecast*, writes that the discovery of proinsulin "has been one of the most exciting and most important scientific discoveries in recent years in the diabetes field."

The Ames Company devises the first solid phase system for measuring blood glucose with a reagent (reacting) strip and a reflectance (measuring) meter. "Solid phase" means that the blood is tested on a solid pad rather than in a test tube. The early machines are generally limited to use in laboratories and physicians' offices. Within a few years, manufacturers on both sides of the Atlantic would be making similar equipment for home blood-glucose testing.

Chapter Eight
Planning Becomes Imperative
1970-75

ADA Presidents

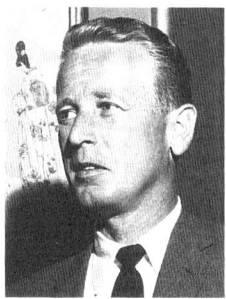 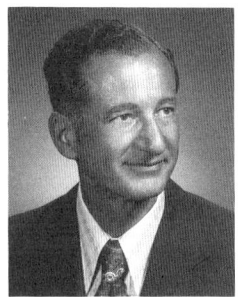

James B. Hurd, M.D.
(1970-71)

Stefan S. Fajans, M.D.
(1971-72)

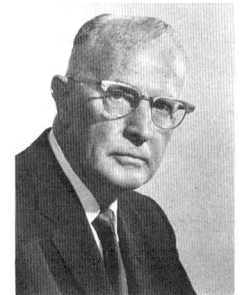 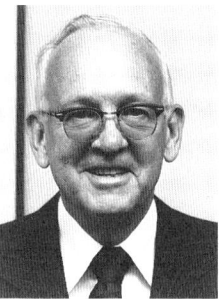 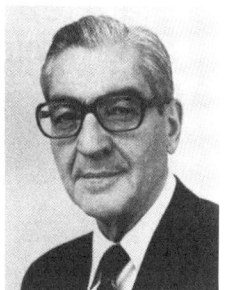

William H. Grishaw, M.D.
(1972-73)

Addison B.
Scoville, Jr., M.D.
(1973-74)

Max Ellenberg, M.D.
(1974-75)

ADA Chairmen of the Board

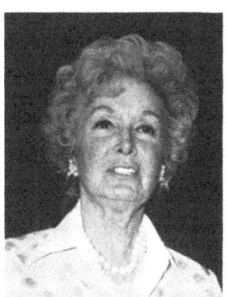 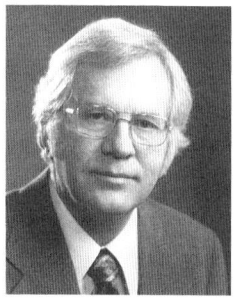

Gail Patrick Jackson
(1973-74)

Wendell Mayes, Jr.
(1974-77)

The early 1970s found the western world reeling under the impact of the OPEC oil embargo and watching helplessly as inflation and unemployment soared. In Munich, Germany, Arab extremists killed 11 Israeli athletes during the Olympic Games, ushering in the era of international terrorism. In Kenya, Africa, Dr. Richard Leakey found a human skull estimated to be 2.3 million years old.

In the United States, 18 year olds became eligible to vote in 1971, and the Equal Rights Amendment (ERA) met opposition in Congress in 1974. Total ratification of the ERA was not achieved, but the impact of the amendment on society was significant, and one that would affect the American Diabetes Association as well. The Watergate hearings riveted the nation, and in 1974 Richard M. Nixon became the first United States President to resign.

In medicine, Earl W. Sutherland, Jr., M.D., of Vanderbilt University, was awarded the Nobel Prize in Physiology and Medicine for his research in the mechanism and action of hormones. Dr. Sutherland was the ADA Banting Lecturer in 1969 and presented a paper on "The Biological Role of Cyclic AMP and its Relation to Carbohydrate Metabolism."

James B. Hurd, M.D., ushered in the new decade as ADA president for 1970-71. A member of the Board since 1962, Dr. Hurd took over at a time when change was clearly in the wind. His election was the culmination of many years of devoted service to diabetes. Since 1952, he had been a member of the Board of Directors of the Chicago Affiliate and was long active as chairman of the affiliate's Camp Committee.

Cigarette advertising was banned from television. This action started a trend in society that would eventually lead to non-smoking sections in restaurants and no smoking on commercial air flights, and culminate in the movement toward a smoke-free society, with federal agencies and industrial concerns cooperating. The Association had long advocated cessation of smoking for people with diabetes because of the deleterious effect smoking has upon the vascular system.

The rights of the handicapped became a national issue in the early 1970s. Section 503 of the Federal Rehabilitation Act of 1973 stated that any employer doing business with the federal government under a contract of more than $2,500 annually must take affirmative action to hire the handicapped. The federal law defined the term "handicapped" according to three criteria: 1) anyone who has a physical or mental impairment that substantially limits one or more of his or her major life activities; 2) anyone who has a record of such impairment; 3) anyone who is regarded as having such as impairment. Under this law, people with diabetes qualified as "handicapped" under the first criterion. This classification was hotly debated. A number of people with diabetes did not want to be considered handicapped, while others had more ambivalent feelings.

Passage of the law presented a philosophical dilemma to the American Diabetes Association. The Association's position had been that people with diabetes can live a normal life and are desirable workers. In 1952, the ADA "Employment Statement" was: "Those with controlled diabetes are good employable risks. They should not be classified as handicapped." Then, in 1972, it was: "Diabetics under adequate medical supervision make excellent employees." The statement went on to delineate three types of people with diabetes: those who controlled their disease with diet, those who used diet and oral agents, and those who used diet and insulin. People in the first two categories should have no employment restrictions, the statement asserted, while people requiring insulin should not be assigned to hazardous jobs, nor do they qualify to drive commercial vehicles in interstate commerce. (The Association's "Employment Policy Statement" was revised again in 1984. See Chapter Ten.)

For people with diabetes and those working in the field of diabetes, 1974 was a banner year. The National Diabetes Research and Education Act was passed by Congress, putting diabetes legislation on the books for the first time in United States history.

Within the American Diabetes Association, there was a feeling of impatience and an eagerness to forge ahead. However, as with past events, important changes within the Association would take time.

An Impetus For Change

Although the vote to reorganize the American Diabetes Association into a voluntary health organization came in 1970, many within the Association felt that reorganization was proceeding at a painfully slow pace. An overworked national staff tried to accommodate new demands, but in so doing found little time to devote to affiliate building, which was a vital part of the reorganization plan. Left to their own resources, many affiliates were struggling for survival.

Frustration arose between some physician Board members and Executive Director J. Richard Connelly over what some perceived as his resistance to the new order. As a result, Mr. Connelly resigned in 1973, after having served as executive director for 24 years. In a struggle of the old versus the new, some of Mr. Connelly's supporters—both staff and volunteer—left the Association as well.

As the first executive director, Mr. Connelly had joined the Association in 1949. From a staff of four and an annual budget of $79,000, he built the organization up to a staff of 23 full-time and 12 part-time employees, two consultants, a legal counsel, and an annual budget of $1,250,000. For some, this record was outstanding; for others, it was not good enough. While Mr. Connelly has often been criticized for being too conservative, several facts should be noted in retrospect. By establishing high standards of excellence, he sowed the seeds of dedication to the cause of diabetes. This dedication has become the hallmark of the American Diabetes Association today. The many able and talented staff members who came to the Association since his departure have built on that foundation of dedication and integrity, acting as the reapers of the good seed sown in those early years.

A Search Committee was established and several months later the Board chose Ernest M. Frost, Ed.D.,

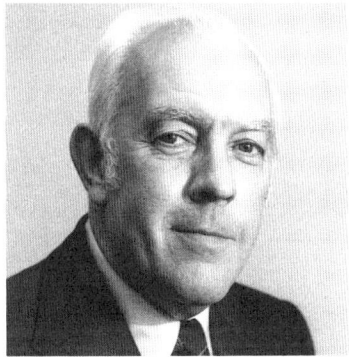

Ernest M. Frost, Ed.D.

as the new executive director (in less than a year the title was changed to executive vice president). Dr. Frost came from the American Heart Association, where he had been on the senior fund-raising staff. Prior to that, he had gained valuable experience working with volunteers and raising funds for the national March of Dimes Birth Defects Foundation.

The contrast in management styles was striking. Mr. Connelly had been a reserved, private person who was at home in the company of professional members but often uncomfortable with lay volunteers. Dr. Frost was an extrovert: outgoing, enthusiastic, expansive, and at ease in any situation. Articulate and a man of action, within a few months he had placed his stamp on the Association. He cultivated volunteers and affiliates, and seized every possible opportunity to speak about the Association.

One of his first major steps was to move the crowded ADA office to larger quarters at 600 Fifth Avenue in Rockefeller Center in New York City.

To establish closer contact with all affiliates, Dr. Frost divided the country into four regions, appointing a regional director to each. These regional directors were to help affiliates in fund-raising and organizational efforts. In addition, he added a talented art director, Patrick Murphy, to the staff. Mr. Murphy gave the Association a new look by redesigning the ADA logo (using a broken triangle, as explained in Chapter Four), letterhead, posters, and public education materials. With Board approval, these innovations were quickly adopted by affiliates; this accelerated the movement toward national unity.

New Diabetes Organizations

In 1970, Leatrice (Lee) Ducat, the mother of a child with diabetes and an active member of the ADA Philadelphia Affiliate, became impatient at what she saw as the Association's apparent lack of interest in research. She made a visit to the national office in New York and was told, "We are working on it." This was not good enough, she decided, and she formed an organization of parents of children with diabetes. Known as the Juvenile Diabetes Foundation (JDF), its primary purpose was—and is—to raise funds for research into insulin-dependent (type I) diabetes. Despite JDF's more limited focus on insulin-dependent diabetes only, the organization found many willing followers. For the American Diabetes Association, this meant competition for dollars and volunteers. Overtures to consolidate the two organizations were made by ADA Presidents Addison B. Scoville, Jr., M.D., (1973-74), Max Ellenberg, M.D., (1974-75), and George F. Cahill, Jr., M.D., (1975-76). At this time, Mrs. Ducat suggested a division of efforts, whereby JDF would concentrate on raising money for research and the American Diabetes Association could concentrate on publications and educational programs. Naturally, this was unacceptable to the Association, because the primary purpose in becoming a voluntary health agency was to increase the funding of research.

Much time and energy has been spent on debating whether the Association could have anticipated this splintering and forestalled the establishment of a competing diabetes organization. In retrospect, it appears that the formation of JDF was inevitable. With growing health consciousness and the Association preoccupied with changing its focus from a professional society to a voluntary health agency, ADA leadership did not fully perceive JDF as the serious challenger it proved to be. In the funding of research and in the legislative field, JDF has made significant contributions, but its efforts remain limited to type I diabetes. The American Diabetes Association, on the other hand, continues to focus on all types of diabetes, in *all* areas of programs and research. The ADA mission—to find the cause and a cure for diabetes, and to improve the lives of people with the disease—continues.

There is no doubt that JDF has spurred the American Diabetes Association into greater action in the quest for research monies and in organizing youth programs. An ADA Committee on Diabetes and Youth was appointed in 1972 by ADA President Stefan S. Fajans, M.D., (1971-72). Donnell D. Etzwiler, M.D., a pediatrician, served as chairman. Dr. Etzwiler, who became ADA president in 1976, was instrumental in getting other pediatricians to join the American Diabetes Association, among them Jay Skyler, M.D., who became the first editor of *Diabetes Care*, and Allan L. Drash, M.D., who became ADA president in 1983.

By the early 1970s, the "team" concept in diabetes—in which the person with diabetes receives education not only from the physician, but from the nurse educator, the dietitian, and other health professionals as well—was an idea whose time had come. This led to the formation of the American Association of Diabetes Educators (AADE) in 1974. Primarily made up of nurses and dietitians working in the field of diabetes, the organization grew rapidly.

Several factors were responsible for this growth: the Equal Rights movement, health consciousness, and,

The Name Game

In a discussion in 1975, William Ferguson, national director of affiliate development, pointed out to G. Rodney Lee, executive director of the Southern California Affiliate, that the American Diabetes Association was handicapped in its national publicity efforts because affiliates were using names that gave only local identification. There was no indication that each affiliate was part of a national diabetes organization. Mr. Lee, who had come to the Association from the American Cancer Society, where all affiliates used the national name, agreed that this presented a problem. They took their idea to have all affiliates adopt the same name to Larry Werner, president of the Southern California Affiliate. Mr. Werner was also enthusiastic about the idea, and introduced it as a proposal at the next ADA Board meeting. It was adopted by the Board, and within a year virtually all affiliates were using the American Diabetes Association name. This simple change served not only to unify the Association, but also to ameliorate some of the "we/they" feelings between affiliates and the national office.

unfortunately, what some saw as the Association's reluctance to fully recognize that nurses and dietitians—a majority of them female—had an important role to play in diabetes education and treatment. Non-physician health professionals were eligible for associate membership in the Association, but there was little incentive for them to belong. Dues were $50 and associate members were not yet permitted to attend physician postgraduate courses or submit abstracts at the Scientific Sessions. It was not until 1974, when the Bylaws were amended to include the position of non-physician vice president, that these professionals received full recognition.

The formation of AADE, like JDF, was perceived by some as inevitable. Efforts to incorporate the groups into the Association have not been successful, but both organizations have acted in concert with the Association on a professional basis—JDF in the legislative arena, and AADE on committees, councils, and professional publications. In partnership, AADE and the American Diabetes Association have undertaken numerous joint efforts over the years. Many AADE members are also members of the American Diabetes Association.

First National Fund-Raising Appeals

One of the most exciting aspects of ADA history is the manner in which ADA affiliates met the challenge of public fund raising once they were given the opportunity. In 1970, a mail appeal to 7,000 homes yielded $70,000, and in 1971, using the slogan "Double Check Diabetes with Detection and Dollars," affiliates raised $1,479,862. In this first year of public fund raising,

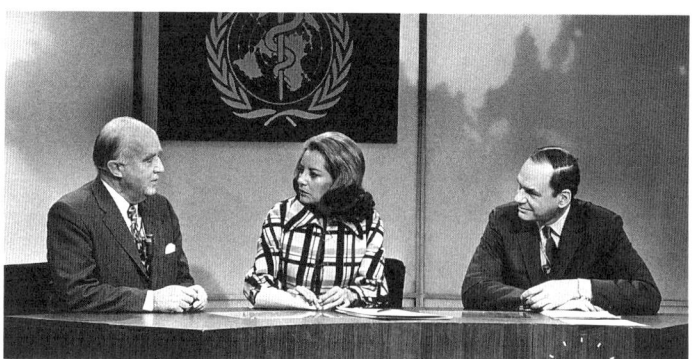

Charles H. Best, M.D., left, describes the experiments leading up to the discovery of insulin in an interview on World Health Day 1971 with Barbara Walters and Edwin Newman on the NBC television "Today" program.

the national office provided promotional materials and public service announcements that, for the first time, made a strong statement: "Diabetes is the fifth leading cause of death from disease."

In 1973, the ADA Southern California Affiliate organized the first Bike-a-thon, demonstrating that an affiliate could raise community awareness as well as big

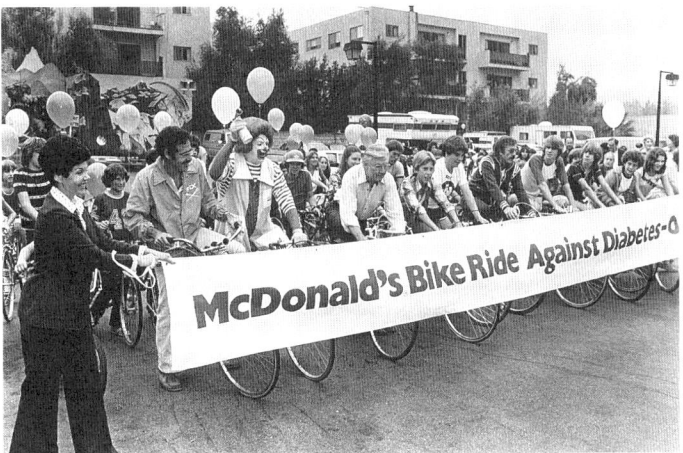

Hundreds of exuberant cyclists prepare to officially kick off the McDonald's Bike Ride Against Diabetes in southern California.

dollars. Affiliate President Larry Werner and Executive Director G. Rodney Lee persuaded the McDonald's Corporation to sponsor the event in the Los Angeles area. The Bike-a-thon was so successful that Mariana Porter, fund-raising director of the Southern California Affiliate, Mr. Lee, and William Ferguson, director of affiliate development at the national office, arranged a meeting at the McDonald's Corporation headquarters in Oak Brook, Illinois, to see if the company would be willing to provide national sponsorship. Interestingly enough, this meeting revealed that McDonald's was operating on rules similar to those used by the Association for organizational fund raising. McDonald's could no more insist that franchises participate in community programs than the Association could get affiliates to sponsor any one program. However, to demonstrate good will and interest, McDonald's published *A Guidebook for ADA Affiliates in Conducting a Bike-a-thon*. This made it easy for affiliates to join in the program, and "a-thons" of all kinds spread rapidly, becoming popular fund-raising events in many affiliates. (For more on McDonald's founder Ray Kroc's contributions to the Association, as well as those of his brother,

Robert, see Chapter Ten.)

Across the country, ADA affiliate-sponsored events expanded to raise needed funds for research and promote public awareness. By 1975, many affiliates were reporting in *Diabetes Forecast* their successful fund-raising events. The Washington, D.C. Affiliate and the *Washington Post* joined forces in 1975 to sponsor a hockey match to benefit diabetes. Bobby Clarke of the Philadelphia Flyers, 1974 National Hockey League most valuable player and insulin-dependent, was there to help. The Washington State Affiliate held its "Day at Long Acres," a fund-raising event held at a local race course. In 1975, 21 affiliates held bike-a-thons, among them the Greater Chicago and Northern Illinois, Oregon, Michigan, and Kansas Affiliates. The Southern California Affiliate sponsored the nation's largest bike ride, with 11,000 participants and more than 59,000 sponsors. Riders pedaled from Santa Barbara to the Mexican Border. Proceeds exceeded $190,000.

Volunteers And The ADA Holiday Sales Program

A dramatic breakthrough in fund raising occurred in the early 1970s, when families involved in a Minnesota parents' support group decided to begin selling holiday cards to raise money for diabetes research. From that dedicated effort grew the American Diabetes Association's National Holiday Sales Program, now one of the Association's single largest sources of revenue. To this day, the program is operated by volunteers and remains a telling example of the power of grass-roots action.

In May 1968, Virginia and Harlan Hanson's 14-month-old son, Mark, developed insulin-dependent (type I) diabetes. Hearing that money for research in diabetes was already inadequate and, with government cut-backs, destined to be further reduced, they decided to take action. "We felt we had to do more than just follow doctor's orders for daily care," said Virginia (Ginny) Hanson-Ullom, one of the project's founders. "There was a future to take care of also."

To Harlan Hanson, the answer seemed natural: sell something. With a little investigation, the groundwork was laid and the local Parents of Young Diabetics group set up a greeting card business in the Hansons' basement. The project was a success in its very first year, bringing in a profit of $5,000. In its second year, profits doubled after the group organized the visit of Charles H. Best, M.D., co-discoverer of insulin, to the second Minnesota Research Dinner.

PLANNING BECOMES IMPERATIVE

William F. Talbert:
An Ace In Diabetes Service
Tennis ace William F. Talbert was one of the first American celebrities to "go public" with

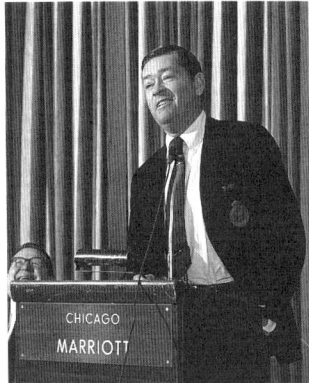

the fact of his own diabetes. But he proved to be far more than a "name." Long after his greatest fame had passed, Talbert remained a dedicated servant to the cause of diabetes and a key member of the American Diabetes Association.

In the world of tennis, Talbert remains one of the best who ever played. Known as Billy during his heyday, Talbert was ranked among the top 10 players in the country for 14 years. He was rated number two in the world in 1949. He played in many Davis Cup tournaments and served as Captain of the United States team for five successive years. In his career, Talbert won 38 national championships. After 25 years of amateur competition, he was elected to the National Lawn Tennis Hall of Fame in 1967.

Talbert's diabetes was diagnosed when he was 10. At the height of his career, he wrote in the May 1950 issue of *ADA Forecast*: "Mine is not a light case. I have had diabetes for 21 years, and at the present time my dosage of insulin is 54 units of U-80 insulin."

Talbert's great success in

At first the group sold cards only in the Twin Cities area. Later, as more and more volunteers came on board, they expanded the sales to the rest of Minnesota.

By 1973, ready to expand the market further and sure that there were others across the country also eager for a cure, the Minnesota volunteers began talking to national ADA leaders, offering to use this vehicle to raise funds nationwide for the cause of diabetes. The market grew as state after state joined the project. And the catalog expanded to other products ranging from calendars to music to a variety of gift items.

The national effort became a great success and was further enhanced when, for seven years, Mary Tyler Moore, a well-known actress with diabetes, graciously

Mary Tyler Moore

served as national chairman for the Holiday Sales Program.

The program experienced tremendous growth over the years. By 1988, the profit (about 50 percent of gross proceeds) had reached $950,000. In its 18 years, the Holiday Sales Program has put more than $7 million to work in diabetes research.

The National Holiday Sales Program is still organized and operated by volunteers in Minnesota. A core group works on the project all year, buying the merchandise, creating the catalog, and organizing promotions. Some 200 volunteers work on order fulfillment each fall.

From 1972 to 1975 the program was operated under the Diabetes Research Fund, Inc. After the Minnesota Affiliate was created in 1974, the Holiday Program and several other fund-raising projects were merged with the new state ADA affiliate. In 1980 it was deemed appropriate that this national program be operated under the auspices of the national ADA budget. Since 1973, all proceeds of this national program have sup-

sports made him a role model for many people with diabetes. He used his celebrity status well, appearing at thousands of diabetes-related events. From the beginning, he participated in every ADA Detection Drive and became increasingly involved in Association projects. He was also active in the New York Diabetes Association and the activities of Camp NYDA, for children with diabetes. He later served on the New York Diabetes Association's Board of Directors.

When the American Diabetes Association changed its membership requirements in 1968, Talbert made history of another sort by being elected to the Board of Directors. He was one of five lay persons elected—the first five ever to serve on the ADA Board.

His value was demonstrated in 1972, when ADA President Stefan S. Fajans, M.D., appointed Talbert chairman of the newly created Committee on Development. The committee spearheaded the Association's first nationwide fund-raising campaign.

Talbert proved an excellent choice. He was already an effective speaker and a tireless campaigner in the cause of diabetes. He often used his sports background to draw analogies. During the period when affiliates and the national office were struggling to reach accord, Talbert spoke of the need for conciliation. "Teamwork doesn't just happen," he said. "It takes compromise, hard work, and aiming for success in terms of a strong national organization. In the beginning, certain problems will arise. But in the end, as in tennis, the national Association and its affiliates will work together as a successful doubles team."

Talbert proved equally adept ported the ADA national diabetes research program.

People who have served as chairpersons of the National Holiday Sales Program are: Harlan Hanson, John Ullom, Tom and Linda Cunningham, Peter St. Peter, John Engdahl, Robert Thompson, Ginny Hanson-Ullom, Diana St. Peter, Susan Greene, John Prestholdt, and Ted Smith. Many have gone on to serve in the ADA Minnesota Affiliate or at the national level.

Staff persons included Dorothy Jacobson, Sandra Hijikata, Nancy Holina Service, and Diane LaFave.

Harlan Hanson served as president of the ADA Minnesota Affiliate in 1978 and as national ADA chairman of the Board from 1981 to 1983. Ginny Hanson-Ullom remains active in the Holiday Sales Program. She also served as a member of the ADA national Board of Directors from 1983 to 1986 and as chairman of the Board of the Minnesota Affiliate from 1987 to 1988.

Fifty Years Of Insulin

The 1972 Annual Meeting, held at the Washington Hilton Hotel in Washington, D.C., was a tribute to Drs. Banting and Best on the fiftieth anniversary of the discovery of insulin. Lady Banting and Dr. and Mrs. Best attended as guests of honor. The meeting was open to the public, and William Talbert, chairman of the Committee on Development, served as master of ceremonies.

ADA President Stefan S. Fajans, M.D., presented commemorative medallions to 14 scientists, five of whom were Nobel Laureates at the time (indicated by * following their name) for their work in insulin research during the preceding five decades. The recipients were the late Dr. Frederick Banting*, the late Dr. Bernardo A. Houssay*, the late Dr. Solomon A. Berson, and Drs. Charles H. Best, Walter R. Campbell, Carl F. Cori*, Dorothy C. Hodgkin*, Panayotis G. Katsoyanis, Rachmiel Levine, Frederick Sanger*, Donald F. Steiner, K.Z. Wang, Rosalyn A. Yalow, and Helmut Zahn.

Dr. Hodgkin delivered the Banting Memorial Lecture, in which she described the use of X-ray beams directed at crystals of insulin to determine its three-dimensional structure. Dr. Hodgkin was responsible for mapping the configuration of the insulin molecule, having received the Nobel Prize for similar work on the structure of penicillin and vitamin B-12.

In his presidential address, Dr. Fajans reviewed the challenges to research, saying, "As we look to the future, let us be realistic. Much progress has been made,

in private business. He rose to the top of the Security-Columbian Banknote Company in New York. On the side, he was a contributing editor to *Sports Illustrated* from its inception in 1954, and co-authored six tennis manuals. His autobiography, *Playing for Life*, was published in 1958.

As the seventies ended, Talbert was honored with the 50-year Joslin Medal in recognition of his long life with diabetes. His pride on that occasion was well-founded. Over the long haul, he had shown himself to be more than the Association's first celebrity spokesman. He had demonstrated that in the boardroom or on the tennis court, a winner is a winner.

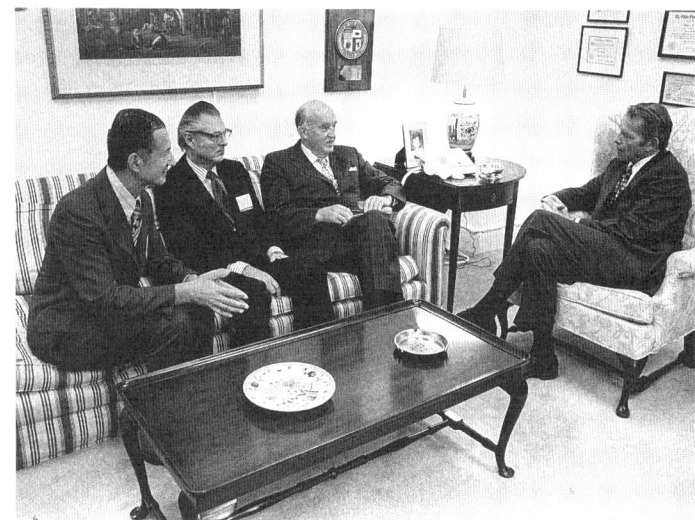

From left, ADA President Stefan S. Fajans, M.D.; G. Donald Whedon, M.D., director of the National Institute of Arthritis, Metabolic Diseases, and Digestive Diseases; Charles H. Best, M.D.; and Robert H. Finch, counselor to President Nixon, June 23, 1972, during a White House visit in honor of the fiftieth anniversary of the discovery of insulin.

but there is a long way to go . . . . If we could reproduce normal delivery of insulin, if we could prevent the ravages of diabetes, and if we could detect diabetes earlier, find the genetic marker . . . all these are questions that must be answered." It is encouraging to note that since 1972, progress has been made in all these areas.

Former ADA President Randall G. Sprague, M.D., (1953-54) and one of the first people with diabetes to receive insulin in 1921, also spoke at the ceremony, saying "Thanks for our health and our lives." These thanks were echoed by others, including Gail Patrick Jackson, secretary of the American Diabetes Association and former actress; baseball player Jackie Robinson; Pastor Jessie O. Gibson; Joan Hoover, the mother of a child with diabetes; and Michael Kaufman, a young man with diabetes. In addition, hundreds of people with diabetes all across the country wrote letters and sent messages for the occasion.

A long-held goal of the American Diabetes Association in the advancement of diabetes treatment was realized in the summer of 1972, when insulin manufacturers in the United States and Canada announced that a new concentration of insulin, U100, was scheduled for release within several months. At the same time, U100 disposable and reusable syringes, capable of accurately delivering varying dosages needed by both children and adults, were to be introduced by syringe manufacturers. In order to acquaint physicians with this new therapy, the ADA Committee on the Use of Therapeutic Agents prepared a statement that was adopted by the Board of Directors on June 23, 1972. (*Diabetes*, Vol. 27:7, 1972)

The goal was to eliminate U40 and U80 insulins and corresponding syringes as quickly as possible to reduce errors in dosages, which were frequent and dangerous. U100 had significant advantages. Besides reducing dosage errors, U100 was compatible with the decimal system. U100 insulin would contain 100 units per milliliter and be available in the usual forms—rapid, intermediate, and long-acting.

Advance notification was given to physician members of the Association to prepare them and their patients for the phasing out of the older insulins. It was planned to have U40 and U80 available for a "reasonable time." (The withdrawal of U80 insulin did not take place until 1980. See Chapter Nine.) In the interim, physicians would be able to educate themselves, and their patients, as to the advantages of the new concentration. When U100 was introduced, an announcement was made in the *Federal Register*, and copies were sent to each member of the ADA professional section, along with the ADA statement.

Diabetes Research: Funding And Legislation

By 1972, 50 years had passed since the discovery of insulin, and many unsolved problems in diabetes treatment remained. While the federal government's attack on heart disease, communicable diseases, and cancer was formidable, diabetes research received only $1 of every $250 in the National Institutes of Health (NIH) budget for research in 1973.

The American Diabetes Association had been concerned for some time that most new diabetes-related research proposals to NIH were not funded and many established research and investigator programs were eliminated. In October 1971, ADA President Stefan S. Fajans, M.D., met with Senator Richard S. Schweiker, of Pennsylvania, to discuss the public health problem of diabetes in the United States. The senator was particularly interested at this time because a friend's daughter had recently become blind due to diabetes. This was a fruitful meeting, as succeeding events testify.

About the same time, two of Senator Schweiker's constituents, Carl Stenzler and Lee Ducat, Juvenile Diabetes Foundation president, started an intensive lobbying effort in Congress. Recognizing the urgency of the problem, Senator Schweiker introduced a diabetes detection and education act in the Senate on August 4, 1972. This bill died, but was revised and later introduced in 1973.

Earlier, a group from the ADA Michigan Affiliate, led by Joyce Kortman and Judge George Benko, had been successful in getting Representative Guy Vander Jagt, of Michigan, to introduce a diabetes bill in February 1972. The purpose of this bill was to give specific emphasis to kidney disease and diabetes, and to remove diabetes from the "other disease" category—a catch-all classification for all diseases not covered by specific legislation. No hearings were held on this bill. Then, on May 3, 1972, Reps. Vander Jagt and William A. Steiger, of Wisconsin, offered an amendment.

Fortunately, this bill—which would change the name of the National Institute of Arthritis and Metabolic Diseases (NIAMD) to the National Institute of Arthritis, Metabolic Diseases and Diabetes (NIAMDD), reflecting the inclusion of diabetes—was supported by the Subcommittee on Public Health and Environment, whose chairman was Representative Paul G. Rogers. In the House debate, Representative Vander Jagt requested that the subcommittee hold hearings on the unmet needs of diabetes. In a compromise, Representative Vander Jagt withdrew his amendment for a name change, in exchange for a pledge that hearings on diabetes would be brought up the following year. (The institute was later renamed the National Institute of Diabetes, Digestive, and Kidney Diseases, or NIDDK.)

One of the supporters of the bill was then-representative Gerald Ford. In a meeting with members of the ADA Michigan Affiliate Legislative Committee in 1972, Representative Ford said, "I personally will devote my best efforts to convincing the committee that the federal government should assume a major role in combating the disease diabetes. Diabetes is a far more serious disease than most Americans recognize it to be. We must end our long years of neglect in this area."

In April 1972, ADA President Stefan S. Fajans, M.D., appointed a Committee on Public Affairs, with Dr. John K. Davidson as chairman. Drs. Buris R. Boshell, George Cahill, Jr., Randall G. Sprague, and Albert Winegrad; Judge George Benko; Gail Patrick Jackson; Joyce Kortman; and Myles Tanenbaum com-

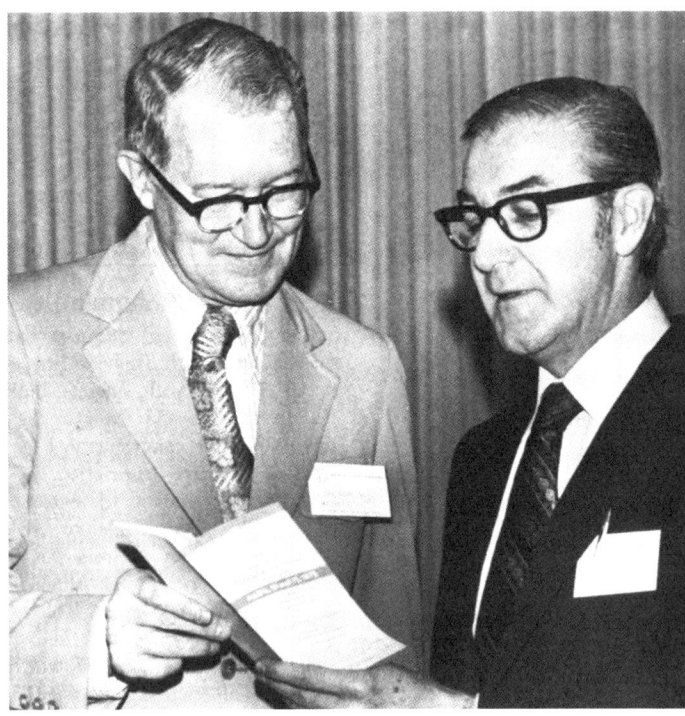

Charles Shuman, M.D., right, reviews the program of the fifth Postgraduate Course with John K. Davidson, M.D., in 1974.

pleted the committee. At its first meeting in Washington, D.C., June 20, 1972, the following objectives were established:

1) expand the authority of NIAMD to advance the attack on diabetes;

2) formulate a long-range program to combat diabetes;

3) implement programs through Diabetes Research and Training Centers (DRTCs) geographically located according to population density; and

4) provide financial support for physicians and allied health professionals training at designated centers.

At the ADA Annual Meeting in June 1972, Wyoming Senator Gale W. McGee, who has diabetes, challenged ADA members "to tell Congress what was needed in the way of legislation to deal effectively with diabetes." From August to December, Dr. Davidson spent hours working with Senator McGee and Robert Bullock, McGee's chief legal assistant, and with members of the Committee on Public Affairs, to formulate a satisfactory diabetes bill. They were assisted in this task by Drs. Donald Whedon and Ronald Lamont-Havers of NIAMD. The bill was introduced to Congress January 21, 1973. Hearings were held before the Senate Subcommittee on Health (of the Committee on Labor and Public Welfare), chaired by Senator Schweiker in February 1973. In the House, representatives Vander Jagt and Steiger introduced the bill and hearings were held by the Subcommittee on Public Health and Environment (of the Interstate and Foreign Commerce Committee), chaired by Representative Paul Rogers, in July and August 1973.

During both hearings, the seriousness of diabetes, its complications, and the need for more federal funds for research to improve treatment and education were stressed. Young people with diabetes—some of them partially or totally blind—provided some of the most effective testimony. Barbara Cavanaugh, of the Delaware Valley Diabetes Association, presented Senator Schweiker with 12,000 signatures representing Pennsylvania citizens interested in diabetes legislation.

Dr. Sprague testified about the bill before the United States Senate Subcommittee on Health, Labor and Public Welfare on February 26, 1973. At the time of his testimony, Dr. Sprague had had insulin-dependent diabetes for nearly 52 years.

"Diabetes is indeed a major health problem in our country," said Dr. Sprague. "Its seriousness as an individual and a national problem is not yet widely appreciated, perhaps because it has relatively low visibility. Diabetes which is, in effect, 'hidden' by being either undetected or well-controlled does not convey an impression of seriousness, which it truly should. In this country diabetes is ranked as the fifth leading cause of death by disease and the second leading cause of new cases of blindness. Heart attacks are at least two and one half times more frequent in diabetics than in nondiabetics of the same age. The overall

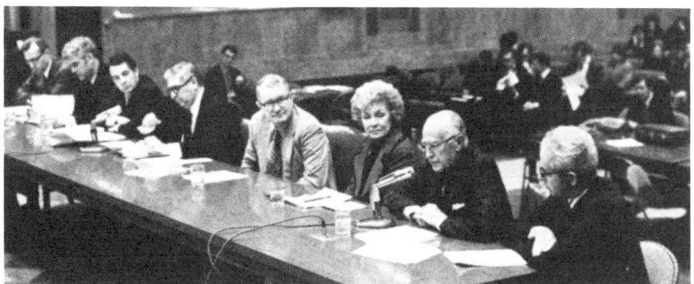

Testifying before the Health Subcommittee of the Senate Committee on Labor and Public Welfare, are left to right: James B. Field, M.D., Oscar B. Crofford, M.D., Donnell D. Etzwiler, M.D., J. Richard Connelly, John K. Davidson, M.D., Gail Patrick Jackson, William H. Grishaw, M.D., and Randall G. Sprague, M.D.

magnitude of diabetes and its complications can be better appreciated when one recognizes that there are close to 5 million diabetics in the United States, and survey data indicate that the prevalence of the disease is steadily increasing.

"Certainly the establishment of a National Diabetes Program merits very high priority and is indeed urgent in view of the large number of people affected by diabetes, their need for care and instruction in self-care, and the overriding need for more research to enhance knowledge of the basic biological mechanisms of diabetes and its complications," said Dr. Sprague.

Meanwhile, ADA affiliates were given frequent progress reports on the legislation through *ADA Forecast* and the *Affiliate Builder*, the ADA publication for affiliates started in 1953. These reports resulted in thousands of letters, telegrams, and phone calls to various senators and representatives. This grass-roots activity was probably the most potent force in passage of the diabetes law, and one in which the entire diabetes community was unified and can take pride.

After the hearings, the provisions of the Senate and House bills had to be fused into a "clean" bill acceptable to all. This required much consultation and compromise between congressional representatives, senators, and legislative assistants, as well as input from members of the ADA Public Affairs Committee. In August 1973, a bill agreeable to both Senators McGee and Schweiker was cleared by the Health Subcommittee and the Committee on Labor and Public Welfare, and passed unanimously by the Senate on December 20, 1973.

The bill, which had acquired 100 cosponsors, seemed well on its way to passage in the House, and committee members breathed a sigh of relief. However, committee members were dismayed to learn in early January 1974 that the bill was about to be buried in the generalized "categorical disease" graveyard: an action that would effectively kill any specific legislation on diabetes alone. It had been rewritten by the Subcommittee on Public Health and Environment with no provision for diabetes centers or expenditures of money and provided only for a commission to study the problems of diabetes. This was totally unacceptable to the Association, and if not changed, in all probability no diabetes law would be enacted that year.

In one of those fortunate accidents of history when events and people come together at an opportune moment, the ADA Committee on Public Affairs met in Philadelphia on January 22, 1974. A new member of

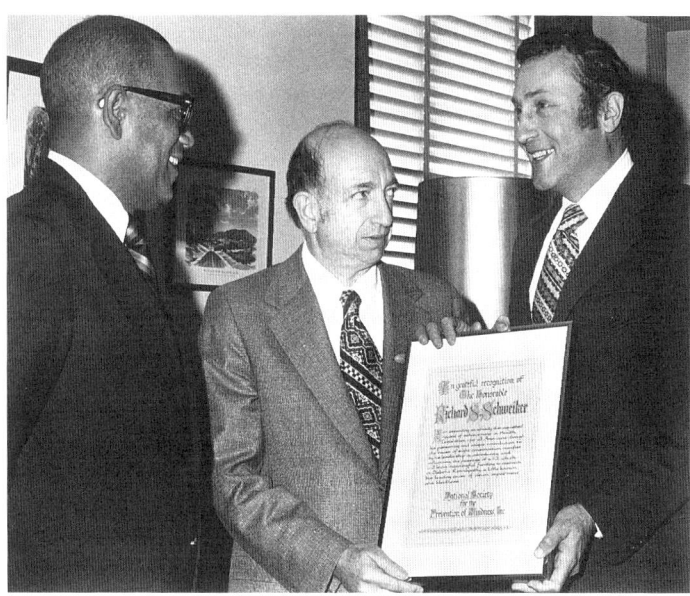

Senator Richard S. Schweiker of Pennsylvania, right, receives a recognition award for his leadership in the campaign against diabetic retinopathy. Arnall Patz, M.D., of the National Society for the Prevention of Blindness presents the award. At left is George T. Brooks, Ph.D., associate director of HEW's National Eye Institute. October 1974

the committee was George Heffner, M.D., a constituent and personal friend of Representative Rogers. The committee agreed that the bill was in serious jeopardy and that something had to be done quickly. ADA President Addison B. Scoville, Jr., M.D., (1973-74) sent Drs. Davidson and Heffner to Washington, D.C., to meet with Representative Rogers immediately. Representative Rogers, in turn, sent them to see Representative Tim Lee Carter, a physician from Kentucky with a long-standing interest in diabetes. Congressman Carter agreed to help, and before the bill was cleared by the Subcommittee, on January 29, 1974, the diabetes centers and some money authority had been restored.

Then, at the eleventh hour, another dilemma developed. The full Committee on Interstate and Foreign Commerce, chaired by Representative Harley O. Staggers of West Virginia, was devoting all of its time to the energy crisis, and it looked as though the diabetes bill didn't stand a chance of being brought up.

Again, the right person appeared at the right moment. John Panza, whose wife had diabetes, was a member of the ADA West Virginia Affiliate and a constituent of Representative Staggers. He contacted Chairman Staggers and persuaded him to give just 30

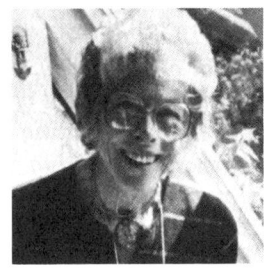

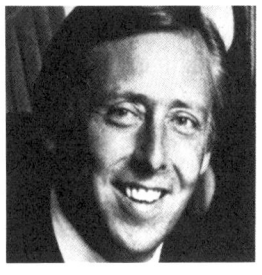

Dorothea Sims and Representative Steny Hoyer, of Maryland. Two of the many dedicated people who helped create and carry through with the Long-Range Plan. Others in this honor roll include: William D. Nelligan; Representative Richard Schweiker, of Pennsylvania; Representative Louis Stokes, of Ohio; Oscar Crofford, M.D.; Senator Lowell Weiker, Jr., of Connecticut; Wendell Mayes, Jr.; Paul Lacy, M.D., Ph.D.; John K. Davidson, M.D., Ph.D.; Lester B. Salans, M.D.; Dorothy Gohdes, M.D.; Representative William Natcher, of Kentucky; Representative Henry Waxman, of California; J. William Flynt, M.D.; George Cahill, M.D.; and S. Douglas Dodd.

minutes to a discussion of diabetes. The Joslin Clinic in Boston, active throughout the legislative process, asked Massachusetts Congressman Thomas P. (Tip) O'Neill, Jr., to encourage a full committee vote, and the combined effort prevailed. The bill passed the Committee on Interstate and Foreign Commerce on February 26, 1974, exactly one year to the day after the Senate hearings and after the bill was introduced in the House. Three weeks later, Representative Carter led the floor fight to a successful conclusion and passage of the diabetes bill by a vote of 380 to 6.

The Senate and House bills were then sent to a conference committee for further reconciliation. At this stage, the money authorized for Diabetes Research and Training Centers (DRTCs) over a three-year period was increased from $22.5 million to $40 million. The conference bill passed in the House 356 to 4 on July 9, 1974, and in the Senate, 94 to 0 on July 10. On July 23, 1974, United States President Richard M. Nixon signed the "National Diabetes Mellitus Research And Education Act," which became Public Law 93-354. This was the first diabetes law in United States history. It is impossible to estimate the time, energy, and commitment of the thousands of volunteers who contributed to the successful passage of the law.

The law required that the director of the National Institutes of Health establish a National Commission on Diabetes. The commission would have nine months to formulate a long-range plan to combat diabetes. The plan would serve the goals of expanding and coordinating national research on diabetes, advancing the education of health professionals, the general public, and people with diabetes, and disseminating updated information about diabetes.

On December 7, 1974, President Gerald Ford signed the Labor-HEW Appropriations Act, which included $1 million for the commission's work. The 17-member Commission on Diabetes was to be composed of seven directors of NIH Institutes, six scientists or physicians, and four members from the general public, two of whom had diabetes or had children with diabetes. Secretary of Health, Education and Welfare Caspar Weinberger, in accordance with the law, appointed the non-NIH members of the commission. Oscar Crofford, M.D., was chosen as chairman, and Drs. Buris R. Boshell, George F. Cahill, Jr., Donnell D. Etzwiler, Paul Lacy, and Lillian Haddock Suarez, all physician members of the Association, were appointed. Lay members included Leatrice Ducat, William D. Nelligan, Dorothea Webb Puckett, and Louinia Mae

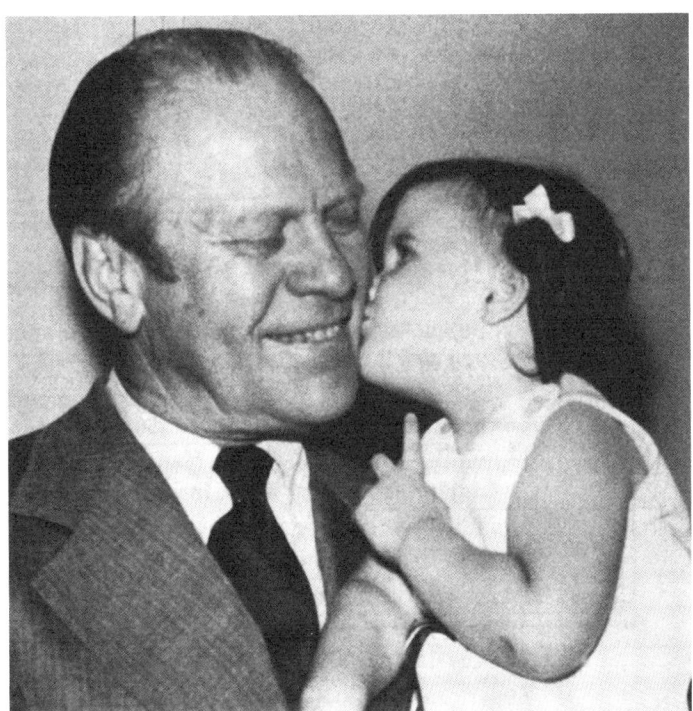

President Gerald R. Ford, an outspoken advocate of the Diabetes Bill that became Public Law 93-354 on July 23, 1974, holds three-year-old Sara Warns.

McKinley Whittlesey.

The commission submitted its report to Congress on December 10, 1975. Details of the commission's long-range plan appear in Chapter Nine. (The story of the law's enactment was reported in "Diabetes Milestone: PL 93-354" by John K. Davidson, M.D., Ph.D., *ADA Forecast*, September/October 1974 issue.)

Insurance Matters

For many years, Jon Hall & Associates had offered a hospital indemnity plan with an open enrollment for people with diabetes. However useful this plan and others like it were, none offered the comprehensive

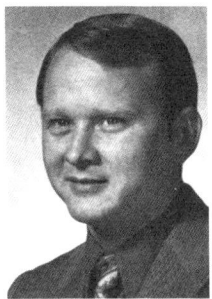

Jon W. Hall received the Outstanding Layman award on June 22, 1972, in recognition of his pioneering efforts to make hospital insurance available to people with diabetes at reasonable rates.

coverage so necessary to individuals with a chronic disease. While ADA committees gave this issue continuous attention over the years, during which time contact with many insurance companies was made, efforts met with only moderate success.

The First Chairman Of The Board

By 1973, the new Bylaws calling for a chairman of the Board "who shall be a layman" had been in place nearly three years, but no chairman had been elected. The Executive Committee was responsible for nominating a chairman from among the members of the Board of Directors; the Board then elected a chairman. This election was supposed to be held at the first Board meeting of each year. At the Board meeting in January 1973, a motion to fill the position of chairman was finally made. It came from Larry Werner, president of the Southern California Affiliate. The motion was followed by a heated debate in which supporters of the motion insisted that there was no reason for further delay in filling the position of chairman of the Board.

The Executive Committee had been reluctant to nominate anyone for this position because, the record indicates, "they had not been able to find the 'right' lay leader; i.e. an outstanding businessman, a community leader, pace setter, a person sensitive to the interests of diabetics and members of the professional and lay sections of the Association." Lay members of the Board and some members of the Central Council interpreted this as resistance to lay leadership.

Wendell Mayes, Jr., (who went on to become chairman of the Board 1974-77) was a member of the ADA Board of Directors during that time. "The January 1973 Board meeting," Mr. Mayes said, "was the first meeting in both the organizational and calendar year. When it was moved that we proceed with the election of the chairman, there was great resistance from the Executive Committee. William H. Grishaw, M.D., ADA president (1972-73), was chairman of the Executive Committee. Finally, after *much* debate, it was agreed that the Executive Committee could have overnight to present a candidate to the Board."

Given this ultimatum, the Executive Committee met and agreed upon Gail Patrick Jackson, who was serving as secretary of the Association. Producer of the "Perry Mason" TV show and a former Hollywood actress, Mrs. Jackson proved to be the right choice at the right time. Her qualifications matched the criteria for leadership that the committee sought and, in addition, she had diabetes.

"Dr. Grishaw may well have done some assisting behind the scenes and at the Executive Committee meeting," said Mr. Mayes about the decision. "Key members of the Executive Committee were the principal ones who resisted the election of anyone as chairman of the Board. William H. Grishaw was Gail Patrick Jackson's physician, and I'm sure that he was responsible for Mrs. Jackson being the one who was nominated."

Mrs. Jackson quickly demonstrated an ability to handle delicate situations with charm and tact. She served until January 1974, and her talent and commitment successfully led the organization through its rebirth into a successful voluntary health agency.

Once a chairman had been elected, a search for more lay persons to serve as Board members began. There were only seven on the Board at that time. One of the first to be contacted was Lee Iacocca, then pres-

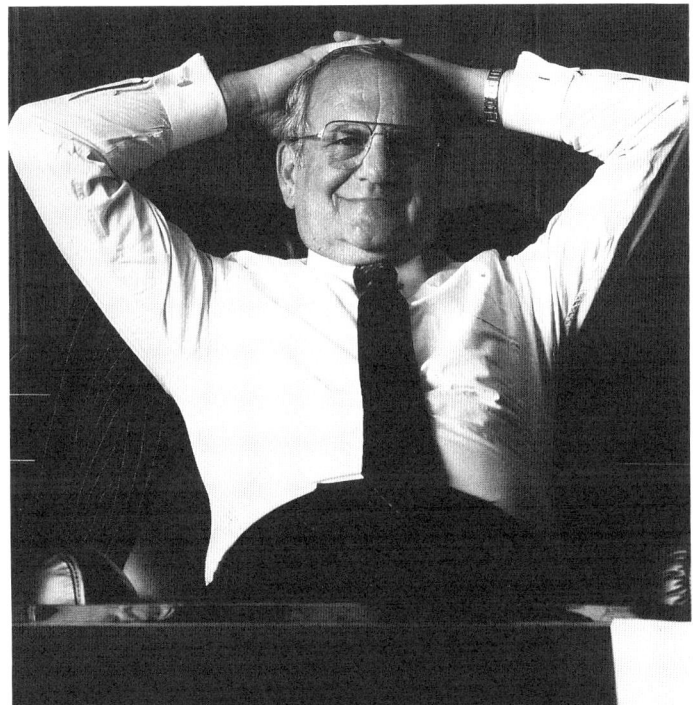

Lee Iacocca as he appears on the front jacket of *IACOCCA: An Autobiography* by Lee Iacocca with William Novak. Photo by Anthony Lowe 1984.

ident of the Ford Motor Company. He agreed to join the Board, although he never attended a meeting. He was invited by Stefan Fajans, M.D., ADA president (1971-72), to visit the national office in 1971. As the story goes, then Executive Director Connelly was a trifle nervous at the prospect of meeting an industrial giant of the stature of Mr. Iacocca and asked Maury Gurin, ADA fund-raising consultant, to join him in the meeting. Mr. Connelly's office was small and modest, piled high with file folders—obviously the office of a working executive.

When Mr. Iacocca entered the office, his eyes swept the room and, turning to Mr. Connelly and Mr. Gurin, he asked, "Where's your five-year plan?" This was a bad moment, as the Association had no plan. Up to that time, planning had been short term.

After his visit, it was reported that Mr. Iacocca had been amazed at the lack of long-term planning and very critical of ADA management, as gleaned from this one meeting. In the eyes of a corporate executive, this judgment was probably fair, but what Mr. Iacocca didn't know about were the pressures of time, space, money, and human resources the national office was subjected during these years. ADA leaders were carrying out all the programs established over the past 30 years and, at the same time, trying to meet the new demands of the changing organization.

At the next Board meeting, each member agreed to raise $10,000. ADA President-Elect Addison B. Scoville, Jr., M.D., apprised Mr. Iacocca of the Board's action and within a week the national office received a check for $10,000 from the Ford Foundation.

At this time, the Board was still dominated by physicians. Mr. Iacocca, however, had made two suggestions for lay members: Donald N. Frey, president of Bell and Howell, and Houston businessman Thomas J. Tierney. Earlier, Dr. Scoville had tried to interest David K. (Pat) Wilson, former chairman of the Republican National Finance Committee, in joining the ADA Board. Unfortunately, all three men lost interest after attending meetings filled with lengthy discussions of medical questions. Apparently, the American Diabetes Association was not yet ready to attract talent from "the big board rooms" of America.

However, the nudge from Mr. Iacocca was not lost on the Executive Committee, and early in 1973, it appointed a Committee on Long Range Plans, which was charged to review and recommend financial needs for programs in patient, professional, and public education, and detection and research. In addition, a Committee on Finance was appointed for the first time. By 1975, this committee was expanded to include budget and finance.

A New Forecast

In 1974, Clifford F. Gastineau, M.D., the editor-in-chief of *ADA Forecast* since January 1965, resigned. Circulation of the magazine had increased during his editorship from 15,000 to 100,000. His ability to sense the needs of people with diabetes and to provide information to them in an attractive, nonthreatening way, unquestionably contributed to his success.

Dr. Gastineau was succeeded by Leo Krall, M.D. In addition to practicing internal medicine, Dr. Krall was director of the Education Division of the Joslin Diabetes Clinic. He had written more than 80 medical articles and sections of textbooks, as well as being involved in clinical research activities.

Dr. Krall, with Patrick Murphy, the new art director, promoted a fresher-looking format for the magazine, and changed its name from *ADA Forecast* to *Diabetes Forecast*. Gone was the old "Reader's Digest"-shaped book. The new *Forecast* was full magazine size, as it is today. The modern layout was more attractive to advertisers, which was important. For 23 years, *Forecast* had accepted no paid advertising—a policy that changed in 1971.

The "new" magazine was mailed with an address label only. The old days of mailing in a brown envelope, to disguise the fact that the recipient had diabetes, were gone. No complaints arose from this change, and it was gratifying to realize that emphasis on "the strong case for diabetes" had made an impact on how people with diabetes felt about the disease.

Dr. Krall would serve as editor-in-chief of *Diabetes Forecast* through 1979.

Youth Activities

Within a year after the forming of the new Committee on Diabetes in Youth in 1972, members—under the direction of Chairman Donnell D. Etzwiler, M.D.—had established a framework of strong objectives and built upon them to serve the growing number of children with diabetes and their parents. These objectives included:

1) to initiate and support research in areas of cause, improved care and ultimate care of diabetes in young people with diabetes;

2) to improve the health, health care, and quality of life in young people with diabetes; and

3) to improve the knowledge and skills of individuals, both professional and nonprofessional, in meeting the physical, psychological, and emotional needs of young people with diabetes.

The May/June 1973 issue of *ADA Forecast* featured a story by Dorothy Kaplan, vice chairman of the Committee on Diabetes in Youth. In her article, entitled "Diabetes in Youth," Mrs. Kaplan said:

"It is the children with diabetes who have the most to gain by adequate care and research . . . . [Children's] concerns are being covered by the Committee on Diabetes in Youth at the national level—and your enthusiasm and work at the local level will see us accomplish our objectives."

Other articles authored by committee members included: "The Child with Diabetes in School," by Allan L. Drash, M.D., in the September/October 1973 *ADA Forecast* and "The Use of U-100 Insulin in Children," by Richard Guthrie, M.D., and Diana W. Guthrie, R.N., in the November/December issue.

A special card, entitled "What School Personnel Should Know about the Student with Diabetes," was prepared by the Committee, and was made available to affiliates.

Actress Dina Merrill made a television announcement for the Association calling on parents of children with diabetes to join their local diabetes association and to help support diabetes research. She was a member of the Committee on Diabetes in Youth and 1973 ADA Parent of the Year.

Across the country, many affiliates already had their own youth committees. Those that did not were urged to start their own. Guidelines were available from the national office to help in the committees' formulation and as an aid in planning programs and activities.

Affiliates continued their dedicated work in sponsoring diabetes camps. ADA President William H. Grishaw, M.D., (1972-73) was honored at a testimonial dinner in February 1973 for his more than 25 years of service in camping. Also honored were his wife, Dorothy Grishaw, and Louise O. Simonson. The Grishaws, according to Chairman of the Board Gail Patrick Jackson, had been at every session of the Uni-Betic Camp's two week summer program, managing the diabetes regimen and being friends and advisers to campers and counselors. The Uni-Betic Camp was located in California's San Bernardino mountains and maintained by the Nonsectarian Conference for Underprivileged Children.

Budgetary Matters

Little attention was devoted to budget planning in the early 1970s, despite the fact that from the early 1960s onward various presidents, Board members, and the executive director had regularly pointed out the Association's precarious financial position.

At the 1975 interim Board meeting, Assistant Treasurer Larry Lapham revealed the extent of the problem. "Let me draw your attention to the fact that we are in a negative fund balance, and, simply speaking, that means we are bankrupt. We are in very serious straits. We no longer have a reserve of CDs to draw on. Our endowment of $175,000 in securities is meager . . . the securities we are holding should be reviewed as some are worthless, but for now we are stuck in a 'bear' market.

"Our problems are accumulated, massive deficits. On the plus side, we are moving forward on advertising for *Forecast*, and we can raise the subscription price. We must reduce administrative costs, which will decelerate staff expansion and, reluctantly, dollars for research. The overall effect of the proposed budget is a $7,500 surplus, meager enough."

In response to Dr. Oscar Crofford's question, "What about the damage to the Association image if we renege on money for research now?" Mr. Lapham replied, "If additional money becomes available during the coming year, research will get first priority."

And, indeed, research did receive funding. In 1974, the Board of Directors had created a five-year Established Investigator Program. This program, created at the recommendation of the Research Committee, would be funded beginning July 1975. It provided financial support for scientists working in the general area of diabetes research and included a $25,000 salary support to foster maximal research productivity, $10,000 for laboratory and travel support, and $1,000 to the department in which the investigator worked. Those chosen for the award were Drs. William L. Chick, Philip Felig, Leonard Jefferson, Joseph Larner, Franz Matschinsky, and Arthur Rubenstein. The 1974 "Annual Report of the American Diabetes Association" dramatized the impressive growth of the diabetes research allocations of the Association and its affiliates. More than $836,000 was allocated to diabetes research, an increase of 130 percent over the previous year.

A Presidential Presence—Almost

In May 1974, ADA President Addison B. Scoville, Jr., M.D., invited United States Vice President Gerald Ford to speak at the Annual Meeting banquet, and the Vice President accepted. As a congressman, Vice President Ford had supported the first diabetes legislation. The American Diabetes Association was grateful and wanted to give its volunteers the opportunity and privilege of meeting him in person. However, as the events of history unfolded, they transcended the Association's plans. The Association received a call that Vice President Ford couldn't appear because of the imminent resignation of President Nixon. As it turned out, the resignation did not take place until August 9, a little less than two months later, but it appears that Vice President Ford had been alerted to stay close to the White House.

Dr. Scoville asked his friend David K. (Pat) Wilson, previous chairman of the Republican Finance Committee, to find a replacement. He did. In the Vice President's place came three United States senators—Richard G. Schweiker of Pennsylvania, later to be a vice-presidential nominee; Gale W. McGee, senior senator from Wyoming; and Howard H. Baker, Jr., of Tennessee.

Dr. Scoville remembered Senator Baker's arrival at the Atlanta airport. "[He] was greeted by newsmen on television," said Dr. Scoville. "When asked why he was in Atlanta, he said he was going to the diabetes meeting. He was then asked if he was a diabetic or if someone in his family was a diabetic. To each he said 'No.' Then why was he here? He replied, 'Because Pat Wilson told me to come!' "

Dr. Best presented each of the senators with the Charles H. Best Medal for Distinguished Service for their efforts on behalf of diabetes legislation. Gail Patrick Jackson, chairman of the Board 1973-74, also received the award. This occasion marked the first time that this prestigious medal had ever been presented.

The meeting in Atlanta was also significant in that it was the last Annual Meeting attended by Dr. Best, co-discoverer of insulin.

At this 1974 Annual Meeting, the Central Council acted unanimously to establish the Addison B. Scoville, Jr., Award for exceptional achievement by a member of the Association, the Board, a committee, or staff. In this way, the Council acknowledged its appreciation to Dr. Scoville for his service and guidance during the critical time of the Association's changeover into a voluntary health agency.

Max Ellenberg, M.D., known as the "father of diabetic neuropathy research," became president of the American Diabetes Association in 1974. For more than two decades Dr. Ellenberg had called for the recognition of neuropathy as a subtle herald of diabetes and as an important cause of suffering in many people with this complication. Through more than 60 published reports—as well as articles, lectures, and teaching activities—Dr. Ellenberg brought neuropathy into far clearer focus than before.

Also in 1974, Wendell Mayes, Jr., was elected chairman of the Board, succeeding Gail Patrick Jackson. The father of a child with diabetes, and an active member in the South Texas Affiliate, Mr. Mayes was the owner of several radio stations. His experience in developing a network of affiliate radio stations would serve him well as he took over the reins as chairman of the Board. He knew and understood the problems facing Association affiliates. He had a rare combination of intelligence, good judgment, common sense, business acumen, and stability under pressure—all of which would serve him well in leading the Association through the turbulent years of reorganization. Always available, always gracious, and selfless in his commitment to the Association, he set an example for all future Board chairmen.

Pieces Of The Puzzle:
What We Knew About Diabetes

1970

ADA Forecast reports in the March-April issue about research findings from a recent international symposium held in Spain. Two separate papers presented at that meeting show a close relationship between blood vessel diseases and hyperglycemia. Abnormal thickening of the basement membranes in capillaries was found in 98 percent of the subjects with diabetes. Only 8 percent of subjects without diabetes showed evidence of thickened membranes.

1971

At the ADA Scientific Sessions held in conjunction with the thirty-first Annual Meeting in San Francisco June 22-23, Roger H. Unger, M.D., of Dallas and his associates demonstrate that intense physical exercise increases the release of glucagon by the alpha cells in the pancreas. In turn, this increases the amount of glucagon in the blood, raising the blood-sugar level. Glucagon is thus shown to be a mechanism for increasing the immediate supply of fuel to the body.

1972

At the 1972 ADA Scientific Sessions in Washington, D.C., Dr. R.A. Camerini-Davalos of New York reports studies of capillary basement membrane thickness in people with diabetes. Results suggests that thickening of the basement membrane (the exterior wall of capillaries in muscles), which is characteristic in diabetes, can be reduced to a minimum in certain circumstances with medications.

1973

The introduction of U100 insulin, in February 1973, ushers in a new era in diabetes therapy. The American Diabetes Association issues a statement regarding U100 insulin. In part, it says: "This advancement in a modality of the therapy of diabetes is the realization of a long-held goal of the American Diabetes Association made possible through the results of research and the cooperation of industry. U100 insulin will have significant advantages. With but this single concentration available and with insulin syringes marked with only a U100 scale, the frequency of errors in dosage should be reduced."

At the twentieth Postgraduate Course in San Francisco, attended by 450 physicians and health-care professionals, Paul E. Lacy, M.D., Ph.D., reports on recent advances in the understanding of islet cell functions. Dr. Lacy, chairman of the Department of Pathology at Washington University School of Medicine in St. Louis, tells attendees that it is imperative the normal ultrastructural and biochemical events of beta cell secretion be clearly understood in order to find the abnormality or abnormalities that might reside in the beta cells of people with diabetes.

1974

Drs. Sidney Cobb and Robert M. Rose examine the possibility that stress may contribute to the development of diabetes. Their findings are published in the *Journal of the American Medical Association*. Their conclusion: If stress is a contributing cause of diabetes, it is a relatively minor one.

David W. Scharp, M.D., of Washington University School of Medicine reports progress in obtaining islets from normal pancreases. Not only can the beta cells be obtained from the normal pancreas, but, as William L. Chick, M.D., of Boston reports, beta cells can be grown in test tubes within bundles of artificial capillaries. The beta cells so produced respond to glucose by producing insulin.

1975

Rachmiel Levine, M.D., sums up the state of recent diabetes research in *Diabetes Forecast*: "The area of great advance in diabetes during the past decade has been the gradual unfolding of the story of how insulin is manufactured, stored, and secreted by the beta cells of the pancreas. This combined effort in understanding the intimate structure of the cell and the controls of insulin secretion will bring with it the practical dividends of our ability to imitate nature in the control of metabolism in people with diabetes. What will follow, at the very least, is a resolution of the question of the exact relationships of the blood-sugar level and the retinal, renal, and neurologic symptoms and signs. Out of such investigations we may hope to set up a rational program of prevention of these 'complications.' "

At the 1975 ADA Annual Meeting Scientific Sessions, Lelio Orci, M.D., of Geneva presents his original work with electron microscopy of the islets of Langerhans. At the same Scientific Sessions, Morton F. Goldberg, M.D., of Chicago presents preliminary reports of the results of laser beams and the new operation, vitrectomy.

Chapter Nine
Opportunity and Momentum
1975-80

ADA Presidents

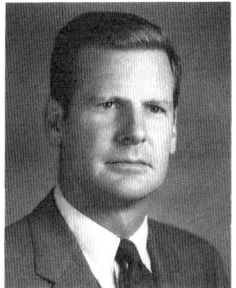 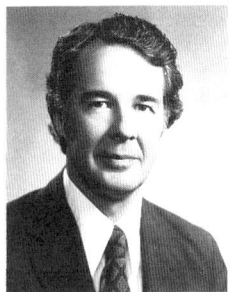

George F. Cahill, Jr., M.D. Donnell D. Etzwiler, M.D.
(1975-76)   (1976-77)

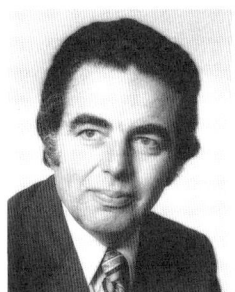 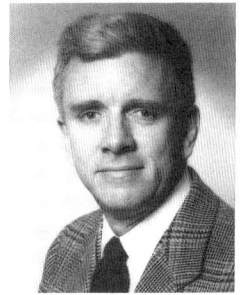 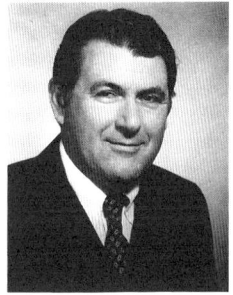

Norbert Freinkel, M.D.   Fred W. Whitehouse, M.D.   Ronald A. Arky, M.D.
(1977-78)   (1978-79)   (1979-80)

ADA Chairmen of the Board

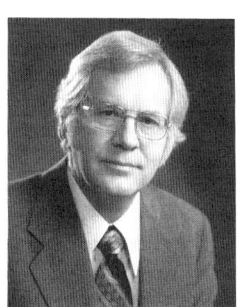 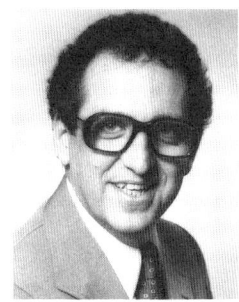 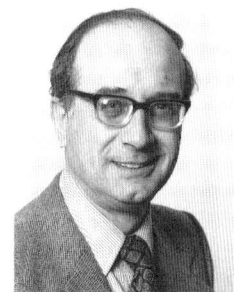

Wendell Mayes, Jr.   Myles H. Tanenbaum   Benjamin Greenspoon
(1974-77)   (1977-79)   (1979-81)

As the Association approached its thirty-sixth year, the United States approached its 200th, and the country celebrated with the birthday party of the century. On July 4, 1976, every city and town in the country observed the occasion. Six million people watched as Tall Ships from around the world sailed into East Coast harbors. Fireworks brightened the night skies as the cheers of millions reverberated across the land. That same year, a man from Plains, Georgia, was elected as the thirty-ninth President of the United States. James Earl Carter walked up Pennsylvania Avenue in the January cold to take his place in the White House, immediately establishing the no-frills style of his presidency. During these years the pace of international terrorism increased and before long, the United States was hopelessly dependent upon events in a far-away country called Iran. Problems culminated in the siege of the United States Embassy in Teheran, Iran. The nation, and the world, watched as 52 Americans were taken hostage, then counted off the 444 days of their captivity.

These events of history, tragic as they were, cast little shadow on the golden years in diabetes treatment and research that lay just ahead. For the American Diabetes Association, 1975 kicked off an era of unprecedented opportunity and growth in the Association. Impetus for this opportunity was the "Long Range Plan to Combat Diabetes," delivered to Congress on December 10, 1975, by the National Commission on Diabetes. That commission, instituted by President Gerald Ford, had been mandated by the National Diabetes Mellitus Research and Education Act, enacted in 1974.

ADA representatives, including commission-member and ADA President George F. Cahill, Jr., M.D., (1975-76) had met with President Ford to discuss the activities of the National Commission on Diabetes. Dr. Cahill was co-chairman (with Paul Lacy, M.D., Ph.D.) of the National Diabetes Commission's Committee on Research. The committee "initiated much of the policy and made the recommendations which led to the dramatic increase in governmental spending on diabetes," Dr. Cahill said.

Those "dramatic" increases were part of a law establishing the National Diabetes Advisory Board (NDAB), which was to advise Congress and the Secretary of Health, Education and Welfare on the implementation of the Long Range Plan. The law provided funds for Diabetes Research and Training Centers (DRTCs). These centers would serve as arenas for scientists from many disciplines to share information, accelerate diabetes research, and translate research progress into better care for people with diabetes.

With regard to ADA research funding, centralization of funding—through national peer review—came in 1977-78. "I actively lobbied for this and was successful in getting most of the affiliates to agree to allot most of their research dollars to the support of research that had been evaluated by peer review at a national level," said ADA President Norbert Freinkel, M.D., (1977-78). "Our volunteer members were the key ingredients in achieving this objective. Once they became convinced that they would get the 'greatest bang for their research buck' by awarding it on a competitive national basis, the implementation became easy."

More Changes To Bylaws

Throughout the history of the Association, Bylaws were changed regularly, often annually. However, in June 1976, important changes were made as the direct result of unprecedented growth. The new Bylaws provided for greater lay participation and reduced physician quotas; made changes in the principal officers and the composition of the Executive Committee; and realigned responsibilities of ADA officers.

Article I of the Bylaws expanded the professional membership to include doctors of medicine and osteopathy, dentists, dietitians, educators, laboratory technologists, nurses, optometrists, pharmacists, podiatrists, physiotherapists, other qualified physicians and scientists, residents, interns, and fellows. This significant change finally eliminated the membership barrier that had spurred nurses to create a separate professional association, the American Association of Diabetes Educators (AADE), in 1974.

Emeritus membership was extended to members of the professional section in good standing who had reached the age of 65, retired from active practice, and had maintained continuous membership in the Association for 20 years or more.

Article II, dealing with affiliate associations, included a new clause whereby the Board could terminate any affiliate not adequately serving its geographic area.

Article III included a new clause whereby the Central Council could override the Board's action with a three-fourths vote if the Central Council proposed an amendment to the ADA Constitution that was voted down by the Board.

Article IV increased participation by expanding the number of Board of Director members to 54, of which seven would be the principal officers of the Association and one the most recent living past president. In addition, the Board was to be made up of 15 members of the professional section, 15 past or present members of the Central Council, and 15 directors-at-large.

Article V concerned officers, their duties, and responsibilities. The seven principal officers were to be: chairman of the board, a non-physician responsible for overall administration of the Association; president, a physician member of the professional section and the principal spokesman for the organization in all medical and scientific matters; president-elect, a physician responsible for professional section programs and activities; a (physician) vice president: professional section to assist the president-elect; a (non-physician) vice president: Central Council to be responsible for the program and activities of the Central Council; a secretary; and a treasurer. The Association could also elect an assistant secretary and an assistant treasurer, and one or more honorary officers.

This change marked a milestone in ADA history. For the first time, the officers of the Association included a non-physician health professional vice president. Patricia Lawrence, R.N., who had been active in advancing greater non-physician involvement in the Association, was the first to hold the position of vice president: Central Council. She brought a great deal of experience and expertise to the office, having been a staff nurse in the 1950s at the New York Hospital (Cornell University Medical Center) and at Newton-Wellesley Hospital in Massachusetts, an education director at the Diabetes Consultation and Education Service of the North Carolina Regional Medical Program, and an instructor and assistant professor at both Duke University School of Nursing and the University of North Carolina Chapel Hill School of Nursing. In 1975, she became associate professor at the Chapel Hill School of Nursing.

The changes also provided for an Executive Committee composed of eight: the principal officers and the most recent living past president.

Other changes in the Bylaws included the addition of an Audit Committee and a clause to ensure continued physician participation. This clause stipulated that physicians shall always account for one-third of the Board, three out of eight on the Executive Committee, and four out of seven on the nominating committees.

Wendell Mayes, Jr., continued to serve as chairman of the Board until 1977. The Bylaws permitted a maximum of three one-year terms for the Board chairman. At the January 1977 Board meeting, an amendment which would have permitted Mr. Mayes to serve an additional term was adopted in principle. He modestly argued against the amendment, but it was passed over his veto. However, it was never fully adopted because the Nominating Committee nominated Myles Tanenbaum to be chairman, and the question of a fourth term was dropped.

Mr. Tanenbaum was a business executive, real estate developer, lawyer, and the father of two children with diabetes. He had worked seven years with both the Delaware Valley Affiliate in Philadelphia and with the national Association. He recognized the need for a broader financial base for the Association and attempted to launch a major national fund-raising event. Unfortunately, the Association was neither administratively nor financially ready to enter into such an initiative.

More Important Changes

The late 1970s and early 1980s marked the establishment of new ADA awards recognizing outstanding service. Five awards were established between 1975 and 1981 through the generosity of Ames Laboratories (later Miles Inc., Diagnostics Division), Becton Dickinson (later Becton Dickinson Consumer Products), Boehringer Mannheim (later Boehringer Mannheim Diagnostics), Roerig (later Roerig, a division of Pfizer Pharmaceuticals), and The Upjohn Company.

The annual awards include:

- Outstanding Health Professional Educator in the Field of Diabetes (Miles Inc., Diagnostic Division);
- Outstanding Contribution to Camping and Diabetes (Becton Dickinson Consumer Products);
- Outstanding Contribution to Diabetes in Youth Award (Boehringer-Mannheim Diagnostics);
- Outstanding Clinician in the Field of Diabetes (Roerig, a division of Pfizer Pharmaceuticals); and
- Outstanding Service in the Field of Diabetes to a Physician Educator (The Upjohn Company).

The Outstanding Affiliate Service Award, started in 1956, came under Squibb-Novo (later to be Novo Nordisk) sponsorship in 1983. The Youth Leadership Award, sponsored by The Nutrasweet Company, originated in 1985. The Outstanding Fund Raising Volunteer Award, sponsored by George Rice & Sons, originated in 1989.

These years saw the formation of professional section councils, whose number gradually increased from year to year. The councils, according to ADA President Fred W. Whitehouse, M.D.,(1978-79) "may be the professional issue of greatest importance to the Association." Their purpose was to provide individuals who had a specific professional interest a forum for expression and involvement.

"On November 17, 1977, Fred Whitehouse, M.D., Patricia Lawrence, R.N., and I formulated the concept of professional councils at a breakfast meeting prior to the Executive Committee session," said ADA President Ronald A. Arky, M.D., (1979-80). "During Dr. Whitehouse's tenure as president, the idea germinated and an experimental Council on Youth was organized by former ADA President Donnell Etzwiler. Under the leadership and urging of Dr. Karl Sussman, the Committee on Planning and Organization proposed the format for professional councils, and the Board of Directors, in June 1980, accepted the concept."

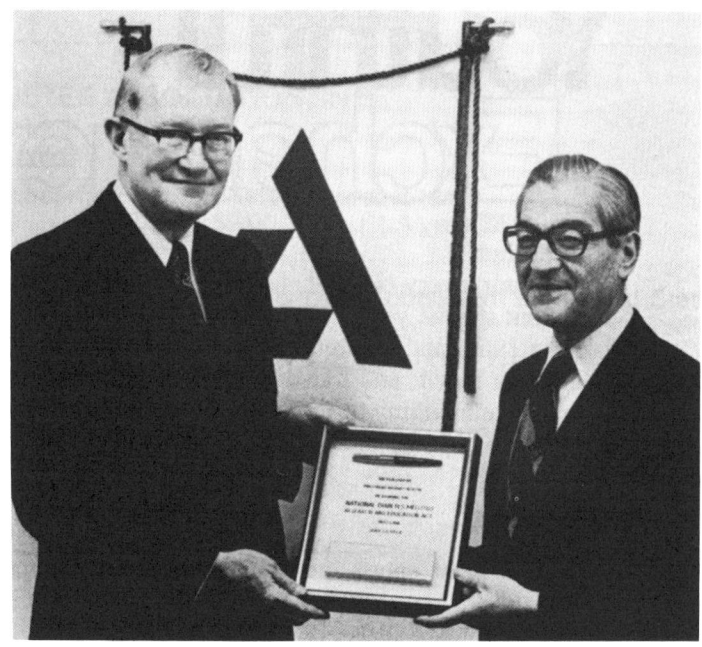

Pen used by President Richard Nixon in signing the National Diabetes Mellitus Research and Education Act (PL 93-354) into law is presented by John K. Davidson, M.D., left, past chairman of the Committee on Public Affairs, to ADA President Max Ellenberg, M.D., (1974-75).

Long Range Plans

In 1974, the National Diabetes Mellitus Research and Education Act mandated the establishment of the National Commission on Diabetes. The commission had nine months to develop a long-range plan to combat diabetes. On December 10, 1975, the 17-member commission submitted its report to Congress.

"This Long-Range Plan," wrote Commission Chairman Oscar B. Crofford, M.D., in letters to Senate President Nelson A. Rockefeller and Speaker of the House Carl Albert, "is based upon a comprehensive study of the magnitude of the disease, its causes, consequences, and the resources available for dealing with it . . . . It establishes the urgent need to address directly and fully the tragedy of diabetes mellitus."

The report confirmed the seriousness of diabetes: "Between 1965 and 1973 the prevalence of diabetes increased by more than 50 percent in the United States. Diabetes now affects 5 percent of the population. In 1974, more than 600,000 new cases of diabetes were diagnosed . . . ."

The plan called for an increase in federal funding from $43 million in fiscal year 1975 to $126 million in fiscal year 1979. It consisted of four major components:

1) a National Diabetes Advisory Board (NDAB) to review, evaluate, and advise with regard to the recommendations of the long range plan, and submit a yearly report to Congress;

2) diabetes research programs to conduct basic research into the causes, cure, and prevention of diabetes as well as research to develop better treatment methods to deal with the disease and its complications;

3) Diabetes Research and Training Centers to research aspects of diabetes' diagnosis and treatment, health-professional training, and continuing medical education. The centers would develop manpower for diabetes research and care and expedite translation of basic research data into clinical practice; and

4) diabetes health-care, education, and control program activities to bring health care to the majority of people with diabetes and to ensure that advances in research and training are available to the health-care system.

The recommendations of the commission that required new legislation and appropriations would be directed to appropriate congressional committees. In other words, the completion of the commission's report did not necessarily mean that its recommendations would be enacted. Congress, and the administration, had first to be convinced that the recommendations should be approved before the plan to combat diabetes could be put into effect.

In June 1979, the ADA Board of Directors approved the Association's own long range plan. It had many priorities, 47 of them rank ordered in an appendix. The number one priority was assigned to a "major nationally coordinated fund-raising event," the very kind of activity that had created so much confusion in 1978. Nevertheless, the 1979 long range plan provided the Association with a clear mission statement and relative ranking of priorities. It was referred to often and remained in effect from 1979 to 1988. (The Association's new, sweeping *Nationwide Comprehensive Long Range Plan*, implemented in 1988, is described in Chapter Eleven.)

Administrative Changes

From June 1973 to September 1980, the Association's national office had three executive directors/vice presidents in rapid succession. Each new leader brought enthusiasm and special expertise to the organization. In this crucial period of growth and change, enthusiastic new people were added to the staff and experienced workers left. These changes took a toll in stability and continuity within the Association.

In June 1976, Ernest Frost, Ed.D., executive vice president (1973-76), resigned. He had come to the Association at the time of the transition to a volunteer health agency and provided dynamic leadership in volunteer and affiliate involvement, particularly in the change that brought all affiliates under the ADA name and logo. Dr. Frost effected many changes that served the Association well. He established the Association as a member of the Combined Federal Campaign, divided the country into four regions and employed field representatives to serve them, developed a public relations campaign that emphasized the need for constant advertising to keep public awareness of diabetes high, initiated interactions with other voluntary health agencies, and presided over significant improvements in *Diabetes Forecast*.

From June 1976 until February 1977, the national office was without an Executive Vice President. William Ferguson, director of development, served as acting executive vice president. To assist in the handling of medical and administrative affairs, Chairman of the Board Wendell Mayes, Jr., and ADA President Donnell D. Etzwiler, M.D., came to the national office on alternate Tuesdays. Each sacrificed time from busy schedules to make the biweekly trip to New York. Their help during the period of transition was invaluable.

John L. Dugan, Jr., succeeded Dr. Frost in February 1977. He had been vice president of finance and

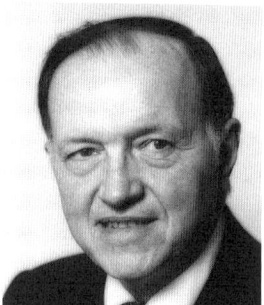

John L. Dugan, Jr.

administration of Chicopee Manufacturing Company (the industrial products division of Johnson & Johnson), assistant to the president of the Grace National Bank, and a consultant with Booz, Allen and Hamilton. Mr. Dugan had a daughter with diabetes and was also a member of the ADA New Jersey Affiliate.

He was enthusiastic, popular, and well respected by

both the Board and volunteers. In one of his first moves, Mr. Dugan brought Caroline Stevens onto the staff as director of publications. Explaining the nature of ADA's publications in the first interview, Mr. Dugan asked Ms. Stevens, "How would you improve the copy and circulation of ADA's magazines?" She quickly replied, "Just because they are medical magazines, does not mean that they have to be dull." Ms. Stevens had a background in consumer magazine publishing and soon found ways to improve the appearance and circulation of publications. New periodicals were added—*Diabetes Care* in 1978, *Clinical Diabetes* in 1984, and a patient newsletter, *Diabetes '83*—and all bore her progressive stamp. Her responsibilities gradually expanded outside the publications area. In 1985 she was named assistant executive vice president.

Mr. Dugan was quick to recognize the Association's limitations in developing and marketing its publications. When it was brought to his attention that the Robert J. Brady Company, a publisher of educational and medical books, would be willing to publish, promote, and distribute books for the Association, he seized the opportunity. He negotiated a contract for *Diabetes Mellitus: Volume V* (1975), and *Diabetes in the Family* (1982), which replaced *Learning About Diabetes*. Both volumes proved profitable for the Association. The Prentice-Hall publishing company purchased the Brady Company at that time and the Association was able to get a similar contract for the *Family Cookbook: Volume I* (1980), which was followed by *Volume II* (1984), *Volume III* (1987), the *Holiday Cookbook* (1987), and *Special Celebrations and Parties Cookbook* (1989).

Mr. Dugan also negotiated an agreement with the National Health and Welfare Retirement Association (NHWRA) for a defined contribution pension plan for national and affiliate staff personnel. A pension plan had been in effect at the national office for some time, but the new arrangement enabled affiliates to participate as well. Funds covering participants in the old plan were transferred into the NHWRA agreement.

Mr. Dugan resigned in June 1980, after three years, but remained on the staff until a new executive vice president was named.

Division of Income

The sharing of divisible receipts between the national office and the affiliates became effective in 1973. The plan strove to eliminate competition in fund raising between the national office and the affiliates. The reasoning was that because the national office and the affiliates each had different, yet coordinated, roles, income would best be shared. This would satisfy the affiliates' strong desire to decentralize all fund raising, while preserving a centralized research and public awareness emphasis. Chairman of the Board Wendell Mayes, Jr. was instrumental in making the plan work properly.

In 1973, the national office was obligated to affiliates for 15 percent of all divisible receipts received. In turn, the affiliates were obligated to the national office in the amount of 5 percent of their total divisible receipts. In 1973, the total amount due to the affiliates was $37,000. The net division of receipts due the national office was $58,273.

The percentage of income due to the National Office from the affiliates increased gradually during the next five years. By 1978, the affiliates were contributing 25 percent of their total divisible receipts to the national office. In turn, the national office was obligated to affiliates for 75 percent of all divisible receipts received.

Though debate about these matters was heated, these years saw the "coming together" of the Association as one organization.

"Much has been said in the past about we and they," said Ernest M. Frost, Ed.D., executive vice president, at the June 10, 1975, Central Council Meeting. "I would like to call to your attention that this philosophy is rapidly disappearing and I have heard throughout my travels in the United States more of the philosophy that we are one organization combating diabetes."

In reality, many affiliates were slow to follow through. Payments from certain affiliates had been deferred for periods of up to 10 years under procedures established by the Association's Board of Directors. At that June Central Council Meeting in 1975, Dr. Frost could single out only a few affiliates—the Greater Chicago and Northern Illinois Affiliate and the New England Diabetes Association—for their acceptance of the division-of-income plan. Outstanding monies from affiliates amounted to $973,667 as of June 30, 1978, and $1,166,757 as of June 30, 1979. A financial crisis was brewing.

Financial Streamlining

Warnings of the Association's precarious financial position were sounded during the 1970s. By 1979, the Association was near the financial breaking point: the treasurer's report to the Board sounded a dire note of impending insolvency.

"In early July 1979," ADA President Ronald Arky, M.D., (1979-80) said, "it became apparent that the ADA was headed for fiscal disaster if organizational changes were not made—in fact, an estimate of an $800,000 deficit was projected by one fiscal officer. By fall of 1979, the situation deteriorated to a point where the Association faced an actual cash shortage within six months."

The years preceding this crisis saw two executive vice presidents, several treasurers, the Budget and Finance Committees, and ADA Boards grapple with the problem—unsuccessfully. The problem was not due to insufficient funds, but rather, according to Executive Vice President John L. Dugan, Jr., to "poor timing of cash flow." Monies flowed into the Association on a cyclical basis through subscriptions, membership fees, and divisible funds provided by affiliates. But because of poor accounting procedures and budgeting practices, these funds were often committed before they were received. In time, as the Association grew and acquired more and more obligations, the gaps between actual and anticipated funds became increasingly acute. Luck had been such that the gaps were often filled with an unexpected contribution or bequest at the last minute. But an organization the size and scope of the American Diabetes Association could no longer afford to operate in this manner.

Several factors entered into the crisis of 1979. In 1975, a study under the guidance of Eric Dunkley, treasurer, began to assess computerizing the accounting department; however, it was many years before the new system became fully operative. In the interim, turnover in the accounting department was high. As a result, reports were late and often incorrect, making budget planning and execution difficult. Concurrent with these problems was the growth of the Association. Volunteers were demanding more committees, more meetings, more services, and more materials. In addition, the staff controller's long-term absence due to illness reduced the quality of information available for decision making, and there were no meetings of the Budget and Finance Committee during the time when the financial crisis was most acute.

Realizing that draconian measures were necessary, in September 1979, Dr. Arky and Benjamin Greenspoon, chairman of the Board, asked Karl E. Sussman, M.D., chairman of the Committee on Planning and Organization, to review and streamline the entire ADA committee structure. The number of committees had increased by almost 50 percent between 1975 and 1979, a cost the Association could no longer afford. Dr. Sussman's task was neither easy nor popular, but his solution produced a more efficient structure and proved beneficial to the Association in the long run. Until the reduced expenditures could have an effect, the Southern California and Washington, D.C. Affiliates agreed to prepay their divisible income for the following year, which enabled the Association to carry on and fulfill its most urgent obligations.

Most committee meetings scheduled for the fall and winter of 1979 were canceled. The only committees permitted to meet were those charged with finding needed fiscal solutions: Budget and Finance, Planning and Organization, and Affiliate Associations. Outside printing was suspended, and special efforts were made to collect payments of divisible income from affiliates on time; delayed payments were a major contributing factor to the 1979 crisis. A freeze on research spending for one year to "catch up" was the most traumatic measure taken. However, in a last minute addition, $600,000 was added to the research budget introduced at the June 1979 Board meeting. That was $600,000 *over* budget. The action was proposed in part to match the growing research funding budget of the Juvenile Diabetes Foundation. This action specifically precipitated the financial crisis.

Again, as had happened before in ADA history, the right person appeared at the right time. Robert S. Bolan, Ph.D., was able to devise a plan to lead the Association out of the quagmire of its financial difficulties. Dr. Bolan was appointed assistant treasurer and vice chairman of the Budget and Finance Committee in 1979. The committee prepared recommendations to the Board that would rectify the faulty accounting practices by providing for a permanent cash flow throughout the year and the collection of affiliate divisible funds on a regular schedule.

Before presenting the committee's report to the Board, Chairman Ben Greenspoon gave a full explanation of the reasons for the recommendations. The report, with its spartan parameters, was accepted by the Board in January 1980 at what has become famous as the shortest Board meeting in ADA history. Mr. Greenspoon was soon renowned for his "bite the bullet" speech, in which he spelled out in blunt language the exact measures the Association would have to take to get back on a sound financial basis.

Mr. Greenspoon fully expected some discussion and was amazed when not a single hand was raised. Board members listened, tightened their belts, and accepted all of the committee's recommendations. In a description of this meeting, Joseph H. Davis, who would later become chairman of the board, said, "I attended my first Board meeting with Ben Greenspoon presiding. And, to say presiding is an understatement. Before I could read the agenda, the meeting was over." As the meeting had progressed so much more rapidly than planned, Mr. Greenspoon received an urgent message from Cathy Ward, ADA's director of national programs, that read, "Please don't end the meeting too soon. Lunch for the Board is ordered and *paid* for and people must stay."

Summarizing the situation in his report on April 30, 1980, then Assistant Treasurer Robert S. Bolan, said,

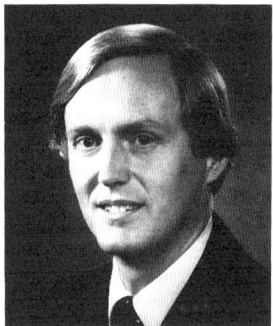

Robert S. Bolan, Ph.D.

"The Association has experienced a severe cash shortage and coped successfully, if not pleasantly, with it."

Increasing Public Awareness And Donations

In the 1970s, the American Diabetes Association began to emerge as a political force. Noting the Association's increasing political activism, Dr. Norbert Freinkel, ADA president (1977-78) said: "Coalescence of the various constituencies suddenly transformed the ADA from a chummy professional group into a weighty political entity and major spokesman for all diabetes-related health issues." This increasing involvement in politics, Dr. Freinkel continued, "coincided with the general activism of that era and the recognition that citizens could muster an effective voice in government."

Under the leadership of Dr. Frost, and later Mr. Dugan, a series of successful national campaign slogans and materials were designed by the advertising agencies of Kenyon and Eckhardt and then Doyle, Dane, Bernbach, at no cost to the Association. In subsequent years, Scali, McCabe, Sloves and then Goldsmith/Jeffrey provided the same *pro bono* service.

Film Premieres Benefit Research

In 1974, the ADA Southern California Affiliate established a new method of fund raising for the Association: the film premiere. This seems only natural, given the affiliate's location in the heart of America's "movie capital." The annual movie premiere was established by a committee that included Frank Wells, president and CEO of Walt Disney Company. By 1988, the film premieres had netted $3.2 million for the American Diabetes Association, all of which was earmarked for research.

In 1974, "Towering Inferno" was the kick off premiere film. The opening, held in Los Angeles on December 16, was attended by more than 1,100 people and raised over $87,000. A black-tie, after-theater dinner was held at the Beverly Hilton in conjunction with the premiere. Many of the film's stars attended, including Paul Newman, Steve McQueen, Fred Astaire, Richard Chamberlain, Jennifer Jones, and Robert Vaughn, as well as dozens of other film notables. Mary Tyler Moore served as Honorary Premiere Chairman. Mrs. Sybil Brand and Ms. Shirley Firestein, both of the ADA Southern California Affiliate, served as executive chairman and chairman, respectively, for this first ever fund-raising event.

The film also premiered in New York City on December 18, drawing a capacity crowd of 1,500 people to the National Theater. The New York premiere, sponsored by the ADA New York Affiliate, raised more than $10,000. Anthony Perkins, Steve Allen, Jayne Meadows, Tony Randall, and Faye Dunaway were among the stars in attendance. Dina Merrill was Honorary Chairman of the New York premiere.

National Diabetes Month was initiated in 1976 with a visit to the White House and President Ford by ADA volunteers. President Ford subsequently served as honorary national ADA chairman from July 1, 1978, through June 30, 1979. The highlight of this period was his appearance before the Central Council, where he was presented with the Charles H. Best Award.

In the fall of 1976, ADA President George F. Cahill, Jr., M.D., (1975-76) was interviewed by the magazine *U.S. News and World Report*. The article, "New Hope for Diabetics" was reprinted and distributed by the Association in the thousands.

New public service announcements and films introduced during this period were "Every 60 Seconds Another American is Diagnosed Diabetic;" "No Sugar Coating," a film depicting the psychosocial problems of adolescents; "You Make the Difference," a film on volunteerism; and "The Other Diabetes," a film on non-insulin-dependent (type II) diabetes.

In 1977, singer Wayne Newton very generously agreed to give four concerts to benefit the Association. The first was held September 8 at the Grand Ole Opry House in Nashville, Tennessee. Three other concerts followed soon after: October 29 at the Music Hall in Kansas City, Missouri; October 30 at the Henry Levitt Arena in Wichita, Kansas; and October 31 at the Civic Auditorium in Omaha, Nebraska. The concerts were a huge success, drawing hundreds of listeners in each city, and adding a total of $500,000 to the four affiliate treasuries.

That same year, the Order of Amaranth expressed interest in helping the Association. The Order was established June 14, 1873 and is a descendant of the Royal and Social Order of the Amaranth in Sweden. Membership today is comprised of wives, widows, mothers, sisters, and daughters of Masons.

A telephone call came in to the national office: "We are considering a charitable cause, could ADA send someone to talk with us?" Dr. Cahill was dispatched immediately.

The first check from the Order of the Amaranth to the Association was for $50,000, raised through a series of local cake sales, pot-luck suppers, and other fund-raising events. The check was presented to ADA President Ronald Arky, M.D., at a formal dinner near Harrisburg, Pennsylvania. Those in the Association who attended will long remember the opening scene at dinner where a Philadelphia Mummer's String Band paraded to the dais, followed by the Order of the Amaranth's Supreme Royal Matron and Dr. Arky doing the "Mummer's Strut." The Amaranth Diabetes

ADA film premiere benefits have been held every year since and include: "Barry Lyndon" (1975); "Nickelodeon" (1976); "The World's Greatest Lover" (1977); "Superman" (1978); "All That Jazz" (1979); "Tribute" (1980); "Buddy, Buddy" (1981); "Six Weeks" (1982); "Two of a Kind" (1983); "City Heat" (1984); 1985 (the film premiere was cancelled at the last minute by the studio. An appeal letter was sent to all those who normally would have attended the event, and $265,000 was raised); "Hoosiers" (1986); "Three Men and a Baby" (1987); "Beaches" (1988); and "Steel Magnolias" (1989).

Foundation was formally created in 1979 under the leadership of Foundation Chairperson, Marie Waters.

There is no doubt that the efforts of ADA Presidents, Drs. Cahill and Arky, helped to build the much valued relationship between the Order of the Amaranth and the American Diabetes Association. Over the first seven years of the Order's fund-raising efforts, close to $1 million was raised for diabetes research.

In 1941, the national office received 250 requests for information. By 1978, the Patient Education Department was receiving 50,000 letters annually—from patients and professionals. Requests for information were handled by a department of two people: a department head and a secretary. A receptionist typed labels and stuffed envelopes as time permitted. Standard packages, consisting of a copy of *Diabetes Forecast*, the booklet "What You Need to Know About Diabetes," and a list of patient education publications, were stockpiled by the hundreds. Other material was added to these standard packages to individualize them as the response required. Inquiries that could not be handled with literature alone were answered by letter, using prepared text that was then edited to provide an appropriate response.

As affiliates grew in size and capability, these letters were forwarded to them for response. In 1980, at the request of ADA President Ronald Arky, M.D., (1979-80) mail received by the Patient Education Department was surveyed. The survey showed that 25,000 letters had been received and handled at the national office during the past year, not including those that had been received at affiliate offices.

Though the funds raised by the Association were rapidly increasing, most of the money was raised at the local level. There was little fund raising done on a coordinated nationwide level. Recognizing the need for a coordinated public relations and fund-raising effort, the Association requested that a film production and publicity firm, Saturday House, develop a proposal for a national fund-raising program.

Saturday House presented its proposal at the January 27-28, 1978, Board of Directors meeting in New York City. Because the proposal called for a large financial commitment—about $500,000—the Board was divided almost evenly on the wisdom of the venture, which was to span several years. The proposal called for a celebrity pool, a youth sports network, invitations to commerce and industry through a President's Advisory Council, a youth campaign, an agreement with the American Contract Bridge League, a national awards dinner, and telethons.

Kid's Corner

Netti Richter began her service to young people with diabetes in 1964, when her daughter Kathy developed diabetes at age 10. She became a prime mover in the Greater Philadelphia Affiliate's fundraising, education, and camping activities.

In 1975, she came up with an idea for a children's page in *Diabetes Forecast*, one that would be fun and teach children with diabetes how to cope with their disease. The first "Kid's Corner" appeared in 1977.

"Children learn best when they are doing something enjoyable. 'Kid's Corner' can provide hours of fun, while encouraging children to be responsible about their diabetes," noted Ms. Richter, a retired teacher.

" 'Kid's Corner' will be a successful learning tool in homes, camps, youth support groups, hospitals, schools . . . where there are children with diabetes and adults interested in their well-being," said Harold Rifkin, M.D., who supervised the publication during his tenure as editor-in-chief of Diabetes Forecast.

For the next 10 years, Ms. Richter's kid's page would appear monthly in the magazine. In 1987, "Kid's Corner" became a quarterly booklet, still printed in *Diabetes Forecast*.

In addition to "Kid's Corner," Ms. Richter authored many other youth-oriented articles, including the first ADA pamphlet specifically about children ("Helping Your Child With Diabetes-Answering Your First Questions") and "A Back to School Guide For Parents," in the September/October 1977 issue of *Diabetes Forecast*.

On the national level, she chaired the Youth Services Committee from 1983-1985. Also, Ms. Richter served on such committees as the Com-

---

ADA affiliate associations, having just fully implemented the ADA policy requiring a 25 percent share of division of income, generally disapproved of this use of money—money they felt they had raised. Ultimately, the Saturday House proposal led to bad feelings and tension between affiliates and the national office that took several years to dispel.

The Saturday House contract was subsequently canceled because the Association did not have the financial resources to see the proposal through. However, many of the proposal ideas were later incorporated into fund-raising plans.

In 1980, the American Contract Bridge League selected the American Diabetes Association as its charity of the year and over a two-year period contributed $250,000 for research and education. In addition to research grants, the ADA film "The Other Diabetes," was developed and funded from this grant.

Devotion To The Cause

Ray Kroc, and his brother, Robert, devoted their lives to the conquest of diabetes and other health problems through the generous use of the resources of the McDonald's Corporation and the Kroc Foundation. The Kroc Foundation, administered by Robert L. Kroc, Ph.D., donated an estimated $15 million to diabetes research.

Among the many research conferences sponsored by the Kroc Foundation were:

- The Conference on Diabetes Microangiopathy held at the Kroc Foundation headquarters in Santa Ynez, California, on April 6-10, 1976. At this meeting, renowned diabetes experts proposed several different hypotheses about the basis for blood-vessel damage in diabetes.

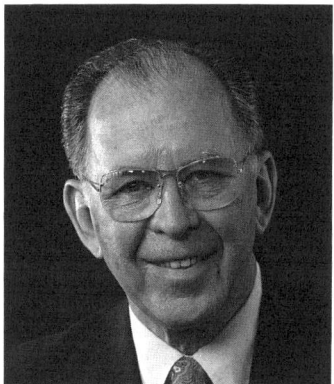

Robert L. Kroc, Ph.D.

mittee on Education of Juvenile Diabetics, Youth Coordinating Committee, and Committee on Planning and Organization.

- The Conference on Pancreas Transplantation held June 8 and 9, 1979, at the Kroc Foundation Headquarters. The stimulus for this meeting was the expressed wish of several participants for a gathering of workers actively engaged in research related to pancreas transplantation to share ideas and results. The Conference addressed the current status of transplantation of adult pancreases and islets in people with diabetes; the problem of rejection; and methods to overcome rejection.

- The Conference on Diabetes and Atherosclerosis held March 2-6, 1981, at the Kroc Foundation Headquarters. The rationale for holding this conference was that accelerated atherogenesis is responsible for a major part of the morbidity and mortality associated with diabetes. The conference brought together leading researchers from a number of disciplines whose work involved the area of atherosclerosis.

- The Conference on Nonenzymatic Glycosylation and Browning Reactions: Their Relevance to Diabetes Mellitus was held on May 4-7, 1981, at the Kroc Foundation Headquarters in Santa Ynez.

- A Workshop on Preventing the Rejection of Transplanted Pancreas Or Islets, held on January 11-14, 1982, at the Kroc Foundation Headquarters. The workshop focused principally on current strategies for dealing with rejection of transplanted pancreases, or of transplanted islets cells.

- The Conference on Diabetic Microangiopathy held May 17-20, 1982. This second conference on diabetic microangiopathy was held six years after the first conference. The meeting provided the opportunity for exchange of new concepts along broad disciplinary lines.

- The Conference on Insulin Pump Therapy in Diabetes, Multicenter Study of Effect on Microvascular Disease, held March 21-25, 1983 at the Kroc Foundation Headquarters.

In 1979, the Kroc Foundation granted funds for a study entitled "Metabolic Normalization and Microvascular Disease." Nine independent groups joined forces to form the Kroc Collaborative Study group. Investigators were from the University of Chicago; Guy's Hospital in London, England; Hammersmith Hospital in London, England; the Mayo Clinic in Rochester, Minnesota; the University of Western Ontario in London, Canada; and Yale University in New Haven, Connecti-

Strengthening The Bond Between Affiliates And The National Organization

Although the Association had been a voluntary health organization for almost a decade, in 1979 the national office had a "weak" public image, according to ADA President Ronald Arky, M.D., (1979-80). "All of our 65 affiliates questioned the authority of the national office. . . .

"The plans and goals of myself and [Chairman] Ben Greenspoon were set late in the spring of 1979, before we assumed office. Although a number of crises arose during the year that compelled some deviation from those plans, we especially strove to strengthen the basic structure of the Association's affiliates and their fiscal base and cited these objectives at the Central Council meeting in June 1979 in Los Angeles as major goals."

A majority of the affiliates did not adhere to the divisible income policy and many questioned the mission of ADA nationally. "A faction favored very strong support of research and competition with Juvenile Diabetes Foundation; another faction pressed for more service and educational activities," Dr. Arky said.

Within this framework, Dr. Arky aimed to boost communication between affiliates and the national organization. "Mr. Greenspoon and I publicly stated that only through functional affiliates could the national organization grow and mature. We appointed Mr. Al Levine of the Southern California Affiliate as Chairman of the Committee on Affiliate Associations with the intent of strengthening the liaison between the affiliates and the national office," Dr. Arky said.

In August 1979, Dr. Arky, Mr. Greenspoon, Mr. Levine, national field staff, regional cut. They held numerous working meetings, and by June 1982 presented to the American Diabetes Association a paper on the feasibility of a multicenter trial of diabetes control and complications. The first major report of the Study group's findings were published in August 1984 in the *New England Journal of Medicine*.

The findings showed that a multicenter, multidisciplinary, multinational study of glycemic control and its relationship to diabetic retinopathy and other small blood-vessel complications of diabetes was indeed possible. The way was paved for the Diabetes Control and Complications Trial (DCCT).

More And More Committees

In 1973, the first national meeting of Diabetes Teaching Nurses was held at the University of North Carolina, School of Nursing, with Patricia Lawrence, R.N., as chairman. At this meeting, members voiced their desire to become more active in the American Diabetes Association as a professional group. They also asked that a third track for nurse educators be added to the Scientific Sessions at the Annual Meeting. (A "track" is a focus or series of presentations targeted for a specific group at the Scientific Sessions. There was a research track and a clinical, or physician, track.) These requests were approved by the Committee on Professional Education and, in 1976, nurses and dietitians were permitted for the first time to present papers, signaling a recognition by the Association of this group as diabetes educators.

With a greater lay voice in the Association and more pressure for action on many fronts, the number of committees grew from 34 in 1975 to 59 in 1979. At one point, in addition to standing committees, there were coordinating committees to which standing committees reported. In an effort to collaborate with other organizations, representatives from the American Association of Diabetes Educators and American Heart Association designated representatives to serve on ADA committees such as Food and Nutrition, Patient Education, and Youth, at ADA expense. While this interaction was useful, it became too expensive for the American Diabetes Association to continue during the financial constraints that came by 1979.

In response to increasing attention to the psychosocial aspects of diabetes, a Committee on Family Behavior was appointed in 1976. Composed of experts in the field, this committee held several meetings and developed plans for a comprehensive program to address these long neglected issues. Unfortunately, the commit-

representatives, and executive directors of many affiliates met in Keystone, Colorado, to review the strengths and weaknesses of existing affiliates and their potential for organizational and fiscal growth. "With the national staff," Dr. Arky said, "we designed a plan to solidify the bridge between affiliates and national, to support floundering affiliates and work for consolidation and strengthening wherever feasible." Consequently, Dr. Arky said, he visited 39 affiliates and traveled about 250,000 miles in the next 11 months, meeting with affiliate officers and members to emphasize the national organization's interest in affiliates and the need for affiliate participation.

"By the spring of 1980," Dr. Arky said, "a number of affiliates that formerly had no organizational structure became functional, areas of the country previously 'uncovered' had newly organized affiliates and discussions for consolidation were initiated." He added, "The leadership of Mr. Levine and Mr. Greenspoon and the Board's willingness to endorse the policies of the Committee on Affiliate Associations and enforce the divisible income provisions were the essential steps that permitted maturation and growth of ADA in the 1980s."

tee also became a victim of the budget crisis of 1979 and was never restored. Yet its ideas and plans did not die; they were subsequently addressed by the Patient Education Committee and the Youth Committee.

Nutrition Guidelines

In 1971, the Food and Nutrition Committee was charged to review new concepts in nutrition, particularly a reduction of fat in the diet, in the prevention of atherosclerosis. Since 1950, when the pamphlet *Exchange Lists for Meal Planning* was published and made available through physicians, the American Diabetes Association had recommended a relatively high-fat diet. A *Cookbook for Diabetics*, published at that time, was also based on the *Exchange List* concept. As a result of this Committee's deliberations, a special report, "Principles of Nutrition and Dietary Recommendations for Patients with Diabetes Mellitus," was developed (*Diabetes*, Vol. 20:9, 1971).

Three points were stressed in this report: 1) the importance of total calories in weight control; 2) regularity of food intake; and 3) alteration of carbohydrate and fat content of the diet. The report went on to say that "important dietary concepts have developed during the last decade which require some alteration in long-held precepts. There no longer appears to be any need to restrict disproportionately the intake of carbohydrates in the diet of most diabetic patients." This was contrary to what many people with diabetes had been taught, and it took many years to break away from the generally accepted concept that "carbohydrates are bad." The report also said, "At the present time there is not enough evidence to determine to what extent restriction of dietary fat and cholesterol is desirable."

After the statement in 1971, it became clear that a revision of the 1950 *Exchange Lists* was necessary. From 1971 to 1976, the Committee discussed, revised, and finally developed a new edition. The new booklet, published in 1976, was prepared by the American Diabetes Association in cooperation with The American Dietetic Association, the National Institute of Arthritis, Metabolism and Digestive Diseases, the National Heart and Lung Institute, the National Institutes of Health, the Public Health Service, and the U.S. Department of Health, Education and Welfare.

Shortly after the 1950 publication of the *Exchange Lists*, the Committee on Food and Nutrition had published a series of diets at specific calorie levels, as well as low-fat, bland, and sodium restrictions. These were originally intended only for use by physicians in prescribing a diet for their patients with diabetes. By 1970, however, diets for people with diabetes, based on the ADA *Exchange Lists*, had proliferated and were even being published by pharmaceutical companies and various other organizations. The foods on these standard diets were often unfamiliar and sometimes too expensive for most people to include in a daily meal plan.

The Food and Nutrition Committee spent many hours discussing the ineffectiveness of these meal plans. The committee decided that because adherence to these diets was poor, the only way to motivate individuals to follow their diet was to tailor meals to individual tastes, keeping in mind nutritional needs and economic means. John K. Davidson, M.D., of the Emory Clinic in Atlanta, had had considerable experience and success in compliance among indigent patients using individualized meal plans. With this concept in mind, the committee included a page for the individual diet prescription in the new *Exchange Lists*.

When the new *Exchange Lists* were published in 1976, the Food and Nutrition Committee recommended discontinuing the old standard meal plans; the Board approved this recommendation. The new idea of individual diet prescriptions was hard to sell to many physicians, who had neither the time nor the nutritional background to provide diet counseling. But dietitians were ready and waiting to step into this gap, as they became a more and more integral part of the diabetes team. By 1980, nutrition had become "big business" in the United States, and dietitians and nutritionists began setting up private practices. This made it easier for people with diabetes to find nutritional counseling for individualized meal plans.

In 1977, the American Diabetes Association published *A Guide for Professionals: The Effective Application of Exchange Lists for Meal Planning*, designed to help physicians, dietitians, and nurse educators in providing individualized diet prescriptions and counseling.

Outreach to The American Dietetic Association increased during Dr. Norbert Freinkel's tenure as ADA president in 1977-78. He initiated a series of regular meetings with that association's officers and staff in their Chicago headquarters.

"Fred Whitehouse and Don Bell [ADA President 1980-81] participated with me in this dialogue, which I believe contributed greatly to a more diabetes-related orientation of The American Dietetic Association and to their more active involvement with programs of the American Diabetes Association," Dr. Freinkel said.

"It served to renew a relationship which had languished following our magnificent collaboration with them during the development of the *Exchange Lists* in the 1950s."

ADA's Food and Nutrition Committee had long advocated a position for a nutritionist on the national staff. Members argued that because diet is a cornerstone of diabetes treatment, a qualified person was needed to address important nutritional issues and represent the American Diabetes Association in these matters. While the recommendation had been made many times, it was consistently rejected until 1976, when Committee Chairman John K. Davidson, M.D., was able to persuade the Board of the benefit to the Association. In September 1977, Mr. Dugan hired Barbara El-Beheri, R.D., a retired army colonel with wide experience and recognition in the field of nutrition. Her immediate assignment was to develop a new cookbook for the Association. *Cookbook for Diabetics* had been withdrawn in 1976 because of the high fat content of its recipes.

Ms. El-Beheri used her expertise in both administration and nutrition to quickly put together a commit-

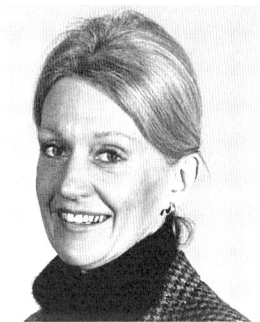

Barbara El-Beheri, R.D.

tee that gathered, analyzed, and tested several hundred recipes. From these, 250 were selected for inclusion in *The ADA/ADA Family Cookbook: Volume I*, which was published in cooperation with The American Dietetic Association in 1980. The recipes in the new cookbook were tailored for family cooking. Recognizing that the person who has diabetes has the same nutritional needs as the person who does not, the new book stressed that it was neither necessary nor desirable to cook special meals for the person with diabetes; doing so sets the person with diabetes apart from his or her family. The public had been waiting for five years for a new ADA cookbook, and although inflation made the new *Family Cookbook* cost about 10 times the price of the old, it was an instant best seller. The second volume, published in 1984, received the same enthusiastic welcome in the marketplace.

In 1979, the "Principles of Nutrition and Dietary Recommendations for People With Diabetes" were on the table again. The Food and Nutrition Committee found it necessary to revise its 1971 statement. A new statement, "Principles of Nutrition and Dietary Recommendations for Individuals with Diabetes Mellitus," was published (*Diabetes*, Vol. 28:11, 1979). Stressing the original concepts of controlling total calories and regulating meals, the new statement said, "Some restriction of saturated fats and foods containing cholesterol are now indicated for persons with diabetes." The report suggested that fat calories comprise 35-38 percent of total calories, a reduction from previous recommendations. Likewise, saturated fat should be decreased to comprise 10 percent of those calories. Carbohydrate should account for 50 to 60 percent of total calories, with the major portion of calories contributed by whole-grain breads and cereals, enriched pasta, vegetables, and some fruits. In general, protein should account for 12 to 20 percent of total calories.

A recommendation on restriction of saturated fat and cholesterol had been advocated for some time by the American Heart Association, but the American Diabetes Association had been slow to come around to this position. In the statement, particular emphasis was placed on complex carbohydrates, and the need for an individual diet prescription was emphasized once again.

In keeping with the times, and to help individuals with diabetes to live in the mainstream, the committee also issued the policy statement "Fast Food Restaurants" (*Diabetes Care*, Vol 3:2, 1980). In this statement, the Association conceded that while fast foods are high in fat and are not always nutritionally complete, they may be eaten by people with diabetes. The key, the statement said, was carefully choosing other foods that day and relying on the advice and direction of the physician or diet counselor.

Developments In Insulin

On July 28, 1978, the *Federal Register* published a proposal to discontinue certification of U80 insulin. A copy of this proposal was mailed to each member of the ADA professional section. Acting upon the recommendation of the Committee on Materials and Therapeutic Agents, which had been on record since 1971 in favor of decertification of U80, the American Diabetes Association continued its education program to keep physicians informed.

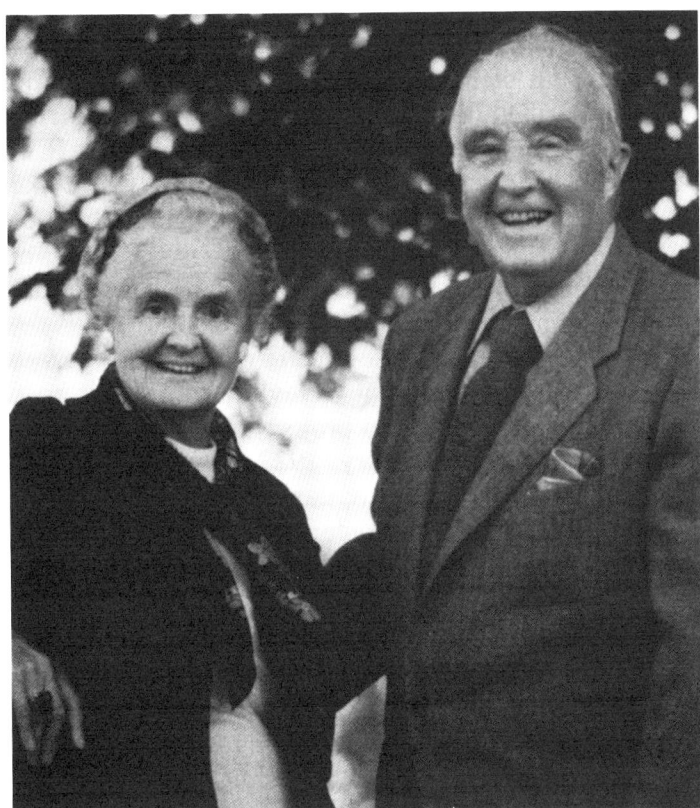

Charles H. Best, M.D., co-discoverer of insulin, and his wife, celebrating their 50th wedding anniversary, September 3, 1974.

In an *Affiliate Builder*, ADA's affiliate newsletter, ADA President Fred Whitehouse, M.D., noted that the Association's position was not binding on individual members, but urged affiliates to publicize the Federal Drug Administration (FDA) proposal and the Association's official position so that members would have a chance to communicate their comments, favorable or unfavorable, to the FDA. He pointed out that if the FDA received no comments, it would proceed with the decertification of U80. "This is an important opportunity for affiliate members to make their views known to the government," he said.

The Association planned a meeting for October 18, 1978, to be attended by representatives from the American Diabetes Association, the Juvenile Diabetes Foundation, the Food and Drug Administration, Eli Lilly and Company, E.R. Squibb and Sons, Becton Dickinson, Sherwood Medical Industries, the American Pharmaceutical Association, the American Society of Hospital Pharmacists, the ADA Committee on Materials and Therapeutic Agents, and the editors of *Diabetes Forecast* and *The Diabetes Educator* (the publication

Diabetes Care From A Nurse's Point Of View

As knowledge about diabetes increased and new technologies became available, changes in diabetes care began to take place. JoAnn Ahern, R.N., of the Yale-New Haven Hospital in New Haven, Connecticut, talks about diabetes care in the early 1980s.

"Most internists did not keep up with advances in diabetes care and patients became more frustrated than ever before," said Ms. Ahern. When people with diabetes "became more educated about diabetes than their physicians, they began to call universities with a specialty in diabetes or other diabetes specialists. They sought educators to answer their questions in a knowledgeable manner.

"The introduction of blood-glucose monitoring made more people with diabetes knowledgeable about blood-glucose control. More local affiliates had meetings dealing with more intensive treatment of diabetes via insulin pumps or multiple injections of insulin. And pure pork insulins began to be used more frequently."

of the American Association of Diabetes Educators). The meeting was held at the Sheraton LaGuardia Hotel in New York City and was presided over by Donald I. Bell, M.D., then ADA vice president. Participants discussed the proposed discontinuance and decertification of U40 and U80 insulins and the meeting proceeded slowly as each participant made a very formal presentation.

At the coffee break, Dr. Bell announced, "To mark this historic occasion the American Diabetes Association has a present for each participant." With that, he produced the new "Pigs Are Precious" T-shirts (which had originated with the North Dakota Affiliate), saying that he had brought them in all sizes. This broke the ice, as participants lined up and Dr. Bell hunted through his boxes for the appropriate size for each person. When the meeting resumed, the formality so prevalent earlier had subsided.

On November 22, 1978, the Executive Committee delivered a copy of the minutes of the October 18th meeting to the FDA's hearing clerk and stated the American Diabetes Association position as follows:

"At a meeting of the Executive Committee three questions posed by the FDA were formally considered and there was unanimous agreement to support our previous position:

1) The ultimate goal should be to have only one strength of insulin available.

2) That one strength of insulin should contain 100 units per milliliter (with the understanding that U500 insulin would continue to be available on a prescription basis).

3) There is no demonstrated need for a low-potency insulin for pediatric use.

"The basis of our position comes as a result of the meeting sponsored by the Association last month to consider the FDA proposal, in which all participants were in unanimous agreement on these points, and also went on record in favor of decertification of U40 at the same time as U80 without any unnecessary delay."

On September 24, 1979, the FDA announced the discontinuance and decertification of U80 insulin within 180 days. The deadline for comments was set for November 27. A review of the comments received revealed very little opposition.

Withdrawal of U80 insulin took place March 24, 1980, as scheduled. Incredible as it may seem, after almost eight years, during which time numerous articles appeared in both *Diabetes Forecast* and the journal *Diabetes*, the Association received a number of complaints from physicians and patients, asking why they had not been warned. They took the stand that U80 worked fine, so why discontinue it?

No action was taken by the FDA to discontinue U40 insulin, and it continues to be distributed by the manufacturers; it is made only from animal sources. The primary market, according to a drug company spokesperson, is the pediatric market.

A National Plan Of Attack

In 1977, the National Diabetes Data Group (NDDG) was established under the provisions of the National Diabetes Research and Education Act of 1974. The NDDG was to gather and analyze all diabetes statistics. From its inception, the American Diabetes Association had a standing Committee on Statistics. The committee's efforts in statistical studies had been remarkable considering the limited means with which it worked. However, with the formation of the NDDG by the federal government, the ADA committee was disbanded.

The following year, the National Diabetes Information Clearinghouse (NDIC) was also created by the federal government and charged with gathering and documenting all diabetes literature and providing a network of information throughout the diabetic community. This relieved the American Diabetes Association of the task of assembling bibliographies, which it had undertaken from time to time in earlier years.

The Diabetes Control Programs (DCP), administered by the Centers for Disease Control (CDC) and established within the federal government in 1977, were charged with reducing illness, death, and costs from preventable complications of diabetes, working through state and local health agencies. The DCP's first director, J. William Flynt, M.D., provided clear vision for

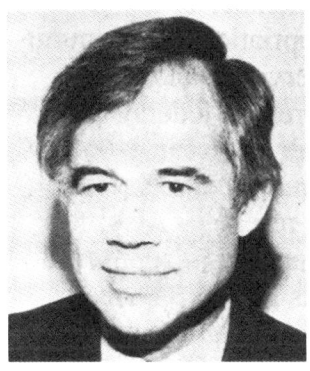

J. William Flynt, M.D.

this nationwide effort to control diabetes and was awarded with the Best Medal for his work. A model diabetes program was established within the Indian Health Service to combat the devastating complications of diabetes suffered by so many Native Americans, among whom diabetes had become epidemic.

For the Association, there was another very important task: continuing the momentum initiated by diabetes legislation. To keep diabetes in front of the public, year-round public education campaigns were planned. In 1972, Senator Gale McGee had told members of the Association, "Tell Congress what is needed." Acting once again on this advice, the Association prepared its first Legislative Position for presentation by volunteers in one-on-one meetings with members of Congress in March 1972. Since then, the preparation and presentation of the ADA Legislative Positions has been an annual activity.

Interestingly enough, while most volunteers applauded the idea of congressional visits, many approached those first visits with some trepidation. To put the volunteers at ease, members of the newly established Government Relations Committee, with the help of Richard Verville, ADA's congressional liaison, developed a humorous role-playing skit, which they enacted at a precongressional visit breakfast. Several members with experience in visiting Capitol Hill assembled a facsimile of a congressman's outer office. The timid volunteer entered and was greeted by an aide, who said cheerily, "Oh yes, Senator So-and-so was planning to see you, but I'm sorry, he's been called to the floor for an important vote." A voice from backstage voice warned, "Don't be put off—talk diabetes to whoever you see in that office. Aides have ways of getting the message to their bosses if your presentation is convincing enough." Much of the tension was relieved by the time volunteers headed for the Hill.

Since that time, congressional visits prior to congressional appropriations meetings have become an important activity for ADA volunteers. These visits have fostered a greater awareness of the seriousness of diabetes among legislators. In addition, ADA's leadership in forming coalitions of academic institutions, professional societies, and voluntary agencies has been a major benefit to all those who seek a fully funded program of high-quality diabetes research at the National Institutes of Health. Recommendations by these coalitions of experts have helped to keep adequate levels of congressional funding for diabetes research.

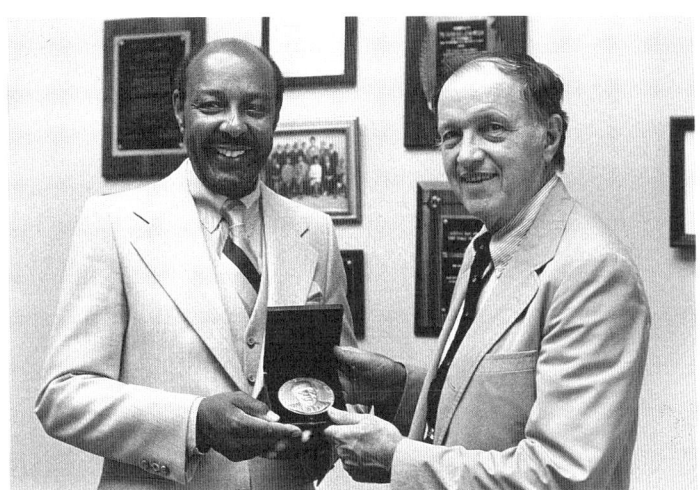

Congressman Louis Stokes, left, of Ohio, receives the Charles H. Best Award in 1978 from Executive Vice President John L. Dugan, Jr.

The Great Saccharin Debate

In July 1970, the Food and Drug Administration (FDA) announced limitations on the use of saccharin, setting off a controversy that continues to this day. Responding to a "limited use of saccharin," recommended by the National Academy of Sciences/National Research Council, the FDA statement, effective February 22, 1972, said, "On the basis of available information, present and projected, use of saccharin does not pose a hazard. Numerous studies are in progress and while these are going on the FDA recommends that the 'average adult consume no more than one gram of saccharin per day, an amount equal to sixty small tablets, or 7 to 12 bottles of a standard diet drink.'" A notice of this announcement appeared in *ADA Forecast* (Vol. 25:5 1972).

Five years later, on April 14, 1977, the FDA announced a ban on the sale of saccharin with a 60-day waiting period to consider arguments. The issue was picked up by the popular press and a debate ensued. Among the consumers who would be affected, people with diabetes were the most threatened by the proposed ban. ADA President Donnell D. Etzwiler, M.D., (1976-77) appointed the Ad Hoc Committee to Study Saccharin and charged it to "make certain that the best possible decision as it relates to both the physical and mental health of those with diabetes is reached."

Dr. Etzwiler presented the Association's case at a hearing before the Subcommittee on Health and the Environment of the House Committee on Interstate and Foreign Commerce, saying, "ADA feels the action of the FDA is premature. Until further data are available, and the human risk is more precisely known, we do not recommend major changes in the use of saccharin by the American public.'' Pointing out the risk versus benefit factor, particularly in the case of people with diabetes, Dr. Etzwiler suggested a revision of the review procedures of the Delaney Clause of the Food and Cosmetic Act—the clause that initiated the ban on cyclamates and the proposed ban on saccharin.

Bills were introduced into the House and Senate in 1977 by Representative Rogers and Senator Edward Kennedy. As these bills were pending in Congress in 1977, Dr. Addison B. Scoville, Jr., Chairman of the ADA Committee on Public Affairs, asked affiliates to write their congressional representatives telling them of the impact a saccharin ban would have upon their lives and asking them to support the ADA position. ADA volunteers rallied by the thousands. According to a July/August 1977 *Diabetes Forecast* article entitled "Saccharin Update," between 800 and 1,000 letters per day poured into Washington, D.C., on the subject—more than were received on the bombing of Cambodia. The American Diabetes Association clearly demonstrated the strength and solidarity of its volunteers with this campaign.

The Association continued to recommend a delay of the FDA ban on saccharin until further study, an analysis of the health/benefit risk factors, and a revision of the Delaney Clause of the Food and Cosmetic Act could be accomplished. Such a revision would give FDA the authority to review food additives with regard to health benefit as well as carcinogenic (cancer-causing) risk. An ADA policy statement, passed by the Board in 1977 (*Diabetes Care*, Vol. 1:4, 1978), said, ". . . based on the evidence now available there appears to be little justification for placing further governmental restrictions on the use of saccharin by the American public at the present time.''

The legislation limiting FDA's action against saccharin was passed. Indeed, Congress postponed FDA's ban on saccharin until 1985, when the controversy again heated up.

In 1985, before the ban was due to expire, the Ad Hoc Committee on Artificial Sweeteners assessed the current data and developed the "Policy Statement on Saccharin," which cited improved quality of life due to saccharin, low cost of saccharin, the *small* risk of bladder cancer in animals *only*, the presence of but one alternative artificial sweetener (aspartame), and insufficient scientific data for a clear-cut ban. The policy statement concluded, "In view of these considerations,

Association Feels Loss Of Leaders

In the mid-1970s, the Association lost five of its most illustrious members: a faithful editor and a hard-working dietitian, the first president, the first executive director, and a co-discoverer of insulin.

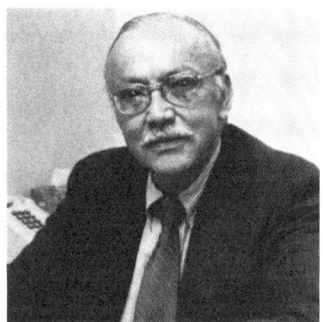

Edward W. Sanderson

On February 16, 1975, Edward L. Sanderson, managing editor of *ADA Forecast* and the journal *Diabetes* for 25 years, died.

Leo P. Krall, M.D., editor-in-chief of *Forecast* at the time, wrote in the March/April 1975 issue, "Ed Sanderson was a quiet and truly gentle man. While the rest talked and talked about educating the patient and his physician, he worked at it. For more than 25 years, editing both journals, he read and corrected untold numbers of words, paragraphs and pages. He strove constantly for perfection. There are many opinions about the hereafter. We would like to believe we know where he went . . . someone just acquired a superb editor."

Sister Maude Behrman, well-known author of *A Cookbook for Diabetics* and consulting dietitian to *Forecast,* died in July 1978. She edited every diet article in *ADA Forecast* from the first issue in 1948 until she left in 1970.

Sister Behrman had been president of the Pennsylvania

we recommend that the ADA support legislation soon to be introduced in Congress, which will extend the limitations on FDA action for another three years. We suggest that such sweeteners be used in a prudent way by children, by pregnant women, and by women in their child-bearing years. Combined use of artificial sweeteners should be encouraged, and continued research into possible risks of long-term use of saccharin and other sweeteners, either alone or in combination should continue." In May 1985, the ban was extended again until May 1, 1987.

Controversy Over Genetic Engineering

In 1978, the American Diabetes Association published the Policy Statement, "Recombinant DNA Research." The statement addressed questions raised in recent years about the possibility of a shortage of insulin from accelerated demands in developed as well as developing countries and inadequate supplies of animal pancreases. The Association felt it imperative that explorations for alternatives in insulin production be pursued, even though no shortage was imminent (*Diabetes Care*, Vol. 1:4, 1978).

Immediately preceding the issuance of this statement, the city of Cambridge, Massachusetts, had proposed a local ordinance that would have severely restricted research in genetics and DNA technology. Because Harvard University and the Massachusetts Institute of Technology (MIT), both leaders in such research, were located in Cambridge, such a law would have had a serious impact. The American Diabetes Association assembled a distinguished panel of scientists headed by Donald F. Steiner, M.D., who was assisted by Drs. Edward R. Arquilla and Donald B. Martin. The panel was supported by the Scientific Advisory Panel of the Executive Committee, which included Drs. Norbert Freinkel, Fred W. Whitehouse, Ronald A. Arky, and Donnell D. Etzwiler. The panel was charged with weighing the risks of recombinant DNA research against the potential benefits for people with diabetes.

Among the panel's findings:
1) There was no indication that serious risks to the population or the environment would accrue from this research.
2) Assessment of the risk/benefit ratio of this research indicated that the potential benefits to be derived far outweighed the identifiable hazards.
3) An important benefit that might accrue would be production of human insulin.

Diabetes Association and in 1955 received a citation for her work from the American Diabetes Association and won the Howard J. Reber medal the following year. It was while teaching dietetics and diet therapy at Lankenau School of Nursing that Sister Behrman, a Lutheran deaconess, first became interested in the dietary problems of people with diabetes. She will long be remembered for her contributions to diabetes.

Dr. Cecil Striker, founder, first president, honorary president, and secretary of the American Diabetes Association from 1941 to 1947, died in April 1976. Dr. Striker was responsible for documenting the history of the first 25 years of the Association, upon which the first four chapters of this book are based.

J. Richard Connelly, who had served as the Association's first executive director from 1949 to 1973, died July 4, 1977. At the time of his death, he was a member of the president's Committee on the Employment of the Handicapped and a member of the National Health Council. He had been treasurer of the International Diabetes Federation (IDF) from 1973 to 1976, an adviser to the Office of Secretariat of IDF, and chairman of the IDF Public Education and Detection Committee.

On April 4, 1978, Charles H. Best, M.D., the co-discoverer of insulin, died. At the time of his death, he was an honorary president of the American Diabetes Association. He had served as ADA president from 1948 to 1949 and as chairman of a number of ADA committees, notably the first Diabetes Detection Committee in 1949. In a tribute to Dr. Best, Dr. Norbert Freinkel said, "Some of the greatness of the 20th century has gone out of our

4) Microbiologically produced insulins might become new research tools that would expand knowledge of the basic mechanisms of insulin action.
5) A better understanding of the genetic basis for the susceptibility to diabetes might lead to possible prevention and yield information on other medically important problems that face society.

The statement concluded, "In view of the many potential benefits for diabetics and society as a whole from recombinant DNA research, the ADA strongly advocates the continuation of this research activity under the guidance of the National Institutes of Health, and without the imposition of any further restrictive measures beyond those already encompassed in the present *NIH Guidelines*, and any further modification that may subsequently be adopted."

It was gratifying to the American Diabetes Association about a year later when a combined team of Harvard and MIT scientists announced the synthesization of rat insulin using DNA technology. Production of human insulin, with its potential for improving diabetes treatment, was achieved a mere six months later.

ADA Camping Program Expands Horizons

In 1970, Donnell Etzwiler, M.D., who would serve as ADA president (1976-77), proposed an International Conference on Camping to the Diabetes and Youth Committee. There was agreement that the idea was valid, but unfortunately, no funds were available. Undeterred, Dr. Etzwiler raised the funds and the First International Conference on Camping and Diabetes was held in 1974. The attendance of 70 people was beyond all expectations, and such workshops became a permanent part of the ADA camping program.

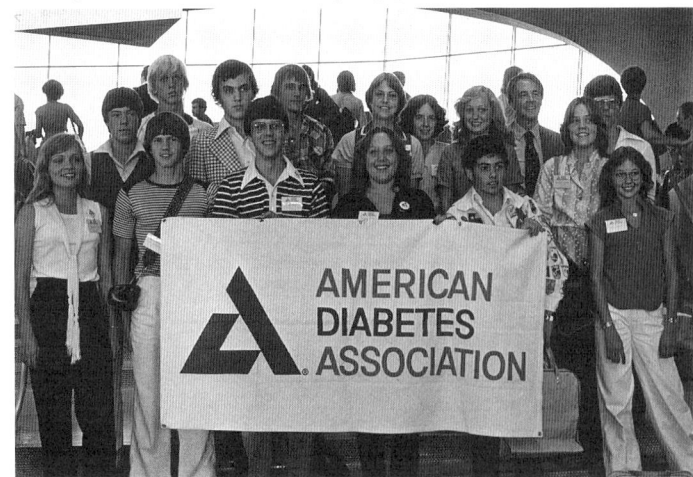

Campers on their way to Egypt at JFK airport.

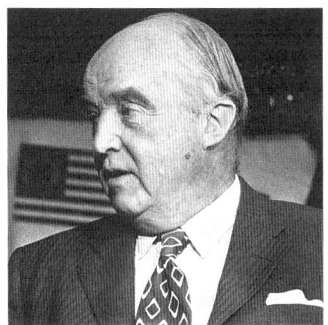

Charles H. Best, M.D.

world with the passing of Charles H. Best . . . Dr. Best translated science into terms that the whole world could understand, and into service that ennobled our efforts. He was a beacon of civilization, typifying the true goals of science and medicine . . . improving and saving human lives."

Dr. Etzwiler, a leader of the Association's "Diabetes and Youth" movement, was instrumental in starting a similar program for the International Diabetes Federation. As a result of this bond, Gamal Gordon, M.D., head of the Summer Camp for Diabetic Children in Egypt, invited 10 American young people, ages 13 to 18, to attend his camp in Alexandria, Egypt, in 1979.

Ted von Eiff, youth coordinator on the ADA national staff, issued an affiliate bulletin asking affiliate executive directors to help locate interested young people. There was no scarcity of applicants, and as the number rose, Mr. von Eiff telephoned Dr. Gordon to ask if he could accommodate five more campers. Dr. Gordon agreed, and the first 15 youths who applied were accepted. At the same time, Mr. von Eiff contacted physicians on the Diabetes and Youth Committee to accompany the group, and Dr. Etzwiler volunteered. No stranger to campers with diabetes, Dr. Etzwiler, a pediatrician, had some years earlier taken a group of youngsters on a wilderness camping trip in Minnesota, no doubt a fitting prologue for the Egyptian camping experience.

Mr. von Eiff made all the travel arrangements for tickets and visas, arranged for in-flight meals to suit the individual requirements of the campers, talked to anxious parents, and met with the boys and girls at Kennedy Airport to see them off. In addition, he arranged with the Ames Company to provide urine-testing materials for all the campers. The campers characterized their experience as both challenging and rewarding.

In other youth-related matters, in 1978 the Coordinating Committee for Juvenile Diabetes became the Coordinating Committee for Youth; the Committee on Education of Juvenile Diabetics changed its name to the Committee on Youth Education. Under the direction of Chairman Netti Richter, the Committee on Youth Education developed a curriculum, or guidelines, to help children with diabetes and their families cope with and learn about the disease.

Pieces Of The Puzzle:
What We Knew About Diabetes

1976

John Najarian, M.D., of the University of Minnesota, implants insulin-producing islet cells in seven patients, all of whom have received kidney transplants and are on immunosuppressive therapy. While six patients reject the cells, the transplant in the seventh is considered successful because the patient's insulin dose is considerably reduced. Dr. Najarian is funded by a grant partially supported by the American Diabetes Association.

The Committee on Materials and Therapeutic Agents asks the U.S. Bureau of Medical Devices to consider ADA syringe specifications calling for a single-space syringe, with dead space of no more than 3 percent; standard black markings; single-unit gradation for low-dose, two-unit gradations for 1 cc, and four-unit gradations for 2 cc syringes; both the package and the needle guard to be color-coded orange. These recommendations are accepted by the bureau and are used by all syringe manufacturers today. Standardization of syringes helps to reduce dosage errors, previously a common cause of poor diabetes control.

ADA President George Cahill, M.D., (1975-76), President-Elect Donnell Etzwiler, M.D., and Vice President Norbert Freinkel, M.D., publish the ADA Policy Statement "Blood Glucose Control in Diabetes." This policy states, "ADA accepts the fact that the overwhelming mass of evidence suggests that controlling blood glucose is of direct value to the patient." (*Diabetes*, Vol. 25:3, 1976) The statement is also published in the *New England Journal of Medicine*, and becomes one of the most quoted medical articles on this issue.

1977

C. Ronald Kahn, M.D., and his colleagues at the Joslin Diabetes Center report the discovery of insulin receptors on the cell membrane. Research shows that both insulin and glucose attach themselves to specific sites on the cell membrane. This discovery raises the possibility that missing, or defective, insulin receptors may be blocking the glucose from entering the cells, thus contributing to the insulin resistance of non-insulin-dependent (type II) diabetes.

The Association and the Committee on Materials and Therapeutic Agents issues a "Statement on Phenformin," supporting the FDA decision to withdraw the drug from the market. "Mounting scientific data from the U.S. and other countries indicated that phenformin may constitute a significant health risk in that lactic acidosis may develop and death may even result in some diabetic patients using this drug.'' (*Diabetes*, Vol. 26:8, 1977)

Glycohemoglobin tests are first reported in 1977 (*Diabetes*, Vol. 30:11, 1977). These are the diabetes "report cards" of the 1980s. When an ad, "Your Red Blood Cells Are Watching You," appears in *Diabetes Forecast* (Vol. 33:1, 1980), patients begin to ask their physicians for the glycosylated hemoglobin test.

Rosalyn Yalow, Ph.D., is awarded the Nobel Prize in Physiology and Medicine for her work in developing a sensitive radioimmunoassay technique used in determining the amount of insulin in biological materials. The Nobel Prize is shared by Drs. Roger Guillemin and Andrew Schally, who identified the hormone, somatostatin (*Diabetes*, Vol. 10:1, 1977).

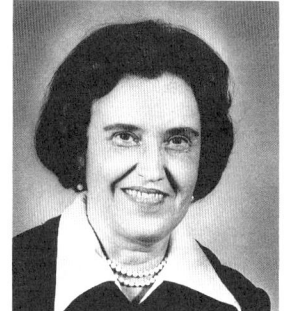

Rosalyn S. Yalow, Ph.D.

1978

In September, researchers at the City of Hope National Medical Center in Duarte, California, and at Genentech, Inc., a private research company in San Francisco, announce they have induced bacteria to produce insulin identical to human insulin. This has long been a goal of scientists working in the field of recombinant DNA research.

The California researchers are able to produce human insulin genes, those small parts of the DNA molecules that direct insulin production. Then they insert the genes into *E. coli* bacteria, where the genetically altered bacteria trigger the production of human insulin.

1979

In June 1979, the Board appoints the ad hoc Committee on Screening, chaired by Irving L. Spratt, M.D., to study mass screening programs. Such programs, carried out by affiliates across the country, were a highlight of National Diabetes Week and continued until the mid-1970s, when questions arose about their effectiveness. Although committee members hold extensive discussions on the effectiveness of mass screening carried out by volunteer health agencies, no consensus is reached. Proponents argue that screening uncovers the undiagnosed cases of diabetes and allows for prompt treatment. Opponents question the reliability and cost effectiveness of these programs and contend that public education is more worthwhile.

At a workshop on screening, "Guidelines for Screening" are developed for use by affiliates and chapters. These are ultimately distilled into the "ADA Policy on Screening for Hyperglycemia 1983," which outlines three basic principles: 1) an intensive public education program encouraging people at risk for diabetes be tested; 2) a test for gestational diabetes in all pregnant women; and 3) specific criteria for affiliates and chapters for scheduling on-site screening programs.

In June 1979, the ADA Board accepts the new "Classifications and Diagnosis of Diabetes and other Categories of Glucose Intolerance," established by the National Diabetes Data Group, and adopts the terms type I or insulin-dependent, type II or non-insulin-dependent, gestational diabetes, and IGT (impaired glucose tolerance) for use in all its publications (*Diabetes*, Vol. 28:12, 1979).

1979

The National Society for the Prevention of Blindness (NSPB) publishes some startling statistics that show there were 46,000 new cases of blindness annually, 5,800 due to diabetes. Incidence is highest in people aged 45 to 65. Prevalence figures show a total blind population in the United States of 498,000, with 7.9 percent, or 39,500, due to diabetes.

By 1979, laser photocoagulation is an effective treatment in certain types of retinopathy, and trials on the benefits of early treatment are started. This ultimately leads to a series of studies begun in 1980 by the National Eye Institute, which prove that early laser treatment is effective. Vitrectomy, a surgical procedure introduced in 1970, has by this time become widely used to restore sight lost as a result of vitreous hemorrhage and retinal detachment (complications affecting the eyes).

1979

The insulin pump is introduced. An 11-year-old boy wearing a pump around his waist appears on ABC-TV with Philip Felig, M.D., who conducted one of the first pump programs. Dr. Felig explains the function and purpose of the pump and discusses types of people who could derive the most benefit from this therapy. This single appearance results in hundreds of calls and letters to the national office and affiliate offices across the country.

1979

An ADA press release in April 1979, "Islet Cell Transplantation Termed Encouraging," cites animal studies in which successful transplantation had been achieved by Paul Lacy, M.D., of the Washington University School of Medicine in St. Louis. At that time, Dr. Lacy was an ADA Board member and chairman of the Coordinating Committee on Scientific Activities.

"I Don't Have Diabetes Anymore," a story by Mary Ellen Baran, appears in *Diabetes Forecast* in 1980 and raises the hopes of hundreds of people with diabetes a little prematurely. In the article, Ms. Baran, who had been the recipient of two pancreas transplants, the first of which was rejected, and the second successful, tells her encouraging story of how wonderful it is to be free from diabetes after 23 years. The article generates hundreds of calls to the national office and affiliate offices (*Diabetes Forecast*, Vol. 33:1, 1980). Unfortunately, not everyone is an eligible candidate for such a transplant, and subsequent studies show that not all such transplants are so successful. Ms. Baran herself acknowledges in speeches at ADA affiliates that she has, in effect, traded the problems of taking insulin for the problems of taking cyclosporin, a drug taken to prevent rejection of the transplanted organ. It is clear, however, that her surgery is a major step forward on the path toward a cure for diabetes.

1980

Paul E. Lacy, M.D., Ph.D., and colleagues at Washington University in St. Louis, Missouri, discover how to surmount the cross-species barrier in the transplantation of beta cells. Insulin-producing cells from healthy laboratory animals are implanted in diabetic animals of another species. The result: diabetes disappears. Such a procedure might eventually be effective in humans.

Chapter Ten
A Corporation Emerges
1980-85

ADA Presidents

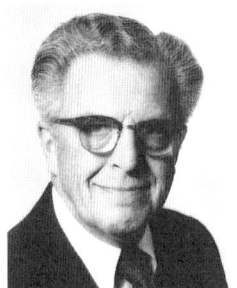
Donald I. Bell, M.D.
(1980-81)

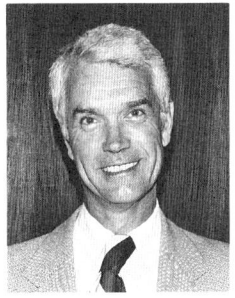
Oscar B. Crofford, M.D.
(1981-82)

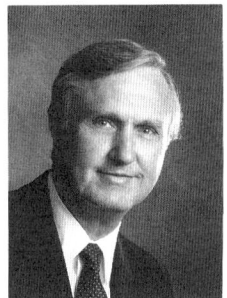
Irving L. Spratt, M.D.
(1982-83)

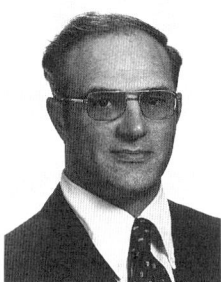
Allan L. Drash, M.D.
(1983-84)

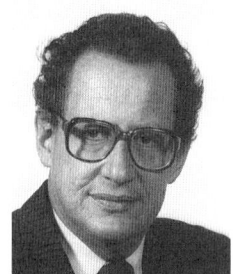
Karl E. Sussman
(1984-85)

ADA Chairmen of the Board

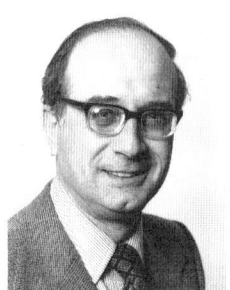
Benjamin Greenspoon
(1980-81)

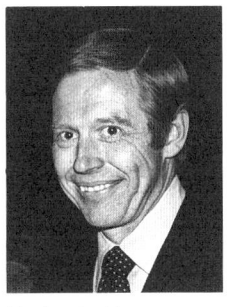
Harlan L. Hanson
(1981-83)

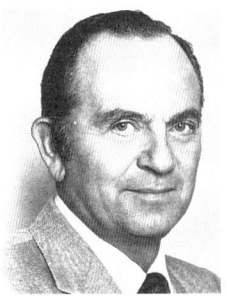
Gordon Stulberg
(1983-84)

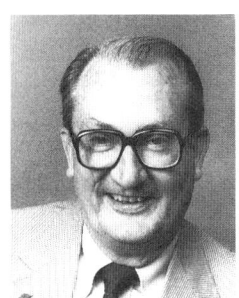
Joseph H. Davis, Esq.
(1984-85)

As the decade began, hostages in the Middle East and American service personnel missing in action in Vietnam and Laos occupied the headlines. In the United States, voters elected their oldest president, Ronald Reagan, then reelected him four years later. A political swing to the right, galloping inflation, and recession early in the decade gave way to rising employment, falling interest rates, single-digit inflation, and a soaring stock market by mid-decade.

Frederick Sanger, M.D., was awarded the Nobel Prize in Physiology and Medicine for isolating the insulin molecule, and Drs. Paul Berg and Walter Gilbert received the Nobel Prize in Chemistry for their work on the structure of DNA. New dread diseases—herpes, acquired immune deficiency syndrome (AIDS), and Alzheimer's disease—were affecting the lives of young and old in alarming numbers. Research was accelerated, but cures remained elusive.

In diabetes, unprecedented advances in research resulted in the production of human insulin and the discovery of the role HLA antigens play in the development of insulin-dependent (type I) diabetes. Cyclosporin, an immunosuppresive drug, was found to halt the destruction of beta cells in type I diabetes, if administered early enough. A second generation of low-dose, high-potency oral drugs was introduced to help treat non-insulin-dependent (type II) diabetes. Researchers studied the use of exercise in the control of diabetes. New areas of nutrition, including the effect of high-fiber diets and the glycemic index, were explored.

In an effort to cut health costs, the federal government—the primary supplier of health care—passed the Omnibus Reconciliation Act in 1981. This act mandated cuts in federal spending for health care and instituted the Prospective Payment Plan through the use of Diagnosis Related Groups (DRGs). This system had an adverse impact on the older person with diabetes. Beginning in 1983, hospitals were reimbursed at a predetermined rate for inpatient services based on a primary diagnosis of diabetes, rather than for the actual cost of care. That actual cost was often much higher than estimated, because hospital stays were often longer than those estimated.

This action by the federal government spawned a revolution in health-care delivery in the private sector that continues to this day. Physicians were urged to freeze their fees for a period of 18 months. This was voluntary and many physicians complied. For-profit hospitals, group medical practices, health maintenance organizations, outpatient surgery, and drug discount plans sprang up all across the country as entrepreneurs recognized their profit potential. All of these innovations gave the individual more choices for improved health care, but these options cost money. As inflation edged these costs upward, many people found themselves unable to buy the kind of care they needed.

People with diabetes were just beginning to benefit from the new technology of glycohemoglobin (GHb) testing, self-monitoring of blood glucose, insulin pumps, pancreas transplants, therapeutic shoes, laser treatment, vitrectomy, fundus photography, and florescein angiopathy. Encouraged by their physicians, they were seeking more self-care education. Unfortunately, technology and education advanced at a faster rate than the willingness of third-party reimbursers to cover the costs.

At issue for people with diabetes were rising costs and a lack of uniform reimbursement policies among the major insurers—the federal government, Medicare and Medicaid, Blue Cross/Blue Shield, and private insurance companies. Clearly, the American Diabetes Association had to take the lead in addressing this problem if people with diabetes were to benefit from improved treatment modalities.

Another important concern of the Association and the Patient Education Committee was the need for continuing, quality patient education for people with diabetes. Studies had shown unequivocally that education in self-care reduced hospital costs, yet in 1980, diabetes cost the nation $4.8 billion, according to Public Health Service statistics. Costs rose to $14 billion by 1984. Hospital care costs accounted for nearly 46 percent of that figure. Obviously, more education in self-care was needed, and to be effective it had to be provided on a continuing basis. In the 1980s, coverage for outpatient diabetes education remained largely inconsistent and was only arbitrarily provided by private insurers. Thus, education was unavailable to many, often those who needed it most.

By 1980, the American Diabetes Association was recognized as the leading authority in the field of diabetes in the United States and throughout the world. This enviable reputation had been earned by thousands of volunteers working countless hours to create and fund programs in education and research. By raising public awareness of the seriousness of diabetes and providing accurate, timely information on every aspect of the disease, the Association was able to attract increasing public support. The fiscal crisis of 1978-79 had taught the need for long-range planning and setting goals, and these now became the main focus of the Association. A corporate mentality emerged as the Association moved into the most fruitful decade of its existence.

The new decade ushered in important staff changes, most notably the appointment of Robert S. Bolan, Ph.D., to executive vice president in August 1980.

Changes At The National Office

Robert S. Bolan, Ph.D., succeeded John L. Dugan as executive vice president. Dr. Bolan came from an academic background that included directorships in Career Planning and Placement at the University of Southern California and Executive Education and Management of Field Studies at the University of California at Los Angeles (UCLA) Graduate School of Management. He had also served as dean of student activities at the Uni-

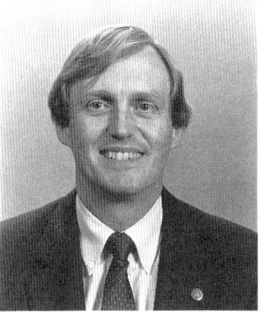

Robert S. Bolan, Ph.D.

versity of Santa Barbara and as director of governmental affairs and assistant to the chancellor at Los Angeles Community College System, and had held teaching appointments in management and business administration at UCLA, West Los Angeles College, the University of San Francisco, and the University at Redlands. Prior to his appointment as ADA treasurer and chairman of the Committee on Budget and Finance, Dr. Bolan served on the Board of the ADA Southern California Affiliate.

A man of vision and singleness of purpose, Dr. Bolan moved the Association forward. Along with Harlan Hanson (chairman of the Board 1981-83), he reaffirmed the Association's mission as first set forth in 1940 by Dr. Striker, putting it into two simple, concise statements: 1) to promote the search for a preventive or cure for diabetes and 2) to improve the well-being of people with diabetes and their families.

To paraphrase an old saying, "You can take the teacher out of the classroom, but you can't take the classroom out of the teacher." Dr. Bolan did what came naturally—he began to teach. Focusing on the mission statement, he held management training sessions and development conferences for all levels of the organization. He encouraged goal-setting and long-range planning in all areas of ADA activities, administration, finance, programs, committees, and departments. He established a weekly management letter, consolidating all communication between the national office and affiliates into one publication.

DCCT Established

There had long been debate over the effectiveness of tight control in preventing or delaying the complications of diabetes. (Tight control means keeping blood glucose as close to "normal" or nondiabetic levels as possible. This is accomplished through diet, exercise, and insulin.) By 1981, new technologies and methods were available to help people with diabetes achieve tight control—blood-glucose meters, self-monitoring of blood glucose, insulin pumps, and the hemoglobin A1c test. These new technologies offered the perfect opportunity for a comparative study between tight, aggressive control of diabetes and the somewhat more relaxed standard treatment.

In 1981, the National Institute of Arthritis, Metabolic, and Digestive Diseases (NIAMDD) established a study known as the Diabetes Control and Complications Trial (DCCT). The ten-year clinical study, funded by the National Institutes of Health (NIH), is an attempt to assess the effects of tight control of blood-glucose levels on the development of complications in people with insulin-dependent (type I) diabetes. The study has four phases: planning, feasibility testing, full-scale collaboration trials, and data analysis. NIAMDD received the grant for the study in 1981, and the study actually got under way in 1982. The first patient was enrolled in 1983.

The DCCT is the most extensive study of its kind. Twenty-seven clinical centers were established in the United States and Canada (two of the clinics have "satellite sites" to assist in recruitment, treatment, and data collection), and approximately 300 health-care practitioners and 1,400 people with insulin-dependent diabetes

Throughout Dr. Bolan's tenure, Caroline Stevens served in several senior positions and became chief operating officer in 1988. She was generally regarded as the most effective manager within the ADA staff and served as principal deputy to Dr. Bolan among the executive staff.

In October 1983, John H. Graham IV, was appointed director of affiliate development. Prior to joining the national staff, Mr. Graham had been the executive director of the ADA Greater Philadelphia Affiliate and from 1971 to 1979 served in several fund-raising and field-service positions with The Boy Scouts of America. Coming from one of the oldest ADA affiliates, Mr. Graham saw that the potential strength of the organization lay in making affiliates more effective and cohesive in raising funds and delivering programs. To achieve this, he instituted regional training programs for affiliate executives and staffs. He was promoted to assistant executive vice president in 1985 and became deputy executive vice president in 1988.

In response to a long-articulated need for a medical director on the national staff, a new department was created to include the research, health-care professional, and patient education programs. Richard Kahn, Ph.D., was appointed assistant executive vice president for scientific and medical affairs in September 1985, later becoming chief science and medical officer.

Before coming to the Association, Dr. Kahn served as chief of scientific affairs of the American Red Cross (ARC), Bi-State Chapter in St. Louis, Missouri, from 1982 to 1985. He was responsible for developing the first organ/tissue bank in the Midwest and the largest research laboratory in the Red Cross system. From 1976 to 1982, he was scientific director of the ARC, Missouri/Illinois Regional Blood Services. He was also an associate professor of pathology at the Washington University School of Medicine.

Internal strengthening of the Association was achieved through a significant number of volunteer and staff training activities carried out both nationally and in communities throughout the country. A new, well-organized system of training and planning, conceived in 1983, was fully operational in 1985. It included these components: a meeting of affiliate Executive Directors in January for training and goal setting for the upcoming fiscal year, which begins July 1; the Annual Meeting in June, where volunteer leaders could formally adopt and dedicate their affiliates to goals for the coming year; and four regional training meetings to provide detailed support to implement those goals, attended by chapter and mid-level affiliate volunteers,

are taking part in the study. Each clinic has ten to fifteen health-care practitioners on staff.

"The origins of the DCCT are grounded in legislation—specifically, the National Diabetes Mellitus Act of 1974," said Oscar Crofford, M.D., chairman of the DCCT and ADA president 1981-82. In 1974, the Long-Range Plan to Combat Diabetes specifically recommended that such a study be carried out, said Dr. Crofford. However, insulin pumps, blood-glucose meters and self-monitoring of blood glucose, and the validation of the hemoglobin A1c test as a measure of metabolic control were still in developmental stages at the time. "All of those technologies had to be developed before the study could begin," Dr. Crofford noted.

Nearly 20 years will have elapsed between when Congress, as urged by the American Diabetes Association, conceived of the idea for such a study and when final results from the study will be available. "This is illustrative of how important long-range planning is in getting something this extensive carried out," Dr. Crofford said. He noted that ADA support was very important in getting the DCCT under way. In addition, support from the public, NIH, and the Juvenile Diabetes Foundation was also essential. "Without support from all of the various constituencies, there's no way it could have been done," Dr. Crofford said.

The trial is scheduled to conclude in 1993; it is estimated that a minimum of two years will be necessary to analyze the data obtained from the study.

staff, and other leaders within the region.

In addition, the Association offered a self-study program to affiliates, in which a group of national staff people would perform an in-depth analysis of an affiliate's operations with the help and cooperation of affiliate staff and volunteers.

After considerable study, plans were completed in 1985 to relocate the national office from New York City to Alexandria, Virginia. The move was undertaken to reduce the long-term occupancy costs and other overhead expenses, as well as to increase the effectiveness with which the Association carried out its programs by assuring close proximity to the United States Congress, many of the federal agencies, and other associations with which we work.

A Time For Professional Councils

During Dr. Whitehouse's presidency (1978-79), the concept of professional section councils began to take shape and a pilot Council on Youth was organized by Donnell Etzwiler, M.D., former ADA president. With the leadership and support of Karl Sussman, M.D., the Committee on Planning and Organization proposed the format for professional councils, and the Board of Directors accepted the concept in June 1980.

In 1981, the Council on Diabetes in Youth was formally established to promote the needs of children and adolescents with diabetes. The council works to emphasize the importance of patient education, teaching, and research. It provides pediatricians and pediatric-related professionals with a forum for the exchange of information on diabetes education and research related to the care of young people with diabetes.

In 1982, two more professional special interest councils were established. ADA's Council on Epidemiology and Statistics strives to stimulate the exchange of information about epidemiology and diabetes and to foster the use of epidemiologic methods in research on the cause of diabetes and the progression of the disease and its complications. The Council on Health Care Delivery and Public Health helps generate, evaluate, and disseminate scientific knowledge about public health, education, and health-care delivery related to diabetes. In addition the Council works to foster interdisciplinary research and education with the goal of achieving the best possible health planning and care for people with diabetes.

Two more councils emerged in 1983: the Council on Nutritional Science and Metabolism—one of the largest special interest councils—and the Council on

Health-Care Professionals: The Changing Roles

From 1983 to 1985, Patricia Schultz, R.N., M.S., C.D.E., was ADA vice president-health professional. She—along with Linda Hurwitz, R.N., M.S., and Barbara Maschak-Carey, M.S.N.—drafted, typed, and circulated a petition at an ADA national meeting to justify the establishment of a professional council for educators. Overnight more than the required number of signatures were obtained. Ms. Schultz became the first chairman of the Council on Education. By 1989, membership in this council was 1,904.

Ms. Schultz is recognized within the American Diabetes Association as being a strong

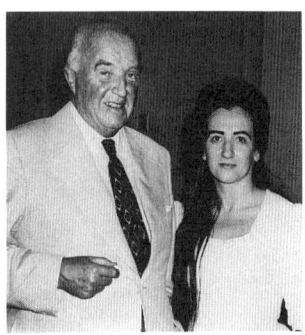

Charles H. Best, M.D., and ADA volunteer Patricia Schultz, Miami, 1972.

advocate for the "non-physician" health professional. To make the point that nurse educators and dietitians do not define themselves solely by their "lack" of an M.D. degree, she once introduced a former ADA president as a "non-nurse."

Ms. Schultz first became involved with the American Diabetes Association in 1970, when she met Dr. Best. Although she was already involved in diabetes care, Dr. Best triggered her interest in the Association.

At that time, Ms. Schultz said, in order to join the Association non-physician health professionals had to have two physicians sign their membership form. One of the physicians who signed her membership form "wasn't even an ADA member—but it didn't matter, as long as it was a doctor," she said. "There were many years when non-physician health professionals struggled to find a place within the ADA," Ms. Schultz added.

In the early 1970s, non-physician health professionals—today called health-care professionals—came to take a more active role in health-care delivery and subsequently became interested in the Association. The Association recognized this increased interest, Ms. Schultz said, by allowing the health-care professionals to develop a steering committee; the committee then developed an "allied health" section. But this recognition did not come quickly enough for some nurse educators and dietitians, and in 1973, the American Association of Diabetes Educators (AADE) was established. Ms. Schultz feels strongly that the formation of AADE was *not* inevitable, but instead resulted from a lack of foresight on the part of the American Diabetes Association. "AADE formed because of a void that ADA hadn't recognized fully," she said.

Health-care professionals began to serve on the ADA Executive Committee in 1977, when the position of vice president-health professional was established; these officers serve a two-year term. And the Task Force on ADA Structure, established in June 1983, "was another turning point with regard to the role of the health-care professional within the Association," Ms. Schultz said.

The health-care team has become a critical part of diabetes management, Ms. Schultz said. "As diabetes management has progressed, the roles of the patient and health-care professional have changed. It used to be that patients would go to the doctor and the doctor told them what to do. Now," she said, "patients come to doctors and sometimes suggest therapy." Ms. Schultz added that health-care professionals have taken on more and more responsibility with regard to providing information and treatments to patients with diabetes, and physicians have increasingly seen the importance of the health-care team working together.

"The expertise of health-care professionals is being recognized," Ms. Schultz said, noting that opportunities for them are increasingly available within the American Diabetes Association. "More and more health-care professionals are getting involved with the organization, as evidenced by increased membership," she said, adding, "There's excellent opportunity within the organization to learn and to provide leadership in a variety of ways. Most times, the limits are only those that are self-determined. We've come a long way, and the path is open for even greater accomplishments," said Ms. Schultz. "Furthermore, it is my firm belief that the potential of the health-care professional in the Association is not yet fully realized."

Health-Care Professionals: More Comments

Diana Guthrie, R.N., Ph.D., received the ADA Outstanding Health Professional Educator Award in 1979. She also commented on the evolution of the role of health-care professionals within the American Diabetes Association.

"Health professionals, other than physicians and biochemists, have come a long way in this association," Dr. Guthrie commented. Initially, she said, the American Diabetes Association "was intended to be a social-intellectual gathering of physicians to share information and frustrations regarding the management of diabetes mellitus." As the needs of people with diabetes grew, she said, the nurses, dietitians, and others responding to physician orders found that they had increasing needs in terms of managing the disease. But at the time, most physicians did not recognize these needs.

"Dietitians were often the instigators of education programs in the hospitals," Dr. Guthrie commented, adding, "Nurses were relegated to giving insulin or teaching about an injection procedure or urine testing procedure.

"As nurses and dietitians started talking with each other, they recognized a need that was not being met by the Association," she continued. "In the 1960s, the American Nurses' Association (ANA) was perhaps ahead of its time, as least as far as the ADA was concerned, in assisting nurses to set up standards of care for particular patient populations. The nurses in the American Diabetes Association would have nothing to do with ANA directives, but I feel that it directed their thinking in regard to the education needs of the person having the disease."

Dr. Guthrie said that many of the health-care professionals who held leadership roles in the American Diabetes Association were also involved in the development of the American Association of Diabetes Educators (AADE). Like the ANA directives, Dr. Guthrie said, the formation of the AADE was directing the American Diabetes Association to examine the needs of allied health professionals. "If the timing had just been delayed by just a few years, the ADA would have recognized the needs of all diabetes educators and perhaps the AADE would not even have been formed," she commented.

In retrospect, Dr. Guthrie said, the formation of the AADE gave just enough impetus to the American Diabetes Association to "recognize the input of such health professionals to the care of the person with diabetes and to the organization as a whole."

"Overall, the quality of health-care professional input into the Association has increased," Dr. Guthrie said, adding, "The recognition by physicians has increased." She cited the establishment of the Outstanding Health Educator Award in 1978 as an example of this recognition.

As the quality of education for health-care professionals has increased, physicians' respect for health-care professionals has increased, said Dr. Guthrie. This, she said, has led to a growing awareness "that knowledgeable dietitians and nurses, especially on the Master's and Ph.D. level, can take their place right along with the physicians and biochemists in fulfilling a particular part in the total picture of diabetes care."

Diabetes In Pregnancy. The Council on Nutritional Science and Metabolism works to disseminate new information, update knowledge, and to promote research in the field of nutrition. The concern of the Council on Pregnancy in Diabetes is to encourage research in the area of diabetes and pregnancy, to develop improved methods of patient care, and to disseminate such information to health professionals involved in the care of pregnant women with diabetes.

Diabetes Becomes Big Business

Self-monitoring of blood glucose—simple, accurate, and more convenient than urine testing—was both a technical triumph and a psychological boon to people with diabetes. An idea whose time had come, it was an instant success. These factors, combined with aggressive marketing on the part of manufacturers, made diabetes big business overnight.

Testing requires lancets, strips, and blood-glucose meters, and there was a rush by entrepreneurs to provide these necessities. Because monitoring blood glucose allowed tighter control of diabetes, the consumer needed more information about insulin, syringes, syringe devices, and products to counteract hypoglycemia, and the manufacturers expanded their marketing to meet this new demand. Diabetes mail-order supply houses sprang up like new grass after a spring rain. Advertisers challenged readers, ''Compare Our Prices,'' and the race was on. It was inevitable that some affiliates would be enticed into this market by eager manufacturers, on the basis of providing a service to their members. This resulted in serious conflict between the national office and affiliates.

In November 1980, the Executive Committee proposed a ''Policy on the Sale of Medical Equipment and Medicines,'' for inclusion in the *Statement of Purposes, Principles and Policies of the ADA*. The policy stated: ''The ADA (National and Affiliates), a voluntary health agency, is prohibited from selling medical equipment or medicines. This policy prohibits acting as a distributor, agent, or in any manner profiting from such transactions.''

An affiliate bulletin from Chairman of the Board Benjamin Greenspoon and President Donald I. Bell, M.D., (1980-81) urged affiliate presidents and executive directors to inform their officers of the recommendation and the reasons for the decision. The Executive Committee had three concerns: 1) that the sale of a product implied ADA endorsement by implication, despite any disclaimers, and was contrary to the *State-*

ment of Purposes, Principles and Policies; 2) that fiscal arrangements, the use of capital, inventory and credit losses, and billing and bookkeeping could have potential tax ramifications; and 3) that professional relationships within the community could be endangered by entering into competition with dealers, pharmacists, hospitals, and manufacturers in the area.

Debate was heated in the Central Council, but agreement was finally reached and the policy was approved by the Board in June 1982.

As the use of continuous infusion insulin pumps (CIIP) and self-monitoring of blood glucose (SMBG) grew in popularity, the Association saw the need to establish guidelines for patients and professionals in order to achieve optimal benefits from these new treatment modalities.

In 1981-82, an ad hoc Committee on Therapeutic Modalities was appointed, comprised of Drs. Harvey C. Knowles, Jr., chairman; Philip Felig; Charles M. Peterson; Philip Raskin; Julio V. Santiago; David S. Schade; O. Peter Schumacher; and Marion Franz, R.D.; Diana Guthrie, R.N., M.N.; and W. Wayne Young, Pharm.D. Under the aegis of the Executive Committee's Scientific Advisory Panel, composed of Drs. Oscar B. Crofford, Irving L. Spratt, Allan L. Drash, Donald I. Bell, and Florence R. Ruhland, R.N., the ad hoc committee developed a policy.

The Board approved a combined policy statement, "Indications for Use of Continuous Insulin Delivery Systems and Self-Measurement of Blood Glucose," which was published in *Diabetes Care* (Vol. 5:2, 1982). The statement described the purpose of CIIPs, identified which people were the best candidates for this type of therapy, and included warnings about the possibility of severe hypoglycemia. With reference to self-monitoring of blood glucose (SMBG), the statement said that it may be desirable for all people with insulin-dependent diabetes, and particularly for pregnant women with diabetes.

Due to the increasing use of SMBG and new research findings on the CIIP, by 1985 the Association saw the need to restate the policies of 1982. An additional issue was third-party reimbursement to cover the cost of pumps and blood-glucose testing materials. Some insurance companies denied reimbursement on the basis that the technology was still experimental. At this time, separate policies on the CIIP and SMBG were developed, and the statements are specific on the point of reimbursement, saying, "These devices are no longer experimental. When prescribed by a physician they are a part of routine treatment, and should be cov-

An Invitation To Young Leaders

In April 1984, the Association held its first national Youth Leadership Congress at the Key Bridge Marriott Hotel, just

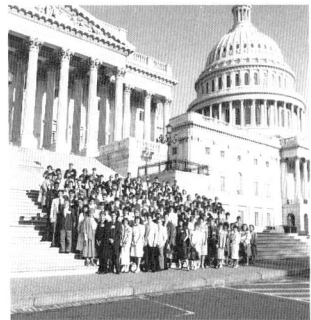

Youth Leadership Congress (1987)

across the Potomac River from Washington, D.C. The congress, whose theme was "Building a Better Tomorrow," brought together teens and young adults from all across the country. Ninety-five young people, ages 16-26, attended workshops and rap sessions and visited the White House. They went to Capitol Hill and carried to their congressional representatives the message that diabetes is a serious disease. They met with ADA officers and discussed living with diabetes with television star Dana Hill and the "Diabetic Ironman," Bill Carlson. They learned about the newest trends in research from scientists of the National Institutes of Health and about the dynamics of volunteerism in leadership sessions.

Delegates to the congress were chosen by their affiliates for their leadership qualities. The young people were encouraged to return to their homes and become involved in the work of their local affiliates and chapters. The Youth Leadership Congress was so enthusiastically received by the young people, their parents,

ered by the usual payment mechanisms.'' The policies were published in *Diabetes* (Vol. 30:9, 1984).

The pump policy contains specific recommendations: use of continuous subcutaneous insulin infusion requires that continuing care by a skilled professional be available; that patients be carefully selected and given meticulous monitoring; and that provisions for recording and reporting experiences be provided. These cautionary remarks were necessitated by reported deaths of several patients using insulin pumps. Each case was investigated by the Centers for Disease Control, and its findings were considered by the Association in developing the policy statement.

Association's Research Program Grows

The early 1980s saw an emphasis on improving the Association's research program through long-range financial planning. The goals of the research program, however, remained the same as before: find a cure for diabetes and a way to prevent its complications.

ADA President Oscar Crofford, M.D., (1981-82) said he felt the most important thing that he achieved as ADA president was to help the Association initiate a stronger diabetes research program than it had had in the past. "During my years on the Executive Committee, and then as president, we gave a great deal of emphasis to research and tried to redirect the focus of the Association toward research," Dr. Crofford said. The research program was a necessary first step in getting the Association to grow and obtain donations from the public, according to Dr. Crofford.

To establish a stronger research program, the Association developed a long-range financial plan emphasizing research. The plan, which for the first time gave the Association some direction in the percentage of expenditures that should be devoted to various programs, was developed while he was on the Executive Committee and culminated during his term as president, Dr. Crofford said. The plan worked on something of a sliding scale. "As revenues increased, an increasing percentage of revenues was channeled to the diabetes research program," he explained. This was important, Dr. Crofford noted, because it "represented not just approving the research plan in principle, but actually acting on the principle by adopting a plan."

"It was important to redirect funds toward research because 1) it was what donors and potential donors want and 2) the community of biomedical researchers was discouraged and perhaps disappointed that ADA was making such a paltry contribution to research,"

and affiliates, that it has become an annual event.

The first congress was supported in part by grants from G.D. Searle, Squibb-Novo, and Eli Lilly and Company. Subsequent youth congresses have been sponsored by The NutraSweet Company whose generous grants paid transportation and expenses for the majority of delegates and made the meeting possible.

The concept of a national youth congress was first raised in 1982 by Patricia Schultz, R.N., M.S., then chairman of the Committee on Youth and Parents Groups. Netti Richter, M.S., who was ADA's Executive Committee liaison to the Youth Committee, presented the concept of a youth convention to the Executive Committee for approval. Her presentation to the Executive Committee was a critical assignment and one that changed the history of the Association tremendously. The Committee on Youth and Parents Groups then began ambitious and extensive planning. Deborah Hinnen, R.N., served as chairman of the committee the year of the first Youth Congress, 1984.

Each year at the Youth Leadership Congress, delegates elect one person to serve for one year as the national youth spokesperson. This person is chosen from among the newly elected Youth Action Committee members. The national youth spokesperson traditionally speaks at the ADA Annual Meeting in June, and serves as a member of the national Committee on Youth Services to represent all youth. The congress elected Tom Smith of the South Carolina Affiliate as ADA's first national youth spokesperson in 1984.

Dr. Crofford said. (The Juvenile Diabetes Foundation, he noted, was making great strides in support of research.) "The long-range financial plan emphasizing research boosted the morale of researchers and helped them understand that ADA was going to be an important agency in funding diabetes research," Dr. Crofford said.

Dr. Crofford's commitment to research carried over into the politics of diabetes research funding. He said he felt it was important "to help the Association be a more influential advocate for the cause of diabetes research at the federal level." Dr. Crofford said he and other ADA members worked with Congressional representatives "to be a more effective voice in lobbying for funds through the National Institutes of Health."

A controversy during his term that has continued, Dr. Crofford said, is whether funds for research should flow from ADA affiliates to the national office and be distributed by the national office (central distribution), or whether affiliates should keep the funds and distribute them as they see fit (local distribution). "The philosophy is that funds should go to where the best research is being done; money should go to where the research is most promising," Dr. Crofford said. "However, some people want to give money to support local researchers and will not give if the money is going to centrally supported researchers," he said. "We tried to restructure the program so that funding could be scientifically sound, and so that it would work both ways (central and local)."

ADA President Irving L. Spratt, M.D., (1982-83) and Chairman of the Board Harlan L. Hanson continued to focus energies on building the research program. In fiscal year 1981, total ADA research grants had totaled about $1 million. By fiscal year 1983, Dr. Spratt and Mr. Hanson announced a jump to $3.7 million. In addition, the Association's year-round national advocacy efforts resulted in expanded federal support of diabetes research, training, and service programs, totaling nearly $190 million in 1983.

By fiscal year 1985, the figure for research grants had climbed to $5 million.

A strong partnership began between the Association and Lions Clubs International (LCI). Dr. James Fowler, 1983-84 LCI president, expressed the commitment in these words: "Striving towards the elimination of diabetes is a goal every Lion should recognize as one deserving the attention of the largest and most active service club organization in the world . . . that is why I am asking Lions the world over to join hands to eliminate diabetes. . . ."

What It's Like To Visit A Congressman

Ilene Larson, of North Dakota, then a member of the ADA national Board of Directors, "campaigned" for diabetes by making congressional visits in Washington, D.C. She recounted some of her experiences in the December 1985 issue of *Diabetes Forecast*.

"I have met for rather lengthy visits and photo sessions, had brief chats in reception rooms, waited at length for a delayed appointment because of a role call vote in the House, spent an entire appointment with a health aide, and once even found myself with no one to speak with.

"From this, I have learned to be prepared for anything. Fortunately, the American Diabetes Association provides training for many of its volunteers, gives them a sense of what to expect and how to behave, and provides complete information to use in preparing for a congressional visit. This information includes a fact sheet about diabetes, copies of the ADA Annual Report, and the all-important ADA legislative position, which includes budget recommendations for the federal government's diabetes efforts. Before each visit, I become familiar with this information. The congressman may be the authority on legislation, but for the time of my visit, I am looked upon as the authority on diabetes and the needs of people who have diabetes.

"Next, I prioritize the points I want to make, In the ideal meeting, a congressman and his health aide (who keeps abreast of health issues and briefs the lawmaker) will be available to talk. However, often the lawmaker is alone and on a tight schedule, which means time is limited. In this case, I emphasize the points I

Dr. Fowler's words were translated into action. Worldwide, Lions Clubs conducted a variety of educational and fund-raising projects, including "Journey to Sight" to help raise money for diabetes-caused blindness and other serious eye disorders.

In 1983, the Lions Clubs International Foundation gave $250,000 to the Association to administer an international diabetes research grants program. Also in 1983, the Supreme Order of the Amaranth contributed $100,000 and increased their four-year commitment to $235,000.

Health Insurance, Health Care, And ADA

In the early 1980's, people hospitalized at the time of diagnosis received diabetes education as an integral part of care, and this was generally reimbursed by third-party payers. However, the vast majority of individuals with diabetes are diagnosed in the doctor's office, and the education provided there was not reimbursed, nor were programs in which the individual was not hospitalized, including those offered by ADA affiliates, hospitals, and other organizations. Third-party payers were reluctant to reimburse for these programs, they said, because "There is no way to measure their effectiveness." While third-party payers supported the idea in principle, they wanted proof that outpatient education did indeed reduce costs.

In 1983, the ADA Council on Education and the Council on Health Care Delivery and Public Health recommended that the Association support and encourage reimbursement of outpatient education. The statement "Third-Party Reimbursement for Outpatient Education and Nutrition Counseling" was approved by the ADA Board June 9, 1984, and published as a Position Statement in *Diabetes Care*, Vol. 7:5, 1984.

Over the years, the Association had tried to obtain a comprehensive major medical plan for its members, but could find no insurance company willing to underwrite people with diabetes as a group. Hospital indemnity plans were offered through *Diabetes Forecast* magazine from 1970 onward. While these plans were limited to in-hospital benefits, for many people with diabetes, they were often all that was available.

By 1982, health-care costs had soared, the public had raised its expectations for health-care entitlements, and the number of calls to the Association for health insurance assistance had increased dramatically. Due to a wealth of new technology, better diagnostic methods, and spiraling inflation, by 1984 the cost of diabetes per year—excluding hospitalizations and complications—

feel are most urgent.

"One of the most important things I have learned throughout my experiences is that health aides can be great allies. On occasions when I find myself meeting with an aide instead of a lawmaker, I present my best case to the aide. These people are often well informed and very respective to the information I have to offer.

"Another lesson I have learned is to take advantage of every opportunity to discuss diabetes; almost everyone (in government or out) has a relative or friend with diabetes. During one visit, for instance, I struck up a conversation with a young congressional intern while I awaited my chance to speak with my congressman. I discovered I had known this man when he was a young child and that we have friends in common, several of whom have diabetes. That young man may well become a friend of diabetes in Congress one day.

"Congressional visits by American Diabetes Association members are well received on Capitol Hill, and that is due to the efforts put forth in good preparation by the visitors. Everyone strives to be informed, prompt, flexible, polite, and appreciative.

"These visits are a bit intimidating at first and unpredictable, but they are also exciting and a great deal of fun!"

ranged from $1,459 to $2,500 for a person with insulin-dependent (type I) diabetes, and an estimated $900 for a person with non-insulin-dependent (type II) diabetes (*Diabetes Forecast*, Vol. 38:3, 1985).

People were frustrated, and they expected the Association to do something.

The patient education department at the national office made a survey of the five states in which pooled risk plans (PRP) were then available. In comparing these plans, two features helpful to individuals with diabetes were standard: 1) no one applying could be refused and 2) the cost of premiums was commensurate with non-risk plans. This information was provided to affiliates in April 1982.

Additional information on the status of these plans and guidelines for starting a PRP were provided to affiliates in May 1984. By this time, nine states had PRPs and the National Association of Insurance Commissioners had published "A Model Pooled Risk Bill" for use by groups interested in initiating legislation.

The Conference on Financing Quality Health Care for People with Diabetes, conceived by the American Diabetes Association and co-sponsored by the Centers for Disease Control (CDC) and the National Diabetes Advisory Board (NDAB), was held October 22-24, 1984, in Airlie, Virginia. More than 120 leaders from the diabetes community, the insurance industry, and government agencies participated. During the three-day conference, nine recommendations for action were developed. The most beneficial outcome of the conference, however, was the opening of a dialogue between providers and consumers of the health-care system. The Conference report identified PRPs as one solution to the health insurance problem, and the Government Relations Committee was charged to interest Congress in introducing legislation.

During the conference, ADA volunteer Dorothea Sims portrayed a day in the life of a person with insulin-dependent diabetes. In a poignant but humorous presentation, Mrs. Sims opened her bulging tote bag, revealing the "tools of her trade": a lancet, syringe, insulin, test strips and a meter for blood-glucose testing, plus candy for treating hypoglycemia, and a snack in case dinner was late. The point of her demonstration was to emphasize that if new technology and adequate education were available to all people with diabetes, better control could be achieved, and the cost in dollars and human suffering due to the complications drastically reduced. To many in the audience, Mrs. Sims' hour-by-hour account of the monitoring necessary for good diabetes control came as a surprise.

Recommendations of the Airlie meeting appear in "Conference on Financing Quality Health Care for Persons with Diabetes," Executive Summary, published by the American Diabetes Association.

Following the conference, ADA President Karl Sussman, M.D., (1984-85) appointed the Task Force

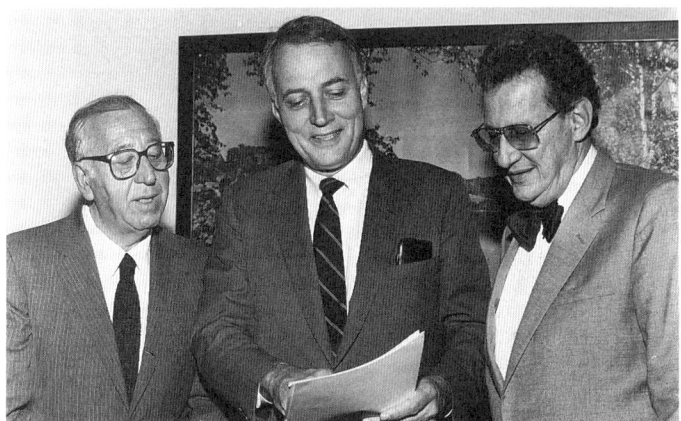

Senator Dave Durenberger (center) with Karl Sussman, M.D., (right) and Harold Rifkin, M.D.

On Financing Quality Health Care For Persons With Diabetes to follow through on these recommendations. The Task Force was charged by the Executive Committee to plan and organize the implementation of the recommendations of the Airlie meeting, and to invite participating organizations to assign an individual for this purpose. "A Report of the Task Force on Financing Quality Health Care for Individuals with Diabetes" was developed with recommendations and submitted to the ADA Executive Committee in June 1986.

The Task Force produced two additional publications: "Diabetes Outpatient Education: The Evidence of Cost Savings," 1986, with documented evidence and supporting statements, and "Third-Party Reimbursement for Diabetes Outpatient Education, A Manual for Health Care Professionals," 1986, to assist health professionals in the use of the health-care system and to provide a model for health benefits.

Diabetes In The News

In the early 1980s, a galaxy of public figures—among them comedian Bob Hope, baseball star Catfish Hunter, and actor Burt Reynolds—helped create greater awareness of diabetes through public statements, television appearances, and radio and television spots. Olympic Gold Medal winner Bruce Jenner and his actress-wife Linda Thompson, who served as ADA

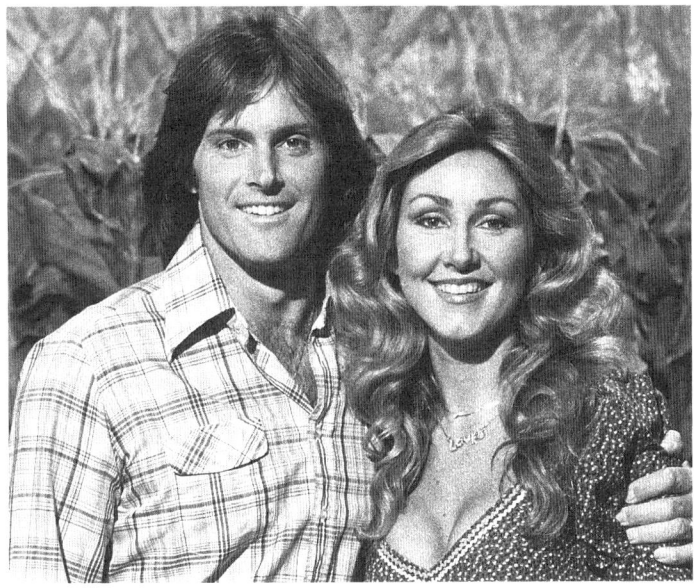

Bruce Jenner and Linda Thompson

national campaign co-chairpersons in 1983, led a national awareness drive. Bill Gullickson, rookie pitcher of the Montreal Expos, recorded public service messages and visited youngsters who have diabetes to help them see that the disease does not have to defeat them. Mike Douglas, Senator John Glenn, Angie Dickinson, Robert Goulet, Olivia Newton-John, Steve Allen and Audrey Meadows, and many others joined Stars War on Diabetes, ADA's attention-getting public awareness and fund-raising program. Actor Scott Baio became the first national youth chairman in 1981.

In June 1981, a five-part series on diabetes was featured on the NBC-TV program "Health Field." Dr.

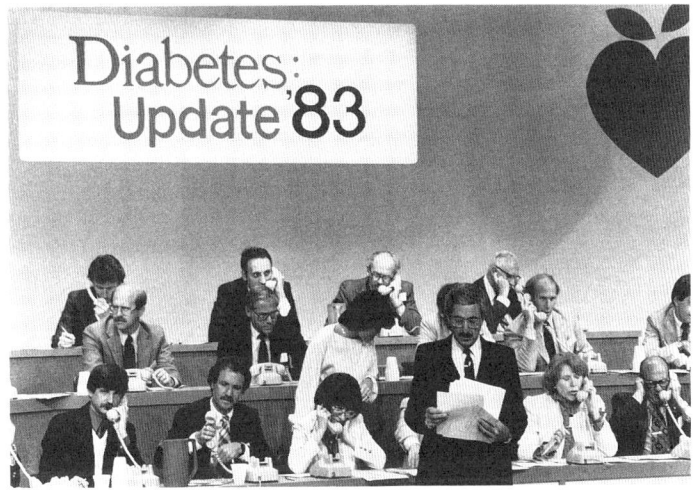

Dr. Art Ulene and Diabetes: Update '83

Frank Field and his daughter, Pamela, served as moderators, with ADA volunteers participating.

The first Diabetes Informathon—Update: Diabetes—was televised in June 1983, with Dr. Art Ulene as moderator. A four-hour, coast-to-coast TV program on the Cable Health Network, the program followed the popular format of a call-in show, giving people a chance to "ask the doctor." ADA physicians selected from all regions of the country took calls, and the phones never stopped ringing. Not everyone could get through on the show, however, and telephones at the national office were set up to take the overflow. The program was so successful that both national and affiliate switchboards were lit up for days after by people seeking information.

To encourage accurate and correct reporting about diabetes in the media, in 1984 the Association established National Media Awards for Excellence in Journalism. The first award was given to Dr. Art Ulene for excellence in communications.

Public awareness of diabetes as a disease jumped tremendously in 1984. When people were asked to list the four most serious diseases in the United States, diabetes came in third place—the most frequently listed disease after cancer and heart disease. Only a few years before in a similar poll, less than half of those interviewed even knew about diabetes. "We have finally reached a level of public awareness about diabetes that reflects the seriousness of its impact upon Americans," said Executive Vice President Robert S. Bolan, Ph.D., in the Association's 1984 "Annual Report."

At the same time public awareness was increasing, so, too, were fund-raising efforts. The majority of ADA support comes from individuals making personal contributions. The 1980s saw an expansion in broad-based fund-raising programs, including outreach to corporations, foundations, and civic organizations.

In 1982, the Association created a coordinated ADA affiliate direct mail program. The program experienced a 300 percent growth in income by 1984, when it generated $1.2 million, almost double the prior year's income.

In communities across the country, volunteers went door-to-door providing their neighbors with important information about diabetes and collecting contributions for the Association.

The National Holiday Sales Program continued its successful annual fund-raising campaign. In addition, the creative efforts of volunteers and staff in ADA affiliates and chapters went full-speed ahead. These pro-

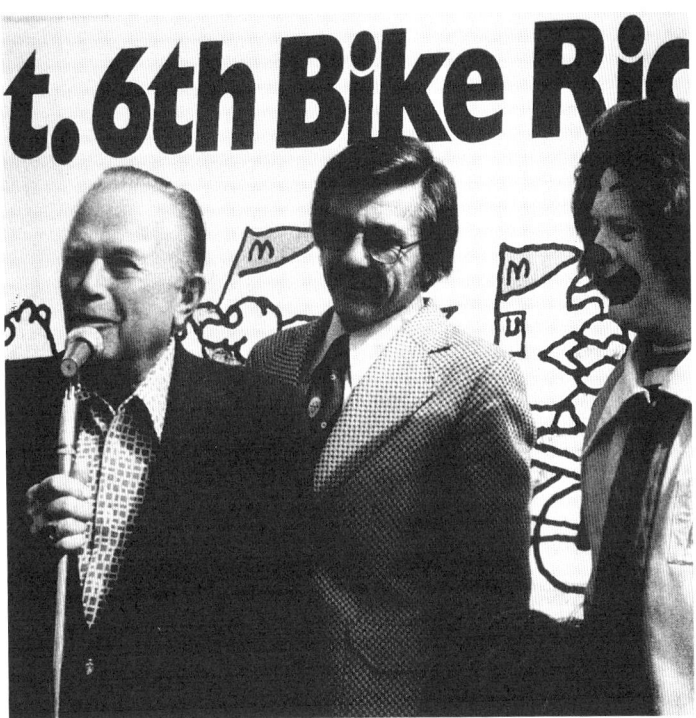

McDonald's founder Ray Kroc, at left, with actor Gary Owens and Ronald McDonald

grams covered a wide range, including: golf tournaments, such as the Pro/Am Two Man Best Ball conducted by the Greater St. Louis Affiliate in June 1983; the Great Catalog Caper, a black-tie adult treasure hunt held in Neiman Marcus stores, which was started by the Washington, D.C. Area Affiliate and also conducted in 1984 by the Texas Affiliate; and Walk-a-Thons, such as "D-Feet Diabetes," which raised $30,000 for the Greater Tennessee Affiliate, and the "DEFEET Diabetes Run," which netted $22,600 for the Kansas Affiliate.

Turning A Page

With the January/February 1980 issue of *Diabetes Forecast*, Harold Rifkin, M.D., assumed the reins of editor-in-chief from Leo P. Krall, M.D. Dr. Krall had served as the magazine's editor for five years and oversaw dramatic changes in *Forecast*'s design, format, and content. In his first editorial (January/February 1980), Dr. Rifkin paid tribute to his predecessor:

"Some of you probably recall the small-sized *Forecast* that Dr. Krall took over in 1974. *Forecast*, even then, was publishing solid, important articles. But Dr. Krall took that small magazine and turned it into the handsome, lively magazine it is today—without sacrificing any scientific accuracy."

In the same editorial, Dr. Rifkin outlined some of his editorial goals for the magazine. He pledged that: "As the times change and new breakthroughs in treatment and prevention emerge, *Forecast* will adapt its reporting to meet your changing needs." He acknowledged that people with diabetes were taking an increasingly active role in self care, and he said "*Forecast* will strive to strengthen its reporting on research developments and treatment alternatives" to help people become well-informed members of their health-care teams. These goals were realized with the creation of fitness, care, food, and research columns during Dr. Rifkin's tenure. With each issue, these columns continue to bring readers the latest information on living well with diabetes.

In the years Dr. Rifkin served as editor-in-chief, *Forecast* readership increased, and the magazine itself grew larger with more pages per issue.

Dr. Rifkin left *Forecast* in 1984, to assume the position of Association vice president. In 1985-86, Dr. Rifkin served as president of the American Diabetes Association.

Dr. Rifkin was ably succeeded in 1984 by Arthur Krosnick, M.D., a diabetes specialist in private practice and clinical associate professor in the Department of Community Medicine at Rutgers Medical School, in New Jersey.

In his first editorial, Dr. Krosnick called *Forecast* a "super publication" and predicted it would "continue to grow and improve." Thanks to his leadership, that prediction came true. *Forecast* took on a fresh new design, expanded its number of pages, and became a monthly (rather than 10 times a year) publication.

In January 1989, Philip Levy, M.D., a clinician in private practice in Phoenix, Arizona, became the next editor-in-chief of *Diabetes Forecast*. "I am honored to be named your new editor-in-chief," Dr. Levy told *Forecast* readers in his first editorial. "Dr. Krosnick's shoes will be difficult to fill, but I will do my best. I will start by repeating Dr. Krosnick's pledge to help *Forecast* grow and improve. With your help, I'm confident we can continue to build on Dr. Krosnick's foundation."

Dr. Levy has long been active in Association activities, both nationally and at the local level, including involvement in government relations, public awareness, and patient education. He is past president and member of the founding Board of Directors of the Arizona Affiliate.

ADA Position On Employment Challenged

In 1982, two young lawyers with insulin-dependent (type I) diabetes—Sandra Polin, of California, and Robert Zagoria, of New Jersey—challenged the Association's position on employment. Ms. Polin and Mr. Zagoria charged that the job guidelines outlined by the American Diabetes Association created unfair employment barriers for people with diabetes. It was Ms. Polin's and Mr. Zagoria's contention that employment should be based solely on an individual's ability to handle a job. After carefully considering the issue, the ADA Board issued a new policy, which said: "Any person with diabetes should be able to accept any employment for which he or she is individually qualified."

In 1984, the Board elaborated, stating: "Diabetes as such should not exclude a person from employment. Individual jobs and individual people with diabetes should be considered, weighing such factors as treatment regimen (diet, oral hypoglycemic agents, insulin) presence of complications, and specific job requirements or hazards."

The Board also urged physicians to examine their patients who had diabetes to identify factors, such as a history of severe insulin reactions or impaired vision, that may limit an individual's capabilities. In addition, the Board urged public education as well as education for employers to optimize opportunities for people with diabetes in the workplace.

People with diabetes still face legal hurdles in some areas of employment. Military careers, for example, are one arena in which obstacles remain. Despite a brief relaxation of regulations during wartime (as mentioned earlier), people with diabetes have always been prohibited from enlistment in all branches of the armed services. And people who develop diabetes while in military service are usually discharged.

The Federal Aviation Administration (FAA) will not issue a pilot's license to a person with type I diabetes, and the Department of Transportation will not issue a license for interstate commerce to a person with type I diabetes. But in light of new developments for diabetes treatment, the American Diabetes Association continues to urge these agencies to relax their regulations and consider each person with diabetes and his or her ability to perform a job on a case-by-case basis.

Heart-Felt Losses

The American Diabetes Association lost two staunch supporters and faithful volunteers in the early 1980s.

Gail Patrick Jackson Velde was one of the first non-physicians to be elected to the ADA Board and among the first to receive the Charles H. Best Medal for Distinguished Service. Although she had insulin-dependent diabetes for many years, this did not deter her from an active life. A movie star, TV producer, and honorary chairman of the National Christmas Seal Campaign in 1970, Mrs. Jackson served on the Advisory Council of the National Institutes of Health, and from 1970 until her death in 1982, was an ADA leader. Mrs. Jackson

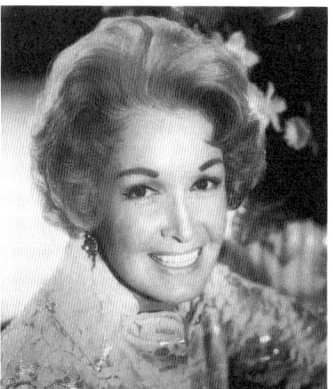

Gail Patrick Jackson Velde

was elected the first chairman of the ADA Board, in 1970. In a tribute to her, Wendell Mayes, Jr., said, "Her ever-present smile and sparkling eyes, smoothed our way as we moved from a professional organization to a voluntary health agency."

Ray Kroc, who devoted his life to the conquest of diabetes and other health problems through the generous use of the resources of the McDonald's Corporation and the Kroc Foundation, succumbed to complications of diabetes in 1984. The Board of Directors commended Mr. Kroc, recipient of the Charles H. Best Medal for Distinguished Service, for his humanitarian concerns on behalf of the interests of the Association in the following resolution: "We mourn the untimely passing of Mr. Ray Kroc, extend sincere sympathy to his wife and family, and commend him for his unique service in the volunteer efforts to fight diabetes and its life-threatening complications."

Identity Crisis

No study of the structure of the Association had been made since 1974, when the Association's Committee on Function and Structure recommended major changes in the Bylaws (covering the election of officers, the Central Council, and the committee structure) required by the conversion to a voluntary health agency.

In 1983, questions and concerns were raised as to the roles, responsibilities, and relationships of these entities within the Association. The specific issues were: 1) the authority, role, and duties of the Central Council; 2) relationships between professionals and lay members; 3) the role of non-physician health professionals in the ADA governing structure; and 4) continuance of service by past officers and Board members.

In June 1983, the Board voted to establish a Task Force on ADA Structure to examine the volunteer organizational structure, make recommendations for changes in the Bylaws to achieve appropriate balance of all membership elements, and work in close cooperation with the Committee on Planning and Organization (P&O). Members from every region of the country were represented on the Task Force: Drs. Charles Clark, Jr., Indiana; John A. Colwell, South Carolina; Messrs. Sam A. Gallo, Louisiana; Benjamin Greenspoon, Maryland (Washington, D.C. Area Affiliate); Eric D. Mayer, California; Wendell Mayes, Jr., Texas; Frank Rosenhoover, Pennsylvania; and Patricia Schultz, R.N., M.S., Florida, were appointed by Chairman of the Board Joseph H. Davis and President Dr. Karl E. Sussman. Caroline Stevens was assigned from the national staff.

The task force studied the Charter, Constitution, Bylaws, Long-range Plan, Committee Goals and Charges, and the Table of Organization. It also reviewed recent minutes of the P&O Committee, and attended regional meetings in the fall of 1984.

For comparative purposes, the task force studied the structure of the American Heart Association. A management consultant with special expertise in organizational structure was asked to review and suggest changes that could be made. Two hundred past and present ADA leaders were contacted for comments. In the 40-percent response received from these volunteers, all expressed an intense interest that the Association continue to be a strong and effective organization.

After four meetings and numerous telephone conferences, the task force issued its "Report of the Task Force on ADA Structure," April 19, 1985. The report contained a total of 50 recommendations that would better delineate the role and responsibilities of the Executive Committee, Board of Directors, officers, Central Council, professional section councils, and committees in the overall structure of the organization. The report was presented to the Board in June 1985 for consideration and was accepted in principle. The major outcome of the work of the task force was a reaffirmation of the Association's existing structure, which was deemed appropriate and effective.

The task force's study revealed a sharp desire among volunteers for more involvement in the decision-making process. It was recognized that the Central Council meeting provides the opportunity for volunteers from around the country to discuss crucial issues and to carry back an understanding to their affiliates. To build consensus, a forum of debate must be provided at Central Council meetings, according to task force members. It was recommended that the Town Meeting be renamed the "Affiliate Assembly." The Affiliate Assembly would improve the consensus-building process of the Association.

The task force recognized that the professional section councils had not been integrated into the structure of the Association and did not have a forum for representation. Therefore, task force members defined the roles of these councils and recommended that a Professional Advisory Panel be established to oversee the operation of ADA's professional section councils—and transmit concerns to the Board of Directors.

The function of the Board of Directors, according to the task force's findings, should be to resolve conflicts, set policy, and provide a nationwide perspective. To be truly representative of the Association, the Board would no longer be required to have one-third of its members as physicians.

Other recommendations included the addition of a new officer position: senior vice president, who would be a leading spokesperson for health-care professionals; and reduction in the size of the Executive Committee from 11 to 10 elected officers. The past chairman of the Board and the past president would no longer serve as members of the Executive Committee.

Committees, traditionally the program-planning arm of the Association, are generally appointed annually by the president and the chairman of the Board. Membership on a committee is from one to two years, and charges are often long-range in nature. In 1979, the number of national committees had reached an all-time high of 59, and clearly had become a burden to the Association in efficiency and cost. When the committee structure was reviewed, it seemed more sensible that the president appoint, from time to time, either an ad hoc committee or a task force to address specific issues that needed attention. This enabled the Association to assemble the most qualified panel of experts, assign the task, and receive recommendations within a reasonable time. This system continues to serve the Association well. It engages the talent of more volunteers, gets the job done, and leaves the long-range planning to a select number of committees.

The work of the Task Force on ADA Structure took three years and required painstaking review, scrutiny, study, and discussion of many documents. It is significant to note that the recommendations and final changes represented a consensus of every element within the Association.

Task Force On Sucrose

In July 1983, the article "Postprandial Glucose and Insulin Responses to Meals . . . " appeared in the *New England Journal of Medicine (NEJM)*. It was heralded in the lay press with headlines, "Ice Cream Instead of a Baked Potato, for Diabetics." The more conservative *Wall Street Journal* carried an article saying that people with diabetes could now eat sweets in moderation, although, it noted, moderation was not defined.

Authors of the *NEJM* article said, "Our data do not support the belief that dietary sucrose aggravates hyperglycemia in diabetic patients. In both Type I and Type II diabetics, we found that sucrose, when consumed in a mixed meal, that also contained protein and fat, did not produce a more rapid rise in plasma glucose levels, than did comparable amounts of potato or wheat starch." The authors went on to say, "We see no reason for diabetics to be denied foods containing sucrose as long as weight reduction is not necessary . . . provided that sucrose is consumed in controlled amounts in nutritionally balanced meals. . . ." And they concluded, "We believe that the inclusion of sucrose in the diabetic diet may increase overall dietary compliance, and thereby help achieve the goals of diet therapy."

This article raised questions from all sectors of the diabetes community, particularly people with diabetes. Taught for many years that "sugar is bad," some asked indignantly why they had been deprived for so long.

In the aftermath of the publicity generated by the article, the Association appointed a Task Force on Sucrose, headed by Ronald A. Arky, M.D., which included Marion Franz, R.D.; David Jenkins, M.D.; Melinda Downie-Maryniuk, R.D.; Frank Nuttall, Ph.D.; Judith Wylie-Rosett, R.D., Ed.D.; and Phyllis Crapo, R.D. The task force met on August 25, 1984, and recommended:

1) that the Association issue a statement on the use of "simple carbohydrates" by individuals with diabetes in the broad area of nutrition, rather than focus primarily on sucrose, and that the statement be widely dis-

seminated in order for its importance to have the proper impact;

2) that an updated, fully referenced position paper on Diabetes and Nutrition be published as soon as possible, introducing new concepts in nutrition; and

3) that the American Diabetes Association revise the *Exchange Lists for Meal Planning* to include the use of modest amounts of sucrose, with "modest" defined.

A Policy Statement, "Glycemic Effects of Carbohydrates," was prepared by the task force and published in *Diabetes Care* (Vol. 7:6, 1984). The statement outlined the American Diabetes Association's position. In summary, the statement says that the goal of diabetes treatment is control of blood sugar; a modest amount of sucrose is acceptable in the diet depending upon metabolic control; carbohydrates that produce the smallest rise in blood sugar should be emphasized; and appraisal of sucrose in mixed meals is imprecise given current knowledge and must await further research.

In a related topic, to prevent a rush to the sugar bowl, the article "The Glycemic Response" was published in *Diabetes Forecast*, Vol. 37:4, 1984. Written by leading dietitians in the field, the article concluded with this cautionary advice: "If you want to include a bit of table sugar in your diet, you *might* be able to do so, especially if your control is good, and if you consume the sugar during a meal when its impact may be blunted by other foods . . . . Talk to your dietitian. This change is *not* acceptable for everyone . . . if you are overweight you do not want to add calories, and you must test carefully to be sure that adding sugar does not disturb your control." By stressing caution in the use of sugar and emphasizing overall control of diabetes, the Association hoped to project a balanced, sensible approach to the use of the glycemic index.

The Clinical Education Program (CEP)

In 1984, the Association launched a far-reaching and innovative program in professional education directed to the primary-care physician. The program, which focused on the treatment of type II diabetes, was financed by a $4.5 million grant from The Upjohn Company, which, like the Association, had recognized the need for physician education in type II diabetes. The Clinical Education Program (CEP) was the largest, most ambitious program ever undertaken by a national voluntary health agency. On April 11, 1984, at the invitation of the American Diabetes Association, 17,000 physicians gathered in 27 cities across the country for a

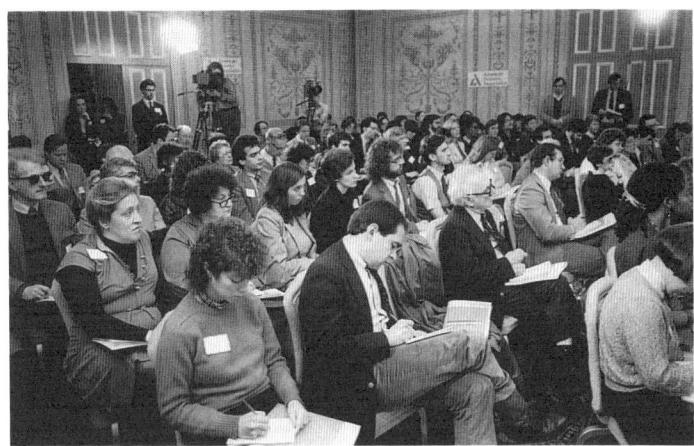

The Clinical Education Program, April 11, 1984

unique learning experience. (In the next two years, 250 CEP programs were sponsored by affiliates. The programs reached a total of 50,000 additional doctors.)

Three physicians, all members of ADA's professional section, were carefully selected for their expertise in the diagnosis, treatment, and complications of type II diabetes, to serve as faculty at each of the 27 sites. Primary text for the course was *The Physician's Guide to Type II Diabetes (NIDDM)* (1984), edited by Harold Rifkin, M.D., with twenty-five contributing editors and consultants.

The *Guide* was endorsed by the American Medical Association, the American Academy of Family Physicians, the American Academy of Ophthalmology, the American Geriatric Society, and the American Society of Internal Medicine. A brief manual, *40 Commonly Asked Questions About Type II Diabetes (NIDDM)*, and a slide presentation prepared for use with the *Guide* completed the curriculum.

Participating in a nationwide teleconference, which was a feature of the program, were editors of the *Guide*, including Drs. Harold Rifkin, George F. Cahill, John A. Colwell, Ralph A. DeFronzo, Sherman M. Holvey, Edward S. Horton, Harold E. Lebovitz, Jerrold M. Olefsky, and Jay S. Skyler.

Outside consultants were used for preconference publicity and for planning the logistics of a meeting of this magnitude. ADA professionals prepared the materials and selected and trained the faculty. Selected members of the ADA staff were assigned to each site to provide any assistance necessary. On April 11, identical programs were delivered with precision and authority at each of the twenty-seven sites. Put together in the record time of nine months, the CEP was a stunning success. It was also a sterling example of support by the pharmaceutical industry; the entire cost of this exceptional program was underwritten by The Upjohn Company.

The Association At Mid-Decade

"All in all," said Executive Vice President Robert S. Bolan, Ph.D., in the 1985 Annual Report, "it has been an extremely challenging and rewarding year for volunteers and staff at all levels of the organization." The Association's commitment to research reached $5 million in fiscal year 1985. Public education was enhanced in the national media by distribution of public service announcements featuring Lee Iacocca, Lena Horne, and Sherman Helmsley. At the local level, affiliate and chapter volunteers not only helped place these announcements in the media, they also created wide audiences for two award-winning educational films, "Josh," which told the story of a small boy with diabetes, and "The Journey and the Dream," which served as inspiration for the title of this book. Professional education reached new heights when more than 2,700 diabetes professionals attended the 1985 Scientific Sessions.

About $20 million was raised from more than one million contributors in an extremely broad-based fund raising program, ranging from film premieres and treasure hunts to golf tournaments, conducted by affiliates and chapters.

Clearly, the Association was moving ahead rapidly and successfully. "The job is not yet done, but we trust you will be with us on the team until it is," wrote ADA President Karl E. Sussman, M.D., and Joseph H. Davis, Esq., in the same 1985 Annual Report. "We are absolutely convinced that affiliate and chapter volunteer efforts are indeed making a tremendous impact on improving the lives of people with diabetes today and bringing closer fulfillment of the promise of a healthier future for them tomorrow."

Pieces Of The Puzzle:
What We Knew About Diabetes

1980

With much fanfare, the Danish companies Novo Laboratories and Nordisk-USA introduce highly purified insulins in the United States. Almost simultaneously, Eli Lilly and Company announces its own line of similarly pure insulins.

Portable insulin pumps receive much attention in the press. But the large size is a major restraint to the portable pump's use.

Michael P. Czech, Ph.D., and colleagues locate the "second messenger" of insulin. This chemical agent facilitates the breakdown of glucose within the cell.

1981

Criteria for diagnosis of type I diabetes, type II diabetes, gestational diabetes, and impaired glucose tolerance are published in *Diabetes Care* (Vol 4. No. 2, 1981) by Irving L. Spratt, M.D., and C.R. Shuman of the ADA Statistics Committee.

Alyne Ricker, M.D., of the Joslin Diabetes Center and William L. Chick, M.D., of the University of Massachusetts, "microencapsulate" islet cells in a covering of polymeric beads. When implanted in the body, these beads permit free passage of glucose, oxygen, and nutrients, as well as the exit of insulin. Destruction of the islet cells by antibodies is prevented.

J. Dupre, M.D., of University Hospital in London, Ontario, and R. Assan, M.D., of Hopital Bichat in Paris show success with the immunosuppressive drug cyclosporin. A significant number of subjects with type I diabetes are able to cut down on their insulin or stop using it altogether. Both researchers urge more large-scale study, especially in lieu of the unwanted side effects of the drug.

Work continues with nasal insulin to help control blood sugar. Robert L. Silver, M.D., of Boston's Beth Israel Hospital, presenting at the 1981 Scientific Sessions, said he feels that nasal insulin may someday be a useful tool but will probably not entirely replace injections.

Penile prostheses—surgically implanted devices that mimic a normal erection—come into wide use for men suffering from diabetic impotence. A simple, nonsurgical device, developed by Perry Nadig, M.D., Richard Becker, M.D., and colleagues in San Antonio, the prosthesis consists of a clear plastic cylinder connected to a hand-operated vacuum pump.

1982

Human insulin produced by genetically altered bacteria is approved by the U.S. Food and Drug Administration on October 29, 1982. The new insulin (called Humulin) is manufactured by Eli Lilly and Company and is the first commercial product of recombinant DNA technology.

"The announcement of the availability in the United States of human insulin . . . is an exciting event in medicine," said ADA President Irving L. Spratt, M.D., (1982-83). "People with insulin-dependent diabetes mellitus will no longer need to rely on animal pancreases as the sole source of insulin."

Approval for a second human insulin, produced by altering purified pork insulin, is granted to Squibb-Novo soon after.

Australian researchers show that a substance known as an aldose reductase inhibitor can improve diabetic neuropathy in rats. Whether such medicines will be safe and effective for humans is still unknown.

Daniel H. Mintz, M.D., and colleagues at the University of Miami School of Medicine report they have found an antigen (tissue protein) that may trigger rejection of transplanted human islets. The antigen, called HLA-DR, is located on the walls of blood vessels in the implanted cells, but not on the beta cells. Based on this finding, the scientists predict that the removal of blood vessels from the implant before transplantation should help to prevent rejection.

1983

Two new oral agents enter the market. The new drugs, dubbed second-generation oral agents, are about 100 to 200 times stronger than the original four sulfonylureas. This means the user can take far smaller doses. In addition, the new drugs are cleared out of the blood fairly rapidly. The advantage of taking smaller doses is that some of the potential side effects could be reduced. There is no clear answer as to when, and in whom, the second-generation oral agents will be appropriate.

1984

Scientists use the immunosuppressive drug cyclosporin to prevent insulin-dependent diabetes in people susceptible to the disease.

1985

George Eisenbarth, M.D., Ph.D., of Harvard Medical School, discusses islet cell antibodies (ICAs) during the 45th Annual Scientific Sessions.

These substances in the blood tend to seek out and attach themselves to insulin-making beta cells. Researchers are not quite sure what ICAs do, but it appears that when someone has certain kinds of ICAs, type I diabetes is virtually inevitable. Dr. Eisenbarth and his colleagues, and other researchers, are testing the potential of ICA testing as a screening tool to identify people whose beta cells are in the process of being destroyed.

Chapter Eleven
Fulfilling Our Mission
1985-90

ADA Presidents

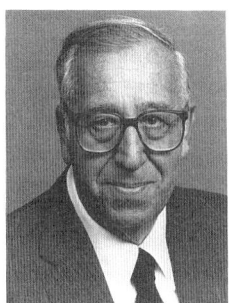
Harold Rifkin, M.D.
(1985-86)

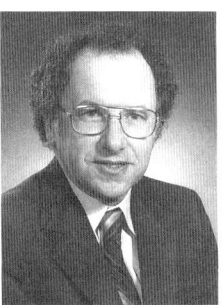
Daniel Porte, Jr., M.D.
(1986-87)

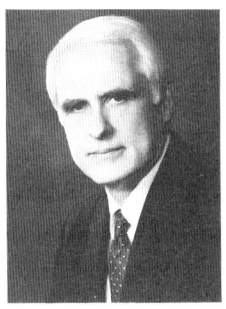
John A. Colwell, M.D.
(1987-88)

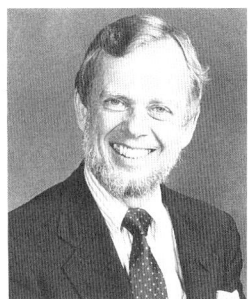
Charles M. Clark, Jr., M.D.
(1988-89)

ADA Chairmen of the Board

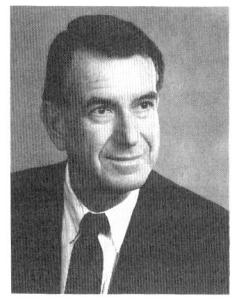
Sherman Holvey, M.D.
(1989-90)

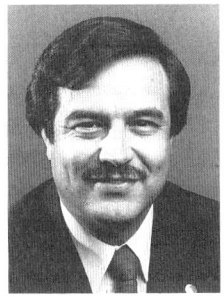
Henry M. Rivera
(1985-86)

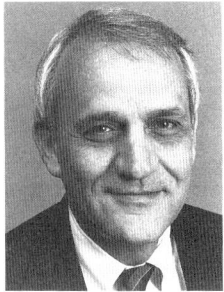
Sam A. Gallo
(1986-87)

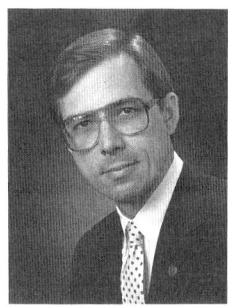
S. Douglas Dodd
(1987-88)

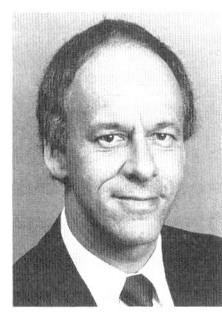
William A. Mamrack
(1988-89)

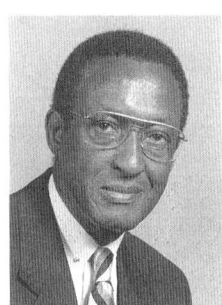
Sterling Tucker
(1989-90)

In January 1986, the space shuttle Challenger exploded just minutes after liftoff. Americans watched the televised launch in horror as six astronauts and a school teacher were killed. The event shocked the world and plunged the United States into a period of grief and soul-searching. A year later, in Iceland, a near thaw in the Soviet-American impasse over nuclear weapons was thwarted by "Star Wars," the theoretical space defense plan held dear by President Reagan. Surprisingly, four months later, Soviet General Secretary Mikhail Gorbachev announced his program of "glasnost" (which translates roughly as "openness"), raising new hope for some solution to the threat of nuclear weapons. In 1988, a tentative step was taken, when the Soviet Union and the United States signed a limited agreement on arms control. The threat of a Soviet/U.S. confrontation further lessened as mostly peaceful revolutions changed the communist face of Eastern Europe in 1989. Each day, it seemed, brought change and optimism.

In the mid-1980s, the American Diabetes Association expanded its international influence. ADA publications are distributed around the world, and monthly periodicals are mailed to 2,000 people or institutions outside the United States. More than 30 countries were represented at the 1989 Annual Meeting. There are more than 850 international professional section members. In addition, the Association has a close working relationship with diabetes associations in Mexico as well as Central and South America and supplies free copies of publications to leaders and offices in Latin America. In 1988, the Association welcomed a new affiliate in Puerto Rico into the ADA network. The affiliate quickly organized to raise funds and provide services to the island.

The American Diabetes Association came to play an increasingly important role in the International Diabetes Federation (IDF). The Association is now the largest member of the IDF and pays the largest amount of dues. The Association publishes the *IDF Bulletin*, a magazine that examines diabetes treatment in different environments and cultures, and is charged with planning and conducting the 14th IDF Congress, June 23-28, 1991. The American Diabetes Association is host for the North American Region, one of the seven regions of the IDF, which as of 1988, boasted 93 full and provisional member associations in 77 countries.

The Association's first Affiliate Volunteer Leadership Conference provided new affiliate leaders the opportunity to discuss plans and priorities for the coming year. And the first orientation program for new Board members was an overwhelming success.

As the decade came to a close, two important initiatives were announced: CURE: American's Fight Against Diabetes and the 50th Anniversary Campaign, led by former Federal Reserve Chairman Paul Volcker. Through these major donor projects, the Association hoped to raise the funds needed to ensure a future free of diabetes.

The National Institutes Of Health

In 1987, the National Institutes of Health (NIH) celebrated its 100th birthday, a century of science for health. The NIH is the U.S. government's principal medical research agency and one of five health agencies that make up the United States Public Health Service. Today, the NIH occupies more than 317 acres in Bethesda, Maryland, and employs about 15,000 people (researchers and staff) nationwide. Some 2,500 researchers work at the Bethesda campus.

The NIH funds nearly 40 percent of U.S. medical research, including more than 90 percent of diabetes research. More than 80 percent of the NIH budget supports scientists in universities, hospitals, and non-federal research institutes across the country. In all, about 1,200 institutions receive NIH funding.

But the NIH—the world's largest biomedical research organization—has come a long way from its humble beginnings. In 1887, infectious diseases such as yellow fever, cholera, and tuberculosis were major health threats in the United States. Because it was thought that immigrants and travelers were bringing these diseases into the country, the federal government attempted to stop these diseases at points of entry—for example, harbors. A laboratory for research on cholera and other infectious diseases was established in the Marine Hospital on Staten Island in New York. Dr. Joseph Kinyoun was the sole staff member of the single room that was called the National Laboratory of Hygiene. In 1891, the lab was renamed the Hygienic Laboratory and was moved to Washington, D.C.

In Washington, the Hygienic

Changes At The National Service Center

In January 1986, the Association opened its National Service Center in Alexandria, Virginia. The question of moving the national office from New York City had risen periodically over the years at Board meetings, but until 1984 it had always been tabled. Four years earlier, the American Diabetes Association had moved to 2 Park Avenue in New York City, with a lease expiring in the spring of 1987. Early in 1984, faced with diminishing space and rising rents in New York, a committee was formed to explore various cities that might be more financially advantageous. Dallas, St. Louis, Indianapolis, Atlanta, and the metropolitan area of Washington, D.C., were considered.

Located just outside of Washington, D.C., Alexandria was ultimately chosen because it offered the best environment for the interests of the Association. The city was close to Washington, D.C., and the federal government was becoming of increased importance to ADA goals; it had a community of other associations; and its location provided access to a good personnel market. What's more, Alexandria provided a very advantageous financing agreement for the Association. Through the purchase of industrial bonds financed by the City of Alexandria, the Association was able to purchase property adequate for its needs and located conveniently to both the Metro (the bus and subway system) and National Airport.

A firm experienced in office relocation was hired to study all aspects of the proposed move. ADA staff was given the choice of reimbursed relocation or a stay bonus for those who remained until the office officially closed. Approximately one-fifth of the staff elected to relocate. While the move was not completely painless, it was accomplished with a minimum of disruption in ADA services. The New York office closed for packing on Thursday, January 24, 1986, moved over the weekend, and opened for business in Alexandria on Monday, January 28.

To introduce the new ADA National Service Center at 1660 Duke Street in Alexandria, a gala open house was held March 9, 1987. A cold March rain coincided with the arrival of the guests at five in the afternoon, but did nothing to dampen the spirit of the occasion. Congressmen, government officials, representatives of voluntary health agencies, and community leaders gathered to see the new headquarters. They were greeted by past and present officers, affiliate volunteers, members of the ADA Board and national staff, ADA National Spokespersons Meredith Baxter Birney and David Birney, and National Bike-Ride Plus Chairman

Laboratory became the National Institute of Health. Mr. and Mrs. Luke Wilson offered to donate 45 acres of their Bethesda estate to the NIH. The offer was accepted, and in 1938, the Institute moved to its current location. The Wilsons later donated additional land, and the NIH also bought adjacent land, increasing the Institute's acreage. As the NIH grew, so did its name. In 1948, in recognition of the Institute's many units, the NIH's name was changed to the plural form: the National Institutes of Health.

Most NIH-sponsored research—into diabetes and other illnesses—is "basic," as opposed to "applied." Basic research focuses on normal aspects of biological processes (for example, the structure of the cell). Applied research uses information obtained in basic research for a specific purpose. Applied research is the type most often used by scientists at pharmaceutical and biomedical engineering companies. In general, the findings of basic research make applied research possible. (For example, the basic research on the genetic makeup of human insulin was largely funded by the NIH; private companies used this information to develop—and sell—the first human insulin.)

The NIH branch that supports research on diabetes was established in 1950 as the National Institute of Arthritis and Metabolic Diseases (NIAMD). In 1972, the name was changed to the National Institute of Arthritis, Metabolic, and Digestive Diseases (NIAMDD), then in 1981, to the National Institute of Arthritis, Diabetes, and Digestive and Kidney Diseases (NIADDK). In 1986, the NIADDK became the National Institute of Diabetes and Digestive and Kidney Diseases

Christopher Atkins. The open house was funded by generous contributions from pharmaceutical companies and friends of the Association and has a place in ADA history as a unique combination of conviviality and good public relations.

National Standards for Diabetes Education

Assuring quality diabetes education for every individual in the United States required rigorous, yet practical, standards. To come up with such standards, in 1983 the National Diabetes Advisory Board (NDAB), following a mandate from Congress, set up a committee to develop and test program standards, which might lead to a national quality assurance plan. To provide a broad-based coalition of experts, the committee included representatives from the entire diabetes community, both public and private. Dorothea Sims and Nina Berlin were appointed co-chairpersons of the steering committee of the National Diabetes Advisory Board.

By 1984, a trial list of standards and review criteria had been developed (and published in *Diabetes Care*, Vol. 7:1, 1984). It was time for a nationwide pilot study to evaluate them. More than 200 patient education programs throughout the United States completed the review process and filled out detailed questionnaires. Responses were carefully reviewed and compared. The Association helped provide pilot test sites for the study. The pilot study showed the need for an official organization to conduct a recognition process and to award recognition to programs meeting the standards.

In January 1986, the National Coalition for Recognition of Diabetes Patient Education Programs (NACOR) was established. The purpose of the national coalition—an independent umbrella group—was to establish an objective review process that would provide recognition of facilities meeting NDAB standards. The American Diabetes Association objected to the creation of a new organization solely for the purpose of recognizing education programs, saying that it was unnecessary and costly, and declined to participate. The ADA Board felt that the American Diabetes Association had both the capability and status to involve all members of the diabetes community and to implement such a program itself. Accordingly, the Association went forward with its plans. In January 1987, NACOR, unwilling to continue without the Association, voluntarily discontinued operations, and the ADA program geared up to serve the entire diabetes community.

(NIDDK).

In the 1950s, NIAMD expanded its programs. The Institute's first grants to researchers were approved, a clinical research center was opened, and Arthur Kornberg, M.D., former chief of the Institute's Enzyme and Metabolism Section, won the Nobel Prize for the first successful synthesis of nucleic acids. In the 1960s, the NIAMD continued to increase its research activity by establishing the Intramural Research Program in Phoenix, Arizona, to study Southwestern Native American populations. The Institute also established the National Pituitary Agency to increase the availability of growth hormone. Marshall W. Nirenberg, M.D., an NIAMD scientist, won the Nobel Prize for his work in partially cracking the genetic code.

In the 1970s, the NIH expanded the resources it devoted to diabetes. A national commission was appointed to develop a long-range plan to combat diabetes. The establishment of Diabetes Research and Training Centers was authorized, and a clearinghouse for information on diabetes was established. In the 1980s, the NIH has continued to devote increased resources to diabetes. The NIH sponsors a variety of diabetes research. A prime example is the Diabetes Control and Complications Trial (DCCT)—a large-scale clinical trial designed to determine whether maintaining near-normal blood-glucose levels will prevent or delay complications of diabetes. NIH researchers are exploring a number of other key questions in diabetes, such as how obesity leads to the development of type II diabetes, how the immune system turns against itself in type I diabetes, and how the success of pancreas and islet cell transplants can be improved.

Rita Nemchik, R.N., M.S., was chosen to be the first chairman of the ADA Committee on Recognition. Members of that committee included Deborah Hinnen, R.N.; Marvin Levin, M.D.; Florence Ruhland, R.N.; Patricia Schultz, R.N.; Irving Spratt, M.D.; and Linda Hurwitz, R.N., M.S. The committee set about determining the best way to set up the recognition process for quality programs.

In a very short time, the committee came up with standards for the recognition process. The National Standards For Diabetes Patient Education and ADA's Review Criteria based on the pilot study were published in *Diabetes Care* in 1986.

The ADA Recognition Program evaluates diabetes education programs across the nation and awards recognition to those that meet ADA's high standards. By June of 1987, as the program geared up, more than 2,000 requests for information on the Recognition Program were received, and 12 programs were recognized. Addressing the ADA's Central Council in June 1987, ADA President Daniel Porte, Jr., M.D., (1986-87) said, "ADA recognition will give professionals a yardstick to measure quality, and help patients identify programs that meet the National Standards." He went on to say that insurance companies had indicated that this process would be a major step in obtaining third-party reimbursement, and to that end, the Association would advise insurers, and state and federal agencies of programs that had been recognized.

The first ADA recognized diabetes education program was at the Diabetes Treatment Center at Georgetown University in Washington, D.C., in May 1987. As of March 1, 1990, 104 programs from 35 states and the District of Columbia had achieved ADA recognition. An additional 51 programs had submitted applications that were in review. Fifty trained reviewers from a cross section of disciplines supported the Recognition Program.

Though some have criticized the review criteria as too restrictive, ADA has basically adhered to the National Standards formulated in 1983. Recognition is based on meeting criteria for ten standards. In summary, they are:

- *Needs assessment.* The program should be flexible enough to meet the needs of the people with diabetes that it serves.

- *Planning.* The program should have a plan that sets goals, establishes teaching methods, and set procedures for patient follow-up. This planning should be developed with the input of patients.

- *Program management.* The program should be effectively managed, with clear lines of authority and communication between an advisory committee and the program coordinator.

- *Communication/coordination.* There should be regular contact between staff and patients.

- *Patient access.* The program should provide information to the community about what the diabetes education program offers and how to enroll.

- *Content/curriculum.* Instructional materials and complete curriculum should be appropriate for each patient and should be reviewed and updated periodically.

- *Instructors.* Instructors should be skilled health-care professionals with recent experience and training in both diabetes and educational principles.

- *Follow-up services.* Such services should include supplemental education, written communication and ongoing interaction between primary care giver and patient, and referral to community resources.

- *Evaluation.* Evaluation should include periodic review of the program and of the patient's progress toward good diabetes management.

- *Documentation.* Program planning and evaluation should be documented. Information about the patient's diabetes education experience should appear in the medical record.

Nutrition Task Forces

Acting on the recommendations of the Task Force on Sucrose, the Executive Committee had appointed a new task force in 1984 to revise the 1979 "Principles of Nutrition and Dietary Recommendations for Patients with Diabetes Mellitus" and the *Exchange Lists for Meal Planning*. Members of the Task Force on Nutrition and Exchange Lists were charged with reviewing a wealth of new information about the effects of diet on the blood-glucose and blood-fat levels of people with diabetes. Questions needed to be answered about the optimal carbohydrate, protein, and fat intake for people with diabetes; the use of fiber; the role of the glycemic index and its relation to food exchanges; and the value of eicosapentanoic acid, or fish oil.

A panel of experts, chaired by Aaron Vinik, M.D., and assisted by Drs. Stuart Brink, Dorothy Gohdes, Barbara Hansen, Edward Horton, Ahmed Kissebah, David Jenkins, and dietitians Phyllis Crapo, Marion

Albert Renold: Mentor To Many

Albert Renold—scholar, traveler, linguist—was one of the world's great diabetologists and researchers. Over a 40-year career, Dr. Renold's scientific contributions covered a

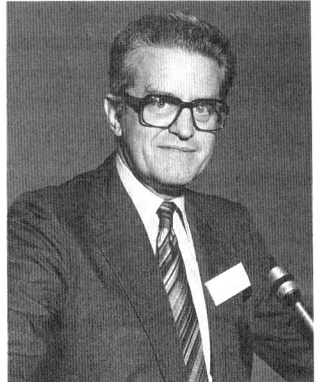

Prof. Albert E. Renold

wide range. He is best remembered as the first man to demonstrate, in 1950, a direct action of insulin on adipose (fatty) tissue. His discoveries led to modern medicine's increased understanding of insulin-dependent (type I) and non-insulin-dependent (type II) diabetes. Dr. Renold also developed a bioassay procedure for measuring plasma insulin, which was used worldwide for many years.

Diabetes was Dr. Renold's field from the start. Born in Karlsruhe, Switzerland in 1923, he received his medical degree in 1947 from the University of Zurich. In his thesis, he examined the biochemical and metabolic aspects of alloxan diabetes. While writing the paper, he was inspired by the work of Drs. Elliott P. Joslin and Alexander Marble of Boston. Upon graduation, he determined to join them, and went to the Harvard Medical Center. There, he spent the first 15 years of his research career.

He became director of the Baker Clinic Research Labora-

Franz, Andrea Lasichak, and Judith Wylie-Rosett, deliberated for two years and published "Nutritional Recommendations and Principles for Individuals with Diabetes Mellitus: 1986," in *Diabetes Care*, Vol. 10:1, 1987.

The recommendations stated that:

1) The amount of carbohydrate in the diet should be liberalized, ideally composing up to 55-60 percent of the total calories, and individualized, with the amount dependent on the impact on blood-glucose and blood-fat levels and individual eating patterns.

2) Foods containing unrefined carbohydrate with fiber should be substituted for highly refined carbohydrates, which are low in fiber.

3) In some individuals, modest amounts of sucrose and other refined sugars may be acceptable, depending on the degree of diabetes control and body weight.

The task force also recommended that people with diabetes monitor their protein intake; that they work to lower their total intake of fats, especially saturated fats; that they watch their salt intake; and that various nutritive and nonnutritive sweeteners were acceptable for people with diabetes.

The task force requested that a committee composed of representatives from both The American Dietetic Association and the American Diabetes Association be formed to revise the *Exchange Lists for Meal Planning*. This expert committee, composed of Patricia Barr and Marion Franz, R.D., M.S., chairman; Harold Holler, R.D.; Margaret Powers, R.D., M.S.; Madelyn Wheeler, R.D., M.S.; and Judith Wylie-Rosett, Ed.D., R.D., produced a revised version of *Exchange Lists for Meal Planning*, which was published in October 1986. Members also produced a pamphlet, "Healthy Food Choices," which is a "survival-level" introduction to the more complicated exchange system. In 1989, the *Exchange Lists* were again updated and revised.

With regard to noncaloric sweeteners, a task force of the Council on Nutritional Science and Metabolism made recommendations in 1987. Council Chairperson Frank Nuttall, M.D., and task force chairperson, Phyllis Crapo, R.D., with help from members of the task force, prepared the "Position Statement: Use of Noncaloric Sweeteners," which was published in *Diabetes Care* (Vol. 10:4, 1987). It states: "Based on available evidence, the American Diabetes Association finds the use of the two commercially available noncaloric sweeteners saccharin and aspartame to be acceptable . . . the dietary needs of people with diabetes vary, and the use of any sweetener should be individualized

tory, later renamed for Dr. Joslin. He worked closely with Joslin, who transmitted to him his concern for the well-being of patients with diabetes.

In 1963, Dr. Renold returned to Switzerland as professor at the Faculty of Medicine of the University of Geneva. He established the Institut de Biochimie Clinique in an old Geneva villa. It was the fulfillment of a lifelong ambition.

At the institute, Dr. Renold created a unique research atmosphere. Many outstanding scientists interested in diabetes had already been trained by Dr. Renold in Boston. With the creation of his Institute, he was able to exert an even greater influence on diabetes-related research around the world. Generations of scientists—many of them ADA members—came to Geneva as research fellows or as visiting professors. They all appreciated the unique freedom given them to carry out their investigations.

Dr. Renold was elected president of the International Diabetes Federation (IDF) in 1975. He guided the IDF through a time of great change. During his term, the organization formulated new bylaws redirecting its structure and activities. He was elected IDF's Honorary President in 1985.

Albert Renold died suddenly on March 21, 1988. He had only recently returned to work on the question of immune mechanisms in diabetes. The world of science mourned his passing.

with consideration to overall diet and nutritional adequacy."

The Nationwide Comprehensive Long-Range Plan

The Association's need for long-range planning became apparent in the early 1970s. By 1973, the Association's Executive Committee had appointed a Committee for Long-Range Plans charged with the responsibility of reviewing and recommending financial needs for programs in patient, professional, and public education, detection, and research.

While the Association had developed an organizational plan for the future in 1979, it suffered from several major failings. Writing in *Association Management* magazine in August 1988, Executive Vice President Robert Bolan, Ph.D., and James F. Wolf associate professor at Virginia Polytechnic Institute & State University, commented that the 1979 plan: ". . . did not rank priorities, point to critical strategies, or translate into operating budgets. In addition, the plan was not comprehensive. ADA derives the majority of its income from the separately incorporated state affiliates. A few state affiliates had long-range plans; most did not. Furthermore, no relationship existed between the ADA national plan and the state plans."

The challenge facing Association leadership was to devise a long-range plan that would include the diverse priorities within the organization. The aim was threefold: to produce a plan that was comprehensive including all facets of the Association, as well as each of the affiliates' structures; to represent a consensus; and to reflect accurately the challenges that the Association would face in the next five years.

A Consensus Development Conference held in December 1987 was the key to the plan's development and ensured that the broadest spectrum of Association interests were voiced. At the Consensus Conference in Dallas, 200 ADA volunteers met to draft a statement that would sum up the concerns of the Association's 225,000 members about how and where its resources should be spent. This was no small feat considering the Association's great diversity. At the end of two-and-a-half days of discussion, participants emerged with a statement that set clear goals for the ADA's future. The Consensus Development Statement was used as a blueprint for crafting the Association's Nationwide Comprehensive Long-Range Plan.

In January 1988, the Consensus Statement developed in Dallas was formally presented to executive di-

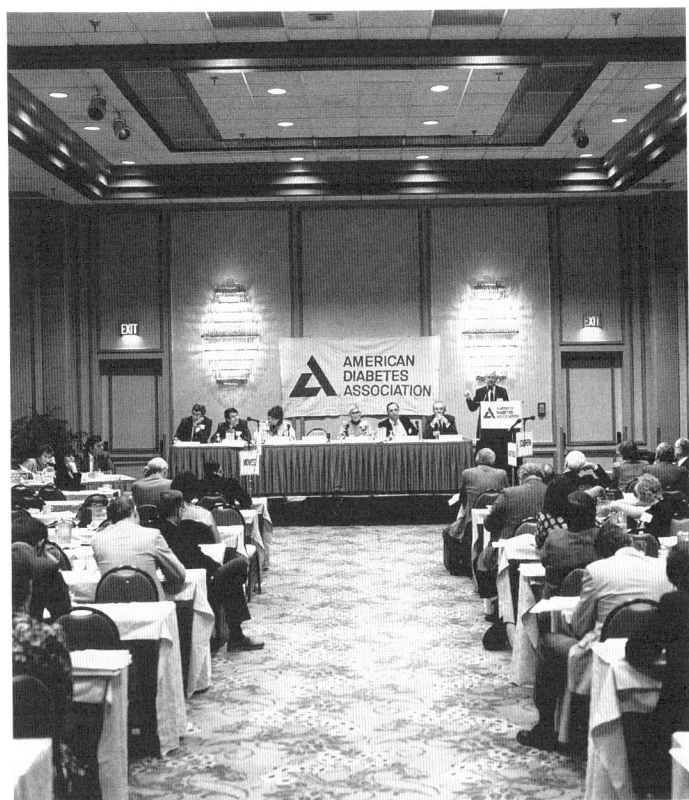

At the Consensus Development Conference, participants from 45 states offered their views on the course the Association should follow.

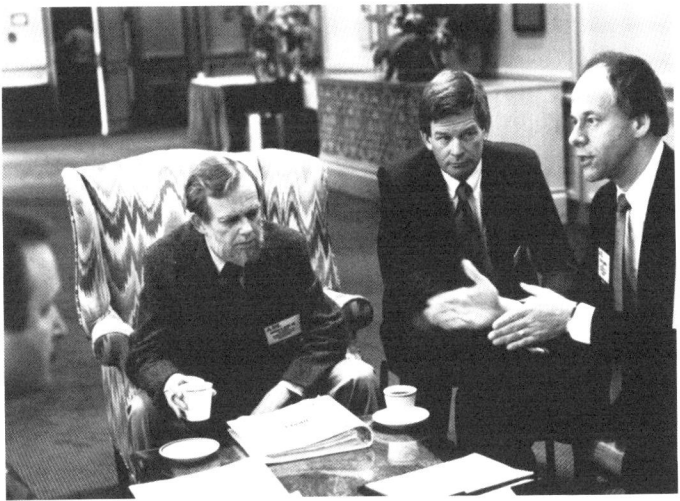

Steering Committee Chairman William A. Mamrack (right) makes a point with (from left) committee member Arnold Bereson, Committee Vice Chairman Charles M. Clark, Jr., M.D., and committee member Todd E. Leigh. They are discussing a draft of the Consensus Statement.

rectors of ADA affiliates, to ADA professional section councils, and to other groups within the Association. These groups had a chance to comment on the document and offer their input on the drafting of the long-range plan. In February 1988, the first draft of that plan was circulated to affiliates, committees, and councils. In March, the ADA's national committees gave their input and the Association's Board of Directors received a status report. The plan was fine-tuned and on June 11, 1988, it was approved by the Association's Board of Directors.

This first Nationwide Comprehensive Long-Range Plan charts the Association's course over a five-year period, from 1989 to 1993. ADA President John A. Colwell, M.D., Ph.D., (1987-88) characterized this plan as ". . . the most important thing . . . in my term as president." He added that the plan, which was developed with maximal input from all segments of the Association, "allows the National Service Center and the affiliates to move together to continue to expand the impressive growth of this Association."

To update and carry forward the plan, an annual review process has been established.

Resource Allocation

The Nationwide Comprehensive Long-Range Plan for the first time provided a blueprint for the nationwide work of the American Diabetes Association. However, the plan did not fully address the issue of how to set priorities and allocate resources among the Association's many programs and activities. As a result, differences of opinion emerged among various ADA constituencies about how the funds raised by affiliates and the national organization should be allocated.

This situation was exacerbated by the fact that growth in public support income had slowed as the Association faced increasing competition for the charitable dollar. The debate centered around the ADA research program, which was designated in the long-range plan to receive a full 30 percent of the total public support generated by affiliates and the national organization.

At the June 1988 Annual Meeting, the Central Council passed a resolution calling for establishment of a task force to study the Association's current system for dividing money between the national organization and affiliates and for supporting the ADA research program. The resolution was adopted a day later by the Board of Directors, and the Task Force on Resource Allocation was appointed soon after. Chaired by Joseph Davis, ADA chairman of the Board (1984-1985), the task force met several times over the next twelve months to consider different resource allocation models.

The resource allocation plan proposed by the task force was widely circulated before it was formally presented to the Central Council at the June 1989 Annual Meeting. It was clear from the discussion that the plan had failed to gain acceptance among a majority of ADA constituencies.

The Central Council passed a resolution calling for continued and expanded examination of the resource allocation issues facing the Association. The resolution also requested the Board of Directors to reconstitute the task force with expanded representation from the affiliate leadership and affiliate executive directors.

The next day, the Board appointed the new task force, known as Task Force Two, to try once again to resolve the issues of resource allocation. In August, the task force, chaired by William Mamrack, ADA chairman of the Board (1988-1989), completed a first-draft proposal that was widely circulated throughout the Association. The proposal was modified based on input received and submitted to the Board of Directors in October 1989. The Board adopted the Task Force Two proposal, effective July 1, 1990.

The proposal made adjustments to existing policies governing the division of income between affiliates and the national organization and how public support income is accounted for. It was hoped that the Task Force Two proposal would restore stability to the ADA Research Program, while providing for continued delivery of services by affiliates and chapters.

ADA Position Statements, Technical Reviews, And Consensus Statements

Between the years 1985 and 1990, the Association acted to produce position statements, technical reviews, and consensus statements, which served as tools to improve the quality of life for those living with diabetes.

Position statements are an official point of view or belief of the American Diabetes Association. Position statements are issued on scientific or medical issues related to diabetes mellitus. They are published in ADA journals and other scientific/medical publications. Position statements must be reviewed and approved by the Committee on Professional Practice and then by the Executive Committee of the Board.

Position statements issued or reviewed during this time period include:

The International Diabetes Federation

In June 1949, the first international meeting on diabetes was held in Brussels. The three-day program included sessions for physicians and laypersons, as well as discussions between the two groups. This was the first international medical meeting to include laypersons as active participants and it established an international network of physicians concerned about diabetes—a network that would eventually form the International Diabetes Federation (IDF).

Due to the success of this first meeting, another international meeting was held in Amsterdam in 1950. The International Federation of Diabetic Associations was established at the Amsterdam meeting, laying the groundwork for the IDF. The principal goal of the IDF's founders was to improve the lives of people with diabetes throughout the world. Today's IDF members also hold this as their primary goal.

Since 1952, IDF has held an International Congress every three years. The number of participants in these meetings has steadily increased. In 1955, there were 500 participants at the Congress in Cambridge, and in 1973, more than 3,000 people from more than 50 countries attended the Congress in Brussels. More than 4,500 people attended the 13th IDF Congress in Sydney in 1988. The IDF also holds regional congresses periodically. In addition the IDF holds joint meetings with the World Health Organization on a periodic basis.

The IDF provides information about the latest developments in diabetes care worldwide to all people in diabetes research, treatment, and education, on all aspects of diabetes, both

- "Nutritional Recommendations and Principles for Individuals with Diabetes Mellitus" (originally approved 10/86);
- "Use of Noncaloric Sweeteners" (originally approved 3/87);
- "Use of Jet Injectors" (originally passed 6/84, reviewed 9/87);
- "Blood-Glucose Control in Diabetes" (originally approved 1975, reviewed 6/87);
- "Bedside Blood-Glucose Monitoring in Hospitals" (originally approved 10/85, reviewed 9/87);
- "Responsible Use of Animals in Research" (originally approved 3/85, reviewed 10/87);
- "Standards of Medical Care for Patients with Diabetes Mellitus" (originally approved 10/88);
- "Eye Care Guidelines for Patients with Diabetes Mellitus" (originally approved 6/88);
- "Concurrent Care" (approved 12/88);
- "Management of Diabetes in Correctional Institutions" (approved 4/89);
- "Use of Human Tissue in Research" (originally passed 12/86, reviewed 4/89);
- "Office Guide to Diagnosis and Classification of Diabetes Mellitus and Other Categories of Glucose Intolerance" (originally approved 1/80, reviewed 4/89);
- "Insulin Administration" (approved 10/89);
- "Continuous Subcutaneous Insulin Infusion" (approved 6/85, reviewed 1989);
- "Third-Party Reimbursement for Outpatient Diabetes Education and Counseling" (originally approved 6/84, revised and approved 10/89); and
- "Screening for Diabetes" (approved 4/89).
- "Gestational Diabetes Mellitus" (originally approved 3/86, reviewed 10/89)

This last position statement advocated screening for gestational diabetes in all pregnancies. "[This statement] has served as an authoritative catalyst in making this a part of public policy," said former ADA President Norbert Freinkel, M.D., 1979 and 1984 chairman of the ADA-International Workshop-Conference on Gestational Diabetes. Gestational diabetes affects

through its meetings and its publications. The *IDF Bulletin*, a magazine published three times a year, examines diabetes treatment in different socioeconomic environments and cultures, previews work in progress, and reports study results from around the world. The *IDF News Bulletin*, a newsletter printed in the intervals between the *IDF Bulletin*, provides an update on events and meetings affecting diabetes research and practice. The IDF also publishes reports, reprints, and resource books, such as *The World Book of Diabetes in Practice* (three volumes) and the *IDF Directory*.

As of 1988, the IDF was comprised of national diabetes associations or sections for diabetes in 76 countries and had more than 1,300 members. In 1991, the American Diabetes Association will host the 14th IDF Congress in Washington, D.C. ADA President Harold Rifkin, M.D., (1985-86) is serving as chairman of the 14th International Diabetes Federation Congress Organizing Committee. He has chaired numerous IDF committees, including the North American Region Committee and the IDF Committee on Professional Education. One IDF activity that Dr. Rifkin thought particularly valuable is the funding of scholarships and fellowships for advanced training of M.D.s and Ph.D.s. By funding such activities, Dr. Rifkin said, IDF has helped advance diabetes training worldwide.

60,000-90,000 women each year in the United States.

"Once again, the unique stature of the ADA has enabled it to impact on nationwide patterns of medical practice by a single decisive enunciation of the 'ADA posture.' It is a heady position of power—and an awesome responsibility—that the ADA has achieved. It makes all of us feel that our lengthy preparatory labors in the ADA vineyards have not been in vain—and that the wines to come will all be of vintage quality," noted Dr. Freinkel.

Technical Reviews are a balanced review and analysis of the literature and state of the art on a scientific or medical topic related to diabetes. Technical reviews are published in ADA journals and other scientific/medical publications as appropriate. A technical review is approved by the Committee on Professional Practice and subsequently by the Executive Committee of the Board of Directors. In March 1988, the Association approved the "Technical Review on Jet Injectors."

Consensus Statements are the result of a comprehensive examination by a panel of experts on a scientific or medical issue related to diabetes. A consensus conference is convened for the purpose of presenting expert opinion on an issue from which a consensus statement is developed. Unlike position statements and technical reviews, consensus statements are not subject to subsequent review or approval. Consensus statements do not represent official ADA opinion. Instead the statements represent the expert panel's collective analysis, evaluation, and opinion.

The first consensus conference in the history of the Association was convened in 1986. By then, self-monitoring of blood glucose (SMBG) had become basic to good diabetes care. In view of its widespread use, the American Diabetes Association, together with the Centers for Disease Control, the Food and Drug Administration, and the National Institute of Arthritis, Diabetes, and Digestive and Kidney Diseases, sponsored a consensus development conference, held November 17-19, 1986. The purpose of the conference was to evaluate medical and technical issues and the impact of SMBG on diabetes care from the perspective of professionals and consumers.

The "Consensus Statement on Self-Monitoring of Blood Glucose" (*Diabetes Care*, Vol. 10:1, 1987), which was a product of that conference, described SMBG as "an exciting addition to our armamentarium to ensure the effective management of patients with diabetes." The statement included nine recommendations

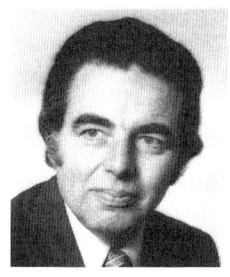

A Noted Passing
On September 5, 1989, ADA President Norbert Freinkel, M.D., (1977-78) died suddenly at age 63. At the time of his death, Dr. Freinkel was C. F. Kettering Professor of Medicine at the Northwestern University Medical School in Chicago, Illinois.

Dr. Freinkel, whose distinguished career spanned four decades, received his medical degree from New York University College of Medicine in 1949. He spent 10 years as a faculty member of the Harvard Medical School, and in 1966 he assumed the position of chief of the Section of Endocrinology, Metabolism, and Nutrition and as the C.F. Kettering Professor of Medicine at Northwestern University Medical School in Chicago. His vigor, enthusiasm, and superb scientific contribution led to the creation of the interdisciplinary Center for Endocrinology, Metabolism, and Nutrition and ultimately to the founding of the Diabetes in Pregnancy Center.

Investigation of metabolic regulation in normal and diabetic pregnancies was the main focus of Dr. Freinkel's research and clinical activities. His work directly led to new strategies and approaches to the management of diabetes in pregnancy. These nutritional and therapeutic programs have become the standard throughout the world and have led to a significant reduction in perinatal mortality in the babies of mothers with diabetes. Dr. Freinkel elucidated the meta-

that would ensure accuracy and precision of data, quality control, and future benefits in diabetes care.

Other consensus statements during this time period included: "Diabetic Neuropathy" (1988) and "Role of Cardiovascular Risk Factors in Prevention and Treatment of Macrovascular Disease in Diabetes" (1989).

More Professional Councils

In 1987, four new professional section councils were formed: the Council on Education, the Council on Complications, the Council on Foot Care, and the Council on Exercise. The Council on Education concerns itself with sound educational principles and practices, as well as with the problems facing diabetes educators and their patients. The Council on Complications provides a venue for discussion among ADA professional section members interested in microvascular, macrovascular, neuropathic, and other complications of diabetes. ADA's Council on Foot Care provides standards for foot care and develops programs in foot-care management for health-care professionals and people with diabetes. Finally, ADA's Council on Exercise brings together professionals interested in the benefits, risks, and practical problems experienced by people with diabetes when they exercise. This council also works to foster research related to diabetes and physical exercise.

Each of the nine ADA professional section councils

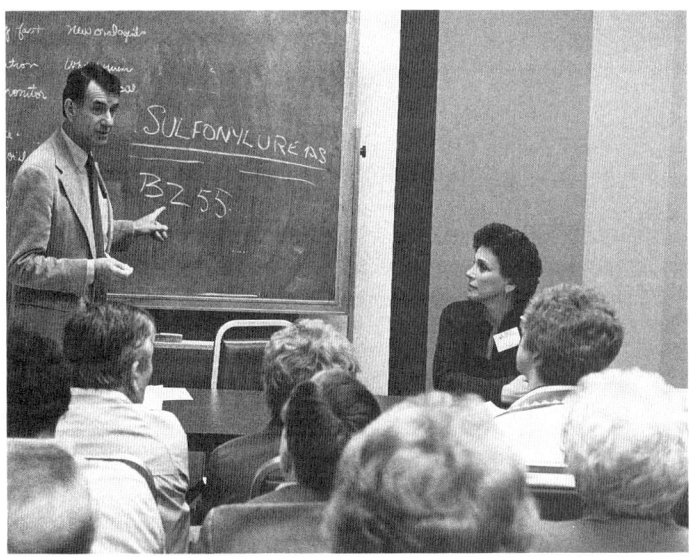

The Association continued its ongoing program of professional education.

bolic basis for the congenital malformations among infants of mothers with diabetes. As a result, the incidence of birth defects among infants born to mothers with diabetes has been reduced almost to the level of risk faced in normal pregnancy.

In later years, Dr. Freinkel focused on the identification and understanding of gestational diabetes. He spearheaded the establishment of the International Workshop Conferences on Gestational Diabetes, and served as co-chairman and chairman, respectively, of the first and second International Workshops. At the time of his death, Dr. Freinkel was chairman-designate for the 1990 Workshop.

Dr. Freinkel received numerous awards and honors during his illustrious career, including the Lilly Award in 1966 and the Banting Medal for Distinguished Scientific Achievement in 1980.

His close friend and colleague Boyd Metzger, M.D., said, "Surely [Dr. Freinkel] was one of the scientific giants of our time and we are tempted to lament for the even greater accomplishments that might have been and over the unfinished manuscripts, and still-open and partially filled notebooks of data and for the new ideas still germinating. However, those of us who had the privilege of be part of his life or even to know his warm smile or jovial greeting share a wonderful heritage which we will cherish and not forget."

contributes to the work of the Association by developing scientific programs for ADA's annual Postgraduate Course and/or Scientific Sessions; periodically reviewing Association medical and scientific policies or position statements that relate to the council's area of expertise; and recommending new policies and statements when necessary.

In noting the changes he'd seen in the Association over the years, ADA President Harold Rifkin, M.D., (1985-86) pointed to the professional section councils as one of the "extraordinary opportunities provided by the Association—a forum for discussion among physicians, diabetes educators, dietitians, other health professionals involved in diabetes care."

ADA Minority Initiative

In 1986, researchers with the National Diabetes Data Group published *Diabetes in America*. Among the disturbing findings were data on the rate of diabetes among minority groups. The publication estimated that diabetes is 30 to 40 percent more common among Blacks than Whites. More than 3 percent of the 27 million Black Americans have diabetes that they know about, while an even greater number—about 4.4 percent, have diabetes and don't know it. Furthermore, Black Americans with diabetes appear to face a greater risk of complications. Among Mexican Americans, 10 to 12 percent have diabetes, and the disease is 2.8 times more common in Mexican American men than in White men. Diabetes appears to be a more common cause of death among Hispanic Americans than among Americans in general. For Native Americans, diabetes and obesity have reached epidemic proportions among many tribes. An incredible 50 percent of all Pima Indians over the age of 35 have diabetes—the highest rate known for any population in the world.

In response to these findings, ADA redoubled its efforts to reach out to minority group members with diabetes. In 1986, the ADA Board of Directors was in touch with key members of the congressional Black and Hispanic caucuses, seeking ways to help those leaders work toward improving the health of their minority constituents. The ADA's public awareness campaign targeted minorities for projects such as Spanish-language public service announcements for print and broadcast media.

The Association provided support for the passage of the Indian Health Care Amendment Act of 1987. Authorized within this Act was Title VIII—Diabetes Prevention and Control Findings and Purpose. This title aimed to broaden the research program of the Department of Health and Human Services relating to diabetes and its complications among Native Americans. In addition, the title strengthened the efforts of the Indian Health Service (IHS) for the treatment of diabetes. A program was implemented for the prevention and control of diabetes and its complications on each Indian reservation and for each Alaskan native village, including five centers of excellence for diabetes care and education programs. The Centers for Excellence program was designed to develop "culturally acceptable" methods for bringing diabetes prevention and treatment services to Native American populations.

In 1987, ADA volunteers continued to focus their energies on the problem of diabetes in minority populations, and the ADA's Task Force on Minority Initiatives was created. Chaired by Jaime Davidson, M.D., of the Texas Affiliate, members of the 1987 task forced included: Dorothy Gohdes, M.D., program director of the Indian Health Service, Carlos Solis, an attorney and member of the California Affiliate, Bronna Lipton, New York Downstate Affiliate, Lillian Tom-Orme, R.N., of the Utah Affiliate, LaDonna Harris of the Washington, D.C. Area Affiliate, and Dolores Gibson of the New Mexico Affiliate. Sterling Tucker, of Washington, D.C., served as Minority Initiative Chair in 1988. Coordinating and chairing the task force's efforts for 1989-90 was P. Preston Reynolds, M.D., Ph.D., of the Greater Philadelphia Affiliate.

The task force works to identify and develop strategies to strengthen the Association's response to diabetes among minorities. In 1987-88, for example, the task force distributed materials on diabetes among minority populations to ADA affiliates, assisting them in developing special outreach programs of public awareness and patient education. Information sent included statistical data, "Diabetes Favors Minorities" public awareness posters, and Spanish-language public service announcements. The task force also worked with ADA's Spanish-Language Materials Editorial Board to help develop patient education materials in Spanish.

Under the leadership of ADA President Charles M. Clark, Jr., M.D., (1988-89) and Chairman of the Board William A. Mamrack, the Association accelerated even further its outreach to minority and underserved populations. The Association worked closely with Representative Albert G. Bustamante, of Texas, to design a bill amending the Public Health Service Act to establish a program for the prevention and control of diabetes and related complications. Jaime Davidson, M.D., in a press conference with Representative

Bustamante, announced the introduction of the bill, to be known as the Diabetes Prevention Act. A hearing on the bill would likely occur in the spring of 1990.

Also in 1989, the Association played an important role in securing five additional model Centers for Excellence, designed to bring diabetes prevention and treatment services to Native American populations. Congress passed new language for the five additional model centers and increased the budget for fiscal year 1990 by $1.5 million, as requested by the Association. A total of $7 million was needed to fully establish the centers.

ADA's Minority Initiative is a major effort to address the serious health problem presented by diabetes in communities that are too often medically underserved. The Minority Initiative works to create networks between the Association and other minority organizations to identify both the diabetes-related needs of minority populations and to help develop program ideas in conjunction with minority communities themselves.

The American Diabetes Alert: A New Phase in Public Awareness

For a number of years, the Committee on Communications had struggled with the idea of establishing a single day when the entire country would participate in an activity that would cause people to think about diabetes. There was a desire to do for diabetes what the Great American Smokeout had done for lung cancer.

In 1986, the committee settled on a "Diabetes

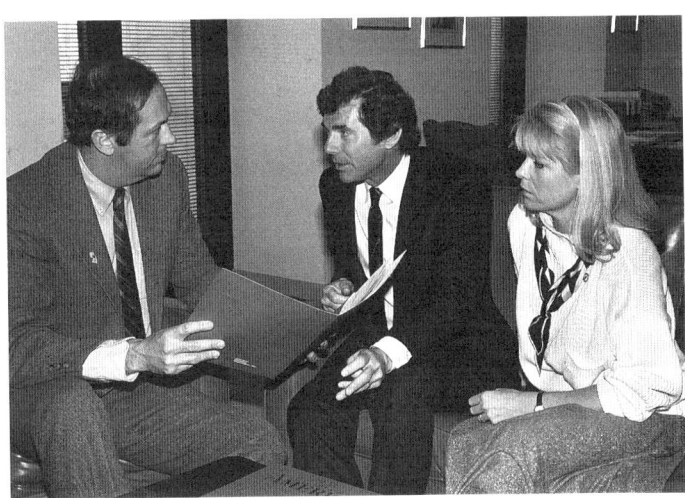

National Campaign Co-Chairpersons David Birney and Meredith Baxter Birney with Senator Bill Bradley, of New Jersey.

Awareness Day," to be held March 12, 1987. March was chosen primarily for two reasons. First, an awareness day in March would coincide with ADA Board and committee meetings scheduled to be held in Washington, D.C. This would help ensure that even if nothing happened elsewhere in the country, at least a few hundred ADA volunteers would be on Capitol Hill, calling on their federal legislators as a part of Diabetes Awareness Day. Second, March was far enough from November—National Diabetes Month—to help make the point that diabetes is a year-round disease and deserves the public's attention year-round.

However, little happened on Diabetes Awareness Day. This can largely be explained by the fact that the program was put together very late in the year and very quickly and only seven affiliates participated. There hadn't been time to develop an activity that could be conducted nationwide. So, the committee went back to the drawing board and worked on finding such an activity. They eventually came up with the idea of encouraging Americans to take a simple, written health quiz to assess their risk of diabetes. A public relations firm suggested the theme: "American Diabetes Alert: Put Your Health to the Test." Diabetes Awareness Day thus became the American Diabetes Alert.

The first American Diabetes Alert took place March 15, 1988, and proved to be the most successful public awareness activity ever undertaken by the Association. Fifty of the 55 ADA affiliates participated, and almost 4 million health quizzes were distributed nationwide. After completing the quiz, people could obtain a score, then call one of two special telephone numbers to get a recorded explanation of their score. Many celebrities, including the Association's National Campaign Co-Chairpersons David Birney and Meredith Baxter Birney, recorded messages for the Alert. Thousands of calls were received on the special lines. ADA affiliates also experienced a tremendous influx of telephone calls on the day of the Alert. In addition, calls to the National Service Center's patient information department increased by about 1,000 a month and maintained that higher level of activity into the summer.

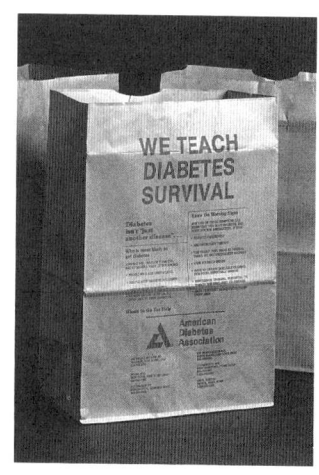

Across the country, ADA affiliates conducted special programs for the American Diabetes Alert. A sampling follows:

In New York City, Mayor Ed Koch issued a proclamation naming March 15 as American Diabetes Alert Day. The ADA New York Downstate Affiliate, gave the mayor a healthy bag lunch, a copy of the newest ADA cookbook, and two low-calorie desserts made from ADA recipes.

The ADA California Affiliate sponsored Legislative Advocacy Day in Sacramento. Volunteers briefed state legislators on important ADA issues. Throughout the state busy volunteers distributed more than 750,000 diabetes tests.

The ADA North Carolina Affiliate sent speakers to four local TV stations and several radio stations to participate in special diabetes programs.

The ADA Tennessee Affiliate helped set up a three-hour cable TV program that featured a panel of doctors and a dietitian who answered viewer questions about diabetes.

Volunteers at the ADA Oregon Affiliate, in Portland, manned the phones to respond to calls for information generated by a lengthy article on diabetes in the area's leading newspaper.

The Alert quizzes were distributed as pamphlets, and were also printed in local newspapers, on place mats, on grocery bags, and in corporate and organizational newsletters. National magazines, such as *Better Homes & Gardens, Weight Watchers,* and *Ladies Home Journal,* carried stories about diabetes and the Alert in their March issues. Stories about the Alert appeared on local evening news programs in many of the country's major television markets.

In addition, the Association hosted a congressional reception as part of American Diabetes Alert activities.

Affiliate participation is the key to the Alert's success. In 1989, all 56 ADA affiliates joined in. The goal of the Alert was to reach the estimated 5 million Americans who suffer from diabetes without knowing it. Just one measure of the 1989 event's success occurred as the result of the ADA Oklahoma Affiliate's efforts. Volunteers distributed nearly 120,000 sets of materials statewide. By the end of the day in one Oklahoma company alone, 10 workers discovered that they might have diabetes and were referred to their physicians.

The 1989 Alert featured a new item—*Be Alert To What You Eat And Do* diaries. The diaries contained calorie information, healthy eating and exercise tips, and space to track daily meals and activities. Eckerd Drugs, Eli Lilly and Company, and Miles Inc., Diagnostics Division, cosponsored Diabetes Alert Seminars in 13 cities. At the national level, American Association of Retired Persons Pharmacies helped distribute Alert materials, as did Walmart Pharmacies, and Medicine Shoppes. Westin Hotels printed 14,000 copies of Alert materials to distribute to its employees.

On March 21, ADA President Charles M. Clark,

Jr., M.D., (1988-89) was interviewed on ABC-TV's popular early morning show, "Good Morning America." That same day, ADA President-Elect Sherman M. Holvey, M.D., was interviewed on "Sonya Live in L.A.," a Cable News Network television show. On Capitol Hill, volunteers and staff distributed Alert materials during their Congressional visits.

Among the creative activities planned by affiliates:

- The ADA New Mexico Affiliate held a telephone-a-thon. Alert brochures in both English and Spanish were distributed.

- The ADA Texas Affiliate provided Alert quizzes to independent pharmacies throughout the state and worked with school systems throughout the state to develop education programs, including poster contests for elementary-aged children and diabetes education programs for junior high and high school students. In addition Texas targeted the minority populations in schools and distributed nearly 75,000 Spanish-language Alert quizzes.

- The ADA Vermont Affiliate reached out to people thanks to a grocery chain and a banking firm. Baggers at Martin's Foods stores throughout the state dropped *Be Alert* diaries into grocery bags. Prescriptions filled in the chain's pharmacies on Alert day were packaged in ADA Alert bags. During March, the Chittenden Trust Company distributed Alert quizzes in all bank statements, reaching nearly 30,000 households.

National Diabetes Month: The Campaign Continues

National Diabetes Month, dedicated to increasing public awareness of the seriousness of diabetes and calling attention to the need for continued research and educational programs about diabetes, was established in 1975. Since 1983, Congress has passed resolutions and the President has signed proclamations naming November National Diabetes Month.

During National Diabetes Month 1987, the Association sponsored the first nationwide "Comedy Crusade Against Diabetes." It was the inspiration of comedian Tom Parks. Mr. Parks, who was diagnosed with insulin-dependent (type I) diabetes in 1985, started mulling over ideas for how he might contribute to the Association's fight for a cure. His father also has insulin-dependent diabetes. "I realized that most of the clubs that I played have a night that they're not open, usually Monday. I got around to asking one of the clubs if

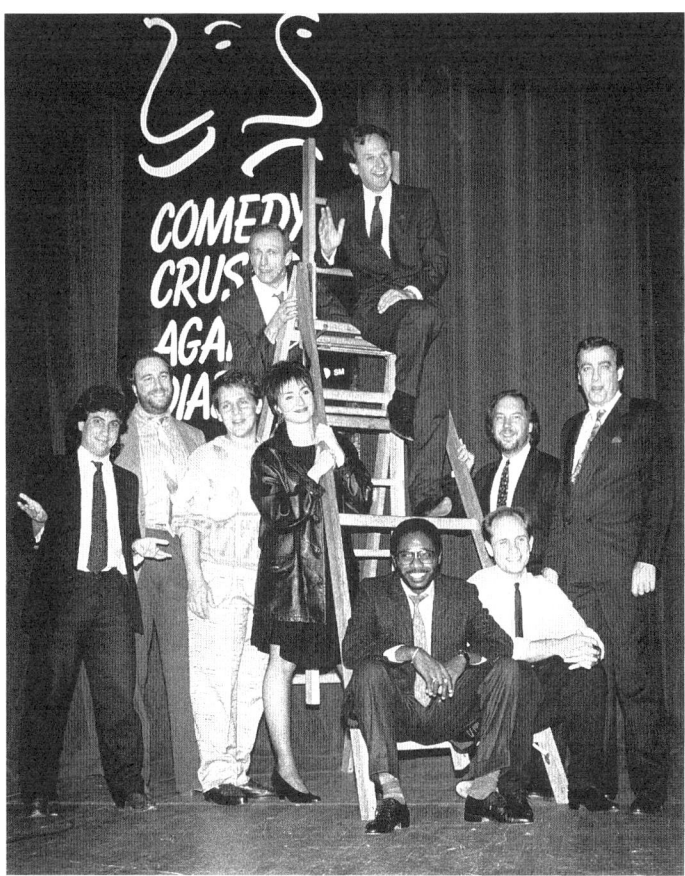

"The Comedy Crusade Against Diabetes," Tom Parks (on top of ladder) and friends.

they'd mind if I did a benefit for the ADA on a dark night. They said sure," said Mr. Parks.

Tom Parks next contacted the ADA Georgia Affiliate to propose his fund-raising idea. "They were grateful, but a little puzzled because no one had done anything exactly like this before."

The first benefit, held at The Punch Line in Atlanta, was a sell-out. Buoyed by that success, Tom Parks started to think about taking his comedy show on the road. He received the backing of the American Diabetes Association, and the program—named the Comedy Crusade Against Diabetes—was born. In addition to local performances, the Comedy Crusade features a nationwide event. The first was held November 2, 1987, with 26 states planning performances and a flagship show occurring in Washington, D.C.

In 1988, the Comedy Crusade's anchor show was held on November 7—again to coincide with National Diabetes Month. The event featured Tom Parks and a host of popular comedians. Held at the Joyce Theater

Diabetes Costs Soar

The years from 1980 to 1990 witnessed unprecedented escalations in health-care costs. The cost of diabetes care was no exception. Each year the cost of diabetes, both to the individual and the nation, increased.

In 1969, it was estimated diabetes cost the nation about $2.6 billion a year. By 1984, that figure had risen to $14 billion. In 1987, just three years later, a study by the Center for Economic Studies in Medicine, which was supported by the American Diabetes Association, estimated that diabetes cost the nation $20.4 billion.

What explained a 46 percent increase over three years? Part of the answer may lie with the study itself. "Direct and Indirect Costs of Diabetes in the United States in 1987," conducted for the Center For Economic Studies in Medicine by Pracon, Inc., of Reston, Virginia, was more comprehensive and accurate than previous estimates of the cost of diabetes care. Prior estimates included only partial costs of treating the complications of diabetes. The 1987 study placed dollar values on such factors as the cardiovascular complications of diabetes as well as the visual, neurological, and renal complications.

The Pracon study also included the costs of extra hospital care that people with diabetes may need. For example, someone with diabetes and pneumonia may need more days of antibiotic therapy than someone without diabetes.

Another factor is the aging of the American people. The incidence of diabetes rises steadily with age. As more and more of the nation's population ages and as lifespans continue to lengthen, a greater percentage of the population is likely

in New York City, the show raised more than $25,000.

The Third Annual Comedy Crusade was held on November 6, 1989, at the Roundabout Theater in New York City, with a predinner show at Caroline's at the Seaport restaurant. Since the program's inception, the Comedy Crusade has raised more than $150,000 to benefit diabetes research and education programs.

Commitments To Professional Education

The years 1985-90 showed increased Association commitment to professional education. Some major events:

- The Clinical Education Program (see Chapter Ten). This program trained many family practitioners, endocrinologists, and health professionals.

In 1990, the Association launched its new Clinical Education Program (CEP), "Managing Diabetes in the 1990s." Funded by a grant from The Upjohn Company, the CEP is a nationwide project that aims to increase public awareness of the seriousness of diabetes; to increase the number of people whose diabetes is under treatment; and to increase the quality of care provided to patients with diabetes. A part of the program is a national public awareness campaign urging high-risk populations to be aware of their blood-glucose value and the seriousness of diabetes.

A series of seminars for primary-care physicians on the diagnosis and management of diabetes is part of the project. Half day seminars, intended for physicians who are not diabetes specialists, provide basic information and focus on the management of type II diabetes. CEP seminars are organized and implemented by ADA affiliates using prepackaged materials. As part of the CEP materials, *Clinical Diabetes Reviews,* Volume 1, published in 1987, gives physicians an overview of the most current information about the diagnosis and pathogenesis of diabetes, as well as the latest treatment approaches.

- *Goals for Diabetes Education*, a key reference for all professionals in the field of diabetes, was published in 1986. The book was written to help the educator plan and evaluate education and counseling programs for people with diabetes. Educational goals in each of 11 content areas were described in detail.

- *Diabetes Care* went from six times a year to ten times a year in 1988. In 1990 it went to 12 times a year.

to face diabetes. In 1987, 38 percent of all people with diabetes were over age 65; 20 percent were over age 80.

Despite the spiralling cost of diabetes care in recent years, study commentator Steven Gambert, M.D., gerontologist at New York Medical College in Valhalla, was optimistic the the nation can lower the bottom line in diabetes costs. What's needed to effect the change, he suggested, is improved follow-up care for those already diagnosed and an increased effort at early identification of those who have the disease without knowing it. Both goals are ones that the American Diabetes Association actively works for in a variety of ways—from programs conducted by professional section councils to affiliate activities and participation in campaigns such as the American Diabetes Alert to consumer information in *Diabetes Forecast*.

- The *Physician's Guide to Insulin-Dependent (Type I) Diabetes* was published and the *Physician's Guide to Non-Insulin-Dependent (Type II) Diabetes* was revised in 1987.

- Four new professional section councils, as mentioned earlier, were established in 1987: councils on complications, education, exercise, and foot care—bringing the total number of councils to nine.

- *Nutrition Guide for Professionals* was published in 1988. The text presented information for physicians, dietitians, nurses, educators, and other health professionals to help in diet counseling for people with diabetes and their families.

- *Diabetes Spectrum*, a bi-monthly magazine for the nonphysician health professionals involved in diabetes care, was launched in 1988 to an enthusiastic welcome. Linda Hurwitz, R.N., M.S., was instrumental in helping to organize the start-up of this publication. Patricia A. Lawrence, R.N., M.A.; Marvin E. Levin, M.D.; and Margaret A. Powers, R.D., M.S. were the first editors.

- The ADA-Endocrine Society Liaison Committee, chaired by ADA President Daniel Porte, M.D., (1986-87) was formed in 1986 and comprised of senior representatives from both organizations. "It is clear that ADA and the Endocrine Society share many common interests, and this Liaison Committee will help both societies meet the concerns of our members," said ADA President John A. Colwell, M.D., (1987-1988).

ADA committee members also showed their commitment to professional education. For example, the Committee on Professional Practice, chaired by Robert Kreisberg, M.D., "developed a superb position paper on comprehensive standards of medical care for people with diabetes mellitus. This extremely important document will undoubtedly serve as the foundation for medical management of diabetes in the future," said Dr. Colwell. Indeed, it did. The position statement "Standards of Care for Patients with Diabetes Mellitus" was approved by the ADA Board of Directors in 1989. These historic standards, for the first time, detailed the kinds of care that people with diabetes should have.

Commitments to Patient Education

Because of the growing need to reach people with diabetes, providing accurate, practical, and up-to-date information has become increasingly important to the

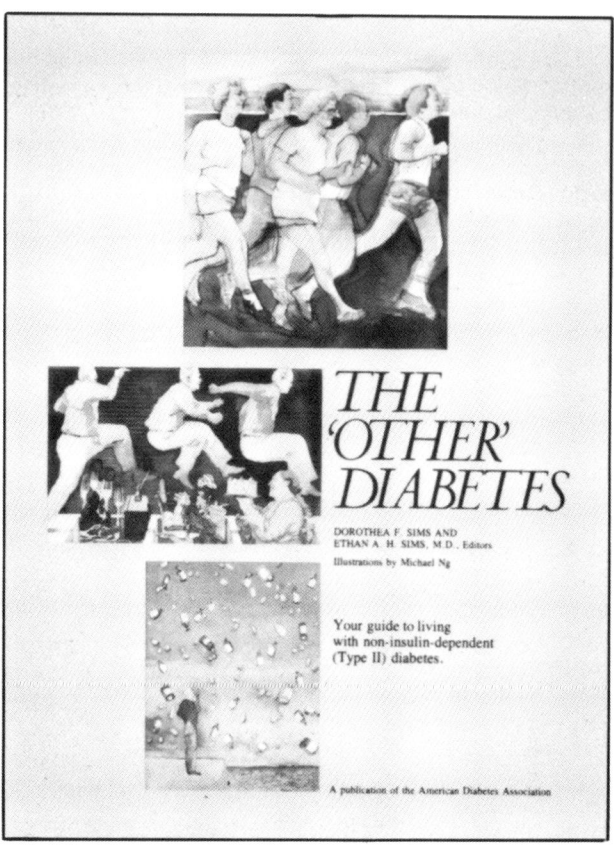

Association. Reaching high-risk populations (members of minority groups, people with low reading levels, and pregnant women) became an especially important goal, and numerous publications targeted for these groups were produced. In 1988, the Association published *Como Escoger Alimentos Saludables,* a Spanish-language version of *Healthy Food Choices.* While an occasional article in Spanish had appeared in *Diabetes Forecast*, this was the first ADA nutrition publication in Spanish. In addition, the "Basic Information Series," 40 pamphlets—one each in English and Spanish—containing essential information about diabetes and diabetes-related topics, was underway in 1989 and completed in 1990.

Many new publications for consumers were published in the latter part of the 1980s:

- *Children With Diabetes* provided a comprehensive look at diabetes management in children and young people for parents, teachers, and others who work with children who have diabetes (1986).

- *The "Other" Diabetes* presented a thorough explanation of non-insulin-dependent (type II) diabetes (revised in 1987).

- The *Diabetes and You* series of booklets dealt with special needs of people with diabetes at different stages of life (1987-88).

- *Diabetes in the Family* addressed both medical and emotional complications that can arise from diabetes, as well as day-to-day issues of diet and self-care (revised in 1987).

- *Diabetes: Reach for Health and Freedom* taught how someone with diabetes can not only survive but excel (1984).

- *Grilled Cheese at Four O'Clock in the Morning*, a novel for children aged eight to 12 with diabetes, was the first publication of this kind for the Association (1988).

- *Diabetes A to Z* offered a revised, expanded and updated version of 1982's *Guide to Good Living* (1988).

- *Kid's Corner* became the mini-magazine for kids and was published four times a year beginning in 1988.

- *Eating Healthy Foods* provided a low-literacy version of the *Exchange Lists For Meal Planning* (1988).

- The *Exchange Lists for Weight Management* and three *Guidelines for Use of the Exchange Lists* offered still more help with diet and nutrition (1989). The three meal planning guides included low-sodium meal planning, low-fat meal planning, and low-sodium, low-fat meal planning.

- *Diabetes in Pregnancy: What to Expect* (1988), designed for women with diabetes who became pregnant or wanted to become pregnant, provided comprehensive information to these "high-risk" groups. *Gestational Diabetes: What to Expect* (1989), was designed for women who developed gestational diabetes.

- ADA's video on coping with diabetes, "Diabetes: A Positive Approach" became available in February 1990. In this video, comedian Tom Parks, national chairman for the ADA's Comedy Crusade Against Diabetes, joined other celebrities with diabetes to teach people how to keep a sense of humor while coping with their disease.

In addition, a variety of successful cookbooks was published: *Family Cookbook, Volume I, Volume II, and Volume III* (1987), *ADA's Holiday Cookbook* (1986), and the *American Diabetes Association Special*

Senator Jake Garn
A Father's Gift

In 1986 U.S. Senator Jake Garn, of Utah, faced a reelection bid for his Senate seat. But his election day victory would not prove his sweetest triumph from that year. Instead,

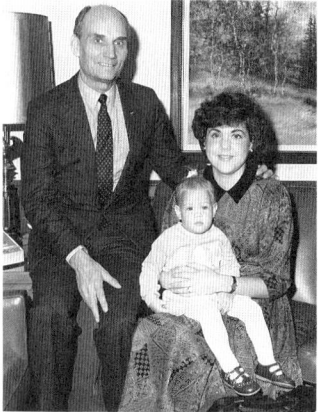

Senator Jake Garn with daughter Sue and granddaughter Allison.

it is a personal victory, one that he and his daughter Sue won together. On September 6, 1986, Senator Garn donated a kidney to his daughter Sue.

Diagnosed with diabetes at the age of 10, Sue began experiencing complications at 24. After the birth of her daughter in 1985, her renal (kidney) function deteriorated. Should her kidneys fail, Sue and her family learned that she had two options: lifelong dialysis or a kidney transplant. Sue determined to try for a transplant operation and her family supported her. When tested, her father and her two brothers, Jake, Jr., 29, and Jeff, 20, proved the closest matches.

Senator Garn determined that he would be the one to donate a kidney to Sue. While her brothers were willing donors, the Senator reasoned that he'd be needing his kidneys for fewer years than they. Also his sons would make ex-

Celebrations and Parties Cookbook (1989). Finally, *Month of Meals* (1989) provided preplanned menus for different calorie levels.

Progress in Research

The growth and scope of the American Diabetes Association's research program is one of the most illustrious pages of the Association's history. From a modest commitment of $5,000 in 1953 for two fellowships, the figure rose to $8.8 million in 1989. In a span of 34 years, the American Diabetes Association awarded more than 1,200 grants and fellowships, and established a clinical research program and a request-for proposal (RFP) mechanism of funding. Included in this figure are 15 grants made through the generosity of the Lions Clubs International Research Fund, established in 1984, which the Association administers.

The ADA research program focuses on helping young researchers enter the field of diabetes research, to pursue their innovative ideas, and to move one day into positions of leadership as established diabetes researchers. The Association research program offers:

- Research and development awards;
- Feasibility grants;
- Mentor-Based Postdoctoral Fellowship Program awards;
- Medical Student Research Fellowship Program awards;
- The Clinical Research Grant Program;
- The Lions Clubs International Foundation Clinical Research Program in Diabetic Eye Disease (formerly known as the Lions Clubs International Research Fund); and
- Local awards made by ADA affiliates.

Research and development awards help promising new researchers make the transition to independent investigators. This support allows investigators the time to start an independent research effort that will result in sufficient accomplishments to qualify them for long-term funding. In other words, the Association supports the growth of mid-level investigators, those in the period after the research felllowship and before totally independent investigation. A critical phase in an investigator's development.

Feasibility grants assist investigators who want to

cellent backup donors should something go wrong with Sue's transplant.

Recalling the eve of surgery, Senator Garn admits experiencing fear—something even a space shuttle ride a year and a half earlier hadn't evoked. Air flight and space missions were something he knew and understood. However, the world of organ transplants and major surgery was unknown and unfamiliar.

In an article reprinted from Encyclopedia Brittanica's *Medical and Health Annual*, and reprinted in Diabetes Forecast, Senator Garn wrote: "I was lying in my darkened hospital room waiting for my eyes to get tired and my mind to get settled so I could sleep. I was getting frustrated with myself for being so restless and for experiencing something that I honestly have not felt a great deal in my life—fear.

"I knew logically and factually, that there was really nothing to worry about—that the operations that Sue and I were to undergo in the morning would be virtually routine, at least so the doctors believed. The physicians involved had been very thorough and reassuring every step of the way. They had shown us facts and figures, and we knew from what they said, for example, that there was an eight times higher mortality rate from appendectomies than from a nephrectomy (removal of a kidney) and transplant procedure."

Post-op the news was good. The transplant was a success. A year and a half after surgery Sue had yet to experience any episodes of rejection.

Interviewed in the hospital several days after the operation, Senator Garn was asked how donating a kidney compared with some of his other notable life experiences. "I did test new and imaginative diabetes-related ideas. The ADA's support offers these investigators the chance to gather the preliminary data that will let them receive future support from the National Institutes of Health or other funding agencies. Feasibility grants support ideas and allow investigators to develop their concepts and plan for further funding.

Mentor-Based Postdoctoral Fellowship Program awards support the training of promising researchers by established diabetes investigators and help to encourage young scientists toward a career in diabetes research. The program is unique in two ways. First, the awards are not given to the postdoctoral fellow, but rather to established and active investigators who will be responsible for selecting and training fellows to work closely with them. Second, although the mentor must be a U.S. citizen or permanent resident, there are no citizenship requirements for the fellow. Thus, this award supports the training of the most promising researchers regardless of nationality.

Medical Student Research Fellowship Program awards help support the training of medical students in clinical investigation or basic research in the field of diabetes.

The Clinical Research Grant Program supports patient-oriented research in diabetes. This program will provide funding for three years to support research involving humans directly.

The Lions Clubs International Foundation Clinical Research Program in Diabetic Eye Disease (LCIF) awards support to research on diabetic retinopathy. The Lions Club program, established in 1983 by a generous contribution from the Lions Clubs, is administered by the American Diabetes Association.

Local awards by ADA affiliates are an important part of the Association's total research effort. These program support research at the local level through grants, pre-and postdoctoral fellowships,and support for medical students. Every application submitted to a local research program receives careful peer review by the affiliate's research committee.

The ADA has two committees that carefully oversee its national research program and make sure that research dollars are used as effectively as possible. The Committee on Research Policy determines broad policy matters on research. Specific proposals for research funding are examined by the Committee on Research Review. The research review committee is composed of scientists selected for their expertise in one or more specific aspects of diabetes research. Each research proposal receives an in-depth review, and the members

not even have to think about the answer. There is simply no other thing I have ever done that has given me greater satisfaction."

Adapted from 1988 Medical and Health Annual, copyright 1987, Encyclopedia Brittanica, reprinted in the May 1988 issue of Diabetes Forecast.

of the committee rate the scientific merit of the proposal. All proposals are then ranked in order of their scientific merit for funding. The ADA's use of the peer-review system ensures that only the highest quality research is funded and that awards are based only the on scientific merit of the proposal.

Another important aspect of the ADA's research effort is providing a forum for scientists and health-care professionals to discuss their ideas, share information, and report their latest findings. In 1988, alone, the Association cosponsored a Consensus Development Conference on Neuropathy with the American Academy of Neurology; held a "Current Issues in Nutrition and Metabolism" symposium; and conducted the Association's International Research Symposium. Every June, the Association holds a Scientific Session in conjunction with its annual meeting. More than 4,000 health professional and research scientists attend these symposia, workshops, and presentations. In addition, the Association sponsors the annual Postgraduate Course for health-care professionals.

A Program For The American Workplace

In the late 1980s, employers were paying more than $10 billion each year for health benefits as well as lost work time for diabetes. Given this dramatic statistic, the Association, under the leadership of ADA President John A. Colwell, M.D., Ph.D., (1987-88) and Chairman of the Board S. Douglas Dodd, developed a multitrack diabetes education program targeted specifically for the American workplace.

Entitled "WORKING ON WINNING: A Corporate Wellness Program of the American Diabetes Association," the new education initiative entered a six-month pilot testing phase in 11 ADA affiliates nationwide in 1988.

The comprehensive program was designed to help employers educate employees about diabetes and reduce the economic impact of the disease in the workplace. By means of multitrack programming, affiliates would be able to offer companies more than one type of program when it comes to educating workers about diabetes. "WORKING ON WINNING" strove not only to deliver general information to employees, but also to provide various additions and alternatives that would make it more "personal" for the employee, and overall, more attractive to the employer as a benefit to his or her employees.

The program finally debuted in May of 1989 and was subsequently implemented by affiliates across the country.

Support For Increased Federal Funding For Medical Research

Since enactment of the Diabetes Research and Education Act in 1974, the Association has taken an active role in encouraging federal funds for diabetes research. ADA presidents and officers have testified before congressional committees and supported annual recommendations for diabetes research appropriations.

In 1987, the continuing battle to increase federal funding for biomedical and behavioral research picked up momentum. The American Diabetes Association joined in a National Health Council (NHC) campaign to bolster public and congressional awareness of the importance of medical research to the nation's health. Working closely with the NHC's 39 voluntary health agency members, the Association took the lead in an event that distributed 1.8 million postcards nationwide so that concerned constituents could express their support for medical research to their representatives on Capitol Hill.

To coincide with the National Institutes of Health's 100th anniversary, October 1, 1987, was designated by Congress as National Medical Research Day. On that day, the American Diabetes Association and other voluntary health agencies went to Capitol Hill to lobby for increased federal support for medical research. ADA spokespersons David Birney and Meredith Baxter Birney met with legislators to urge their support and brought the case for medical research to the public through a major press briefing.

While the presidential campaigns of George Bush and Michael Dukakis swept the nation in 1988, the Association continued its campaign to increase federal support for medical research funding. Once again the efforts of the American Diabetes Association and the NHC resulted in a congressional declaration, this time targeting September 14, 1988, as National Medical Research Day. And for a second year, the Association helped spearhead events spotlighting the need for a stronger federal commitment to medical research.

Medicare Reimbursement for Therapeutic Shoes

The ADA Committee on Therapeutic Agents recommended in April 1977 that the American Diabetes Association endorse Medicare reimbursement for therapeutic shoes for people with diabetes who have severe foot problems. The recommendation, which was endorsed by the Board, pointed out that Medicare reimbursement would save thousands of dollars in lengthy hospital stays and great human suffering in lost limbs.

It was not until July 1985—a decade later—that a corresponding bill was introduced in the House of Representatives. At the same time, ADA affiliates were urging their senators to introduce similar legislation in the Senate.

In the summer of 1987, the House passed the shoes bill as part of a budget "package" of legislation. Expectation was high that the bill also would pass in the Senate. The Office of Management and Budget (OMB), however, erroneously decided that the shoes bill would increase costs, rather than offer savings under the Medicare program. At the same time, several news articles appeared that implied the bill was not a responsible piece of legislation. These articles and the OMB stand reflected negatively on the bill and despite intensive efforts to correct the misinformation, the bill did not pass.

Instead, the Department of Health and Human Services (HHS) was instructed to undertake a demonstration project with a sample group of Medicare beneficiaries to determine the cost effectiveness of providing therapeutic shoes. The study began in October 1988 and will last two to four years, at the discretion of the secretary of HHS. The secretary is required to make an initial report on the results of the demonstration no later than October 1, 1990. If the use of therapeutic shoes is found to be cost effective, the demonstration project will be discontinued and the shoes bill will be fully implemented on November 1, 1990. However, if the secretary believes additional time is needed to determine the cost effectiveness of providing shoes, the demonstration project will continue for another two years. In this case, a final report from the secretary to Congress will be required by April 1, 1993.

Combating Employment Discrimination

In 1989, ADA affiliates and chapters generated more than 400 public comments to support a change in the U.S. Department of Transportation (DOT), Federal Highway Administration's blanket prohibition against certification of people treated with insulin as drivers of commercial motor vehicles. More than 97 percent of the approximately 500 public comments favored allowing case-by-case consideration of interstate truck drivers, as recommended by the petition filed by the Association in 1986.

To date, no decision has been made by the DOT on the Association's petition. The Association is pressing for a decision through letter-writing campaigns and media coverage, while it continues advocacy involvement with other diabetes-related employment discrimination cases, working to ensure equal access to employment opportunities for people with diabetes.

Another way ADA affiliates help combat discrimination is through the Association's Attorneys Network. Established in 1986, the network has grown to include 64 attorneys in 33 states. These attorneys (who are not endorsed by the Association) have indicated an interest in representing people with diabetes or helping them find counsel. ADA affiliates in participating states put people in touch with Network attorneys.

In addition, the Association helps keep people with diabetes informed of their rights through articles on employment discrimination in its consumer magazine, *Diabetes Forecast*, and through the work of the Government Relations Committee.

For a time in 1989, it seemed likely that unprecedented legislation against discrimination might pass into law. Currently, the only federal protection for people with disabilities is that included under the Rehabilitation Act of 1973. However, the 1973 Act only covers employees who work for the federal government or for employers that receive federal financial assistance or have federal contracts. The Americans With Disabilities Act of 1989 would protect individuals who work for any employer, private or public, with 15 or more employees. Under this bill diabetes is legally considered a disability.

The Association worked to support the Act as a means of protecting people with diabetes against employment discrimination in the private sector.

While the bill passed the Senate in September of 1989, it did not pass the House because it had to first be reviewed by several House Committees. The Association hopes these reviews will be completed in 1990 and the Act will be passed into law before the end of the year.

ADA's Support for Animal Research

From the pioneering days of Drs. Banting and Best, whose efforts led to the discovery of insulin and gave life to millions of people with diabetes, laboratory research animals have played a crucial role in the fight for a cure. In the late 1980s, animal rights activists began urging federal legislation that would severely restrict animal research. If such legislation were to pass into law, it would pose a significant threat to medical research and to diabetes research, in particular.

Many recent advances that have led to improved quality of life for people with diabetes—development of the insulin infusion pump and transplantation of islet cells, as just two examples—depended on studies using research animals. The Association took an active role in ensuring that such studies continue despite efforts by animal rights activists to eliminate animal research.

ADA's position statement on the "Responsible Use of Animals in Research," passed in 1985 and reviewed in October 1987, states:

"The American Diabetes Association takes the position that the responsible use of animals is essential to biomedical research and education in the treatment and ultimate cure or preventive of diabetes mellitus." The statement continues to say that the Association requires assurances of the responsible use of animals in research and requires that the institutions receiving ADA grants must meet standards equivalent to those of the U.S. Public Health Service.

During 1988, animal rights activists promoted legislation that would ban or restrict the use of animals in medical research. In the U.S. House of Representatives, Representative Robert Mrazek, of New York, authored the "Pet Protection Act," which garnered more than 110 cosponsors.

In the Senate, Senator Wendell Ford, of Kentucky, introduced the "Pet Theft Act," which went through a number of modifications before being passed by the Senate. Although the final version of the Ford bill was a substantial improvement over previous versions, like the Mrazek bill, it would have placed significant restriction the use of "random source" (pound- and shelter-derived) animals in medical research. Fortunately, the House did not pass such a bill, so the Ford bill was not enacted into law.

In 1989, the Association continued to play a leadership role among voluntary health agencies that are united in their opposition to restrictive legislation like the Ford and Mrazek bills. One example of the Association's proactive stance was its support for The Animal Research Facilities Protection Act of 1989. Introduced by Senator Howell T. Heflin, of Alabama, the act was passed by the Senate in November 1989. This legislation, if enacted, would make it a federal crime to break into research facilities, steal laboratory animals, and destroy data and equipment.

As of 1989, members of the animal research community are supporting two other bills aimed at protecting animal research facilities from break-ins. These bills were introduced in the U.S. House of Representatives in 1989. Representative Charles Stenholm, of

Stepping Into High-Tech
Cynthia Mason, of Santa Cruz, California, told what it was like to live with diabetes during the 1980s. Her story is adapted from the March 1988 issue of *Diabetes Forecast*.

The Diabetes Dark Ages ended just six months ago for me. But it took years for the darkness to lift.

Back in 1981, my pancreas first showed signs of going haywire. I was 26. I spent the next difficult year learning about my diabetes, instructing family and friends, understanding Food Exchanges, and acquiring a new consciousness of health—and sickness. I believed that all I needed for good control was a reasonable diet, urine tests for sugar, and an understanding doctor.

Soon, I had to start using insulin. I started using blood-testing strips as I struggled to improve control. It took a few years to break old habits, but I began feeling better and settled into what I thought was good control.

My first peek at the new age came in 1986. I relocated and had to find a new physician. I was lucky to find an understanding and patient doctor. In her office, she had a glucose meter. At first, I was afraid of this complicated (so I thought) high-tech machine and afraid of making a serious commitment to wresting my blood sugars to the ground.

Soon, however, my frustration with reading test strips and my desire for a journey into a new age of improved control led me to buy one of these newfangled machines. I quickly discovered this new-age device was worth every penny. I was able to pinpoint problem hours of the day.

A few months later, my doctor talked to me about some new ideas appearing in medi-

Texas, introduced H.R. 3270, the "Farm Animal and Research Facilities Protection Act of 1989," which seeks to amend the Food Security Act of 1985 to protect all animal research facilities, including those not federally funded. Representative Henry Waxman, of California, introduced H.R. 3349 to amend the Public Health Service (PHS) Act to protect certain health facilities from illegal activities.

ADA's Government Relations Committee in 1989-1990 took a very vocal role in promoting the responsible use of animals in research. The Association was helping the Foundation for Biomedical Research compile a "Family Album" of personal letters, photographs, and children's drawings from individuals with diabetes and their families who count on animal research for a better life and who hope that responsible animal research will lead to the development of new medical treatments for their children, husbands, wives, parents, friends, and neighbors. The Foundation will devote a whole section to the American Diabetes Association and our responses. The album was presented to President Bush in the spring of 1990, and a selection of letters was sent to each member of Congress.

Organizational Development

In the latter part of the 1980s, the national organization expanded the training opportunities available to affiliate volunteers and staff. In September 1988, a Board of Directors Orientation was launched to acquaint newly elected national board members with the policies, plans and operations of the national organization. In February 1989, the first-ever Affiliate Volunteer Leadership Conference was convened at ADA headquarters in Alexandria for the incoming presidents and chairmen of the board of affiliates. This conference offered participants the opportunity to engage in dialogue with the national ADA officers, receive training, and learn firsthand about the operations of the national organization. A highlight of the program, according to participants, was the orientation session and tour of the National Service Center. Both conferences have since been established as annual events.

Also in 1989, the national organization established the Board Mentor Program, which offered affiliate boards of directors consulting services provided by members of the national Board of Directors.

In addition, the national organization established a comprehensive schedule of training programs for affiliate staff. Courses on chapter development, fund raising, accounting, computer operations, public relations,

cal journals. Careful not to overwhelm me, she fed me information slowly. We discussed how my current therapy of one or two injections a day often didn't cover the ups and downs of blood sugar that occurred in the course of my average day. No matter how scheduled I tried to be, my glucose meter made it clear I wasn't achieving good control with one or two shots. It was important to me that I be in charge of my life—not my diabetes—I wanted to eat when I felt hungry, exercise when I felt like it, and just live like anyone else while keeping in mind the general guidelines for living with diabetes.

So I started using an insulin delivery device—an insulin pen.

One change led to another in my quest to achieve the kind of control right for me. I added ultra long-acting insulin to my regimen of Regular insulin. At long last, I could tailor my insulin delivery to my lifestyle instead of living my life around my insulin injections.

With the setting of the Diabetes Dark Ages and the rising of the High-Tech Age, I have achieved a complete reversal of my old ideas of diabetes maintenance.

I never thought I would be thankful for one cent of research money not spent on a cure. Bitterness and despair might have caused me to deny myself the freedom to live as unhampered by diabetes as possible. But these fruits of diabetes research and technology have encouraged me to overcome the limitations of diabetes. The digital readout in the window of my glucose meter tells the story: a gradual improvement in my blood-sugar control that is giving me growing confidence in a healthy future.

and government relations, plus several new staff orientation programs, were conducted in 1989.

Money Matters

In the late 1980s, the Association laid the groundwork for a strengthened fund-raising capability. New staff were hired at the national level to provide direct consulting services to individual affiliates and to broaden campaign development.

New special events packages were developed for use by affiliates, including a Bike Ride Plus program built around various sporting events and Citizen's Arrest, in which local celebrities are "arrested" and must raise "bail money," which then is donated to diabetes research and education. At the same time, affiliates continued to develop innovative special events, from black-tie galas to "Kiss A Pig" contests.

On the national level, the Board of Directors instituted a "Give and Get" program of incentives to encourage volunteer leaders to support ADA fund-raising efforts. The Association also launched a "cause-related marketing" program in which ADA contributions are linked to the purchase of carefully selected products.

Perhaps the most important new initiative was a major donor program begun in 1989. Known as

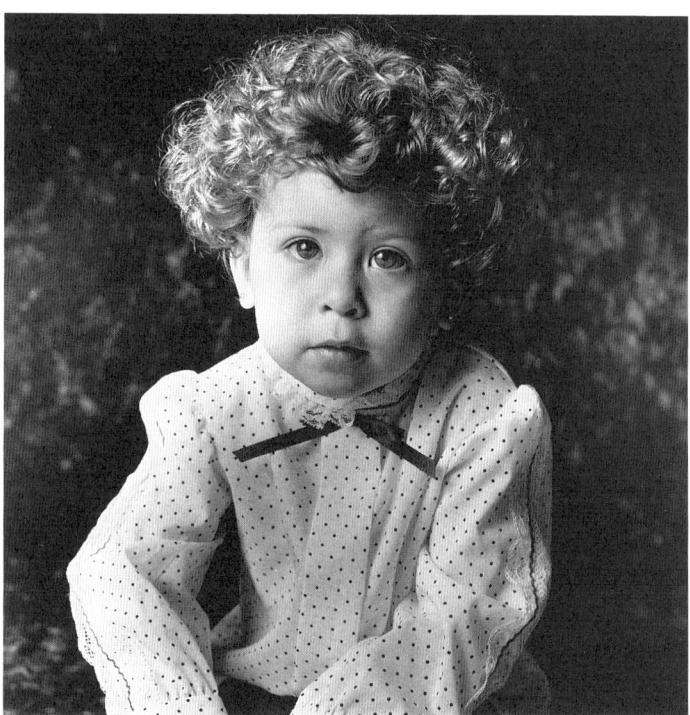

Her hope is for a world without diabetes.

CURE: America's Fight Against Diabetes, the campaign seeks to build a network of major donors working through ADA affiliates. CURE Campaign Chairman Richard Wayne Parker of Mississippi was successful in recruiting a group of nationally recognized civic, professional and industry leaders to spearhead the nationally coordinated major gifts program during its first year of operation.

At the same time, a special 50th Anniversary Campaign, chaired by former Federal Reserve Chairman Paul Volcker, was launched with the ambitious goal of raising $5 million for the fight against diabetes.

As the Association stood poised to enter the 1990s, a sense of renewed energy and vitality had begun to emerge. The creation of the Nationwide Comprehensive Long-Range Plan and the resulting organizational self-assessment that subsequently occurred had refocused attention on the importance of the Association's overriding mission to achieve a world without diabetes. Policies were being formulated to cultivate accelerated affiliate and community development. Mechanisms were in place to revitalize the ADA Research Program. The Association's patient and public education and awareness programs continued to expand. The stature of the ADA Professional Section continued to grow at home and abroad. The American Diabetes Association could look toward its 50th Anniversary with pride in the past and confidence in the future.

Pieces Of The Puzzle: What We Knew About Diabetes

1985

Paul Lacy, M.D., Ph.D., and David Scharp, M.D., of Washington University School of Medicine in St. Louis, report that their first human islet transplants have met with only lukewarm success. None of the six insulin-dependent subjects who recently received islet transplants were able to stop taking insulin injections. The transplants did produce some insulin in three test subjects, who were able to cut back on their insulin needs by 50 to 90 percent. However, after producing insulin for up to eight weeks, those transplants all eventually stopped making the hormone.

Two studies demonstrate that keeping blood-glucose levels near normal is better than "looser" control for eyes with background (mild) retinopathy. This news comes as a relief to physicians who in 1983 heard a more worrisome report. At that time, the Kroc Collaborative Study Group, a multi-centered study, reported that subjects who maintained near-normal blood-glucose levels for eight months (using insulin pumps) unexpectedly had a faster progression of background retinopathy than did those subjects who controlled blood sugar less well. Apparently the dramatic worsening in the pump group was temporary. When the researchers re-examined patients at two years, they found that both groups had experienced some worsening of eye changes compared to the very start, but the pump group showed marked reversal of the changes seen at the eight-month mark, while the other ("conventional therapy") group showed continued worsening. Neither group had changes severe enough to affect vision. The important thing about these studies is that the intensive treatment did no harm.

1986

A series of publications from many laboratories suggests that tight control of blood-glucose levels prevents or retards the onset of diabetic complications. The studies done in both animals and humans provide good but inconclusive evidence that high blood-glucose levels should be avoided. As a result of these reports, the government launches the largest, most detailed study ever—the Diabetes Control and Complications Trial—which is aimed at conclusively proving that tight control is essential. This same year, the American Diabetes Association holds its first Consensus Development Conference on Self-Monitoring of Blood Glucose.

1987

Approximately 300 pancreas transplants are performed in the United States.

Michael Brownlee, Ph.D., and his colleagues at Rockefeller University develop a compound, aminoguanide, which prevents "sticky" glucose from narrowing or blocking blood vessels.

Scientists have been looking for a reliable marker to predict who will develop insulin-dependent (type I) diabetes. Mark A. Atkinson, Ph.D., and colleagues Noel Maclaren, M.D., and William Riley, M.D., at the University of Florida College of Medicine in Gainesville report finding a particular antibody that is highly predictive. It's called the 64K autoantibody because it attacks a 64,000 molecular-weight protein on the surface of beta cells. At this point, a simpler and cheaper test to detect the 64K antibody would have to be developed before mass population screening for diabetes could begin.

At the ADA Scientific Sessions in June, the consensus of an international panel that addressed the ADA's Council on Diabetes in Pregnancy is that having a healthy baby means tight control of the mother's blood-glucose levels—not only during, but also before pregnancy. Researchers continue to study how diabetes increases the risk for birth defects and to assess the level of control needed to minimize the risk for birth defects.

1988

Massimo Trucco, M.D., of the University of Pittsburgh, working with John A. Todd, Ph.D., describes a specific gene abnormality that gives rise to type I diabetes. Subsequent studies on families with multiple members having diabetes reveal that individuals with this genetic abnormality have more than a 100-fold risk of developing the disease. With this discovery, the nature of the genetic defect predisposing diabetes becomes clearer.

Researchers at the University of Wisconsin and the Barbara Davis Center in Colorado conduct clinical trials on fetal cell transplants. The trials record some limited successes in a small number of people with diabetes. Problems remain: First, a method is needed to gather and preserve enough cells for transplantation. Second, there is a shortage of available fetal tissue. And lastly, and perhaps most important, are the ethical questions involved in using fetal cell tissue.

Metformin, which belongs to a group of blood glucose-lowering drugs called biguanides, is under clinical investigation for use in the

United States. It is already being used to treat diabetes in Canada and Europe.

Studies show that angiotensin converting enzyme (ACE) inhibitors not only lower blood pressure but also can reduce the amount of protein in the urine as well as slow the progression of kidney disease. ACE inhibitors block the production of a hormone that raises the pressure in kidney filters.

1989

Investigators develop a glucose-sensing device that offers hope of being implantable. If it could be coupled with the recently developed implantable insulin pump, then, at last an artificial pancreas will have been developed. This advance offers hope that technology will provide an alternative to transplantation.

At the 1989 Scientific Sessions, an international panel of experts discuss how the body keeps its balance between hyper- and hypoglyccmia. Important questions are raised about hypoglycemic unawareness in people with type I diabetes, when the first signs of hypoglycemia are reduced intellectual ability, confusion, seizures, and even coma. Why the condition occurs in some people and not others remains unknown.

Metformin, a biguanide drug, continues to show promise as a new option for lowering blood-glucose levels in people with type II diabetes. If remaining clinical trials go well, metformin could be available for widespread use within several years.

Chapter Twelve
American Diabetes Association Affiliates

Every day, people with diabetes, their families, and health-care professionals turn to state affiliates and local chapters of the American Diabetes Association for their programs of service, education, and research. Today, volunteers and staff at 56 ADA affiliates—serving more than 800 communities nationwide—provide a vital lifeline of information. Here, briefly, is their story.

Alabama Affiliate

In 1947, a group of physicians within the state of Alabama designated themselves the Alabama Diabetes Association and elected their first officers: Drs. Seale Harris, Leon Smelo, and Samuel Eichold. Nearly 14 years later, the group was incorporated by Dr. Smelo, S.K. Selikoff, and Buris Boshell. In 1968, as the organization gained momentum in its fight against diabetes, a lay society developed to aid its cause. By 1974, the Alabama Diabetes Association was the ADA Alabama Affiliate.

As the Alabama Affiliate's first President, Dr. Lloyd F. Pennington, Jr., worked with Executive Director Harry Vincent to build this affiliate. An office was established in Huntsville and remained there until 1987, when it relocated to Birmingham. Today, the affiliate has six chapters.

Alaska Affiliate

Buried in the history of Alaska—a history that is deeply intertwined with the gold rush—are many secrets, including the origins of the ADA Alaska Affiliate. While some volunteers in the Land of the Midnight Sun believe Alaska was an ADA affiliate during the pipeline years of the early 1970s, records are sketchy.

What is remembered is the sometimes painful growth this affiliate has achieved. In 1976, the affiliate needed a helping hand. Having raised less than $500 the previous year, its leaders suspended affiliate status to reorganize and pick themselves up by the bootstraps. Their decisive action brought swift results. After operating under the auspices of the Washington Affiliate for just three years, Alaskans showed revenues totaling $68,000 for the calendar year 1979. The following year, they were back on their feet and ready to resume affiliate status.

For this affiliate, the 1980s were marked by growth and financial stabilization. Chapters began to develop, and today, Alaska has eight.

The Alaska Affiliate regained its proper place in the American Diabetes Association thanks to the guidance and dedication of the following people: Dr. Maynard Falconer, Al Bramstedt, Jr., Chris Hedberg, Donna Lind, R.N., Rick Mystrom, Vincent Casey, Dan Robinson, Kay Sorenson, Duane Lyon, Jeanne Woods, Mel Kalkowski, and Audrey Lee.

Arizona Affiliate

A handful of citizens from Phoenix pooled their talents in 1972 to form the Arizona Diabetes Association. Over the next 15 years, this organization faced many hurdles as volunteers and staff struggled to build the affiliate. Their diligence was rewarded in 1985, when the affiliate achieved an annual budget of $500,000.

This affiliate's greatest achievements include a free eye examination program that reached 4,000 residents of the Grand Canyon State. The affiliate also waged a successful fight against the state's attempt to withhold driver's licenses from people with diabetes, and finally, the Arizona Affiliate helped develop a Diabetes Awareness initiative in the Hispanic community.

Today, with offices in Flagstaff, Tucson, Sun City, and Phoenix, 10 staff members assist the activities of the six chapters and various support groups. Five chapters are in the development stage, including one in the Navajo Nation. Currently, the ADA Arizona Affiliate has more than 5,000 members and will soon launch a program to double its membership.

Arkansas Affiliate

In 1974, a group of nurse-educators recognized the need for an organization devoted to improving the quality of life for people with diabetes and their families. They also knew the importance of increasing the public's understanding of the seriousness of the disease through public awareness and education programs. Together they established the Arkansas Affiliate and set out to accomplish these goals.

The newly formed organization generated a broad base of support from health professionals, community groups, and dedicated volunteers. Over 15 years later, this affiliate continues to build on the volunteer support developed by its founders and to strengthen the role of volunteers in the Association. Five active and two developing chapters provide the basis of fund-raising support, public and professional education and public awareness programs that delivers the ADA message throughout the state.

Annually, the Arkansas Affiliate sponsors professional education programs in partnership with health professionals throughout the state and provides a variety of outdoor activities and patient education programs at Camp Yorktown Bay in Hot Springs for youngsters with diabetes. Support groups are active in a number of communities within the state and a one-to-one referral network is in the planning states. Fund-raising activities include bike rides, golf tournaments, special gifts campaigns, concerts, and theater events and dinner series.

California Affiliate

July 1, 1987 marked the merger of the Northern and Southern California Affiliates. The ADA, California Affiliate, Inc. opened its headquarters office in Sacramento that month to serve the administrative, training and support needs of the original 16 chapters.

The new affiliate rapidly began to fulfill one of the major goals of the merger. Within the first year and a half of operation, four new chapters were added to better serve the state.

Not only has growth in chapter development been rapid, but fund raising and program activities have grown dramatically since the merger. Affiliate level direction, training, and management have resulted in foundation support of over $250,000 and Special Gifts revenues of almost $250,000 in three years. The direct mail program, Special Activities, such as the new Fall Cycle Tour and Spring Ride and Stride programs, and a cultivation program designed to move selected donors into Special Gifts campaigns are all part of the bright fund-raising future. Since the merger, the affiliate camp program has two sites serving over 450 children through seven sessions.

There is now an active "telegram bank," a program with over 400 participants who generate immediate responses to state and national leaders about timely diabetes issues. A Legislative Advocacy Day is held annually at the state Capitol.

The affiliate has seen rapid growth in both public and patient education programs because of emphasis and training placed on the Speakers Bureaus, Corporate Wellness Programs, One-To-One Programs, and media involvement activities. The affiliate has reached health-care professionals effectively through the annual meetings of the California Dietetic Association and the California Academy of Family Physicians.

No discussion or article about the short history of the California Affiliate would be complete without the recognition of Mr. Todd Leigh, who not only served as the chair of the Merger Committee, but also as the chairman of the Board for the first two years of the affiliate's existence. His wise and mature leadership, along with that of the first president, Dr. David Estrich, enabled the California Affiliate to become firmly established as a powerful source in the battle against diabetes.

Colorado Affiliate

Founded on February 11, 1954, the Colorado Affiliate started primarily as a physician's group. As the affiliate grew, it started to involve patients with diabetes and support groups were formed.

These small groups became the beginning of the present day affiliate. There has been a trend in recent years to develop strong chapters to fully serve the entire state. This concept has been slow in coming, but as more volunteers are recruited and understand the mission of the American Diabetes Association, the closer the affiliate is to establishing full service chapters.

An important note in this affiliate's history is that in the late 1970's, affiliate volunteers formed a committee to raise funds for the present office. The office, as it now stands, was dedicated in 1980 and is the center of operations in Colorado.

Since 1978, the affiliate has grown from slightly over $100,000 to over $400,000 in income. This 400 percent increase came despite the fact that Colorado was in a recession because of the oil and gas industries and the fact that the state had a low population growth.

Connecticut Affiliate

The transition from a professional society to a voluntary health organization was a long and slow process in the Constitution State, but it was well worth the efforts of those who created the ADA Connecticut Affiliate.

This affiliate traces its roots to the Connecticut Diabetes Association for physicians, which was established in 1949. The decision to change over to a lay organization came nearly 20 years later, on March 27, 1968. At that time, the Connecticut association had an account balance of $1,817. Over the next five years, lay volunteers enlisted in the fight against diabetes and in 1974, the organization became an ADA affiliate.

Highlights of this affiliate's vast array of programs

include a summer camp for children with diabetes, established in 1975; an annual golf tournament, established in 1978; and a toll-free hot line for state residents. In 1987, the affiliate held more than 110 patient education meetings across the state.

Currently, the Connecticut Affiliate has four chapters and six clubs, a membership of 5,000, and an annual operating budget of $750,000, in addition to hundreds of volunteers. Listed on its "Pioneer Honor Roll" are Dr. Neil Auerbach, Geoffrey H. Dale, James Dull, Dr. William F. Eckhardt, Jr., Dr. Edward L. Etkind, Edith Goldberg, Dr. Barnett Greenhouse, Dr. James C. Hart, Ira V. Hiscock, Philip E. Nelbach, John O. Newell, Dr. William F. Van Eck, and Dr. David S. Wilcox.

Delaware Affiliate

Incorporated in 1959, the Delaware Affiliate continues to prosper. The current slate of officers and board members compliments health care and business communities throughout the state.

This affiliate strives to serve the needs of both the professional and lay community and is dedicated to fund raising for research and education programs.

The Kent/Sussex Chapter was formed in 1985, and within a year, split into separate county chapters. Each county offers educational programs to individuals with diabetes and participating in fund-raising activities.

Recently, the affiliate changed its membership policy to allow anyone in the state to become a member of the Delaware Affiliate at no charge. Members receive "The Monitor", the affiliate newsletter, chapter newsletters, as well as updates on affiliate and chapter activities.

This affiliate faces the 1990's with a challenge of meeting the needs of the entire population of Delaware, estimated now to be 34,000 diagnosed and undiagnosed. Plans include establishing a Task Force on Diabetes, and an initiation of program services through the Department of Public Health.

The affiliate is moving forward and is committed to elevating the level of diabetes knowledge, management, and care to all persons at all stages of diabetes involvement.

District of Columbia (Washington, D.C. Area Affiliate)

This affiliate is unique in that today it serves people in Maryland, Virginia, and the District of Columbia. Montgomery and Prince George's Counties in Maryland, and Northern Virginia were given to the affiliate through agreements with the respective affiliates.

When Drs. Louis Alpert, Maurice Protas, and E. Clarence Rice formed the Diabetes Association of the District of Columbia in 1946, a tradition of education began. In 1964 the organization became the ADA, Washington, D.C. Area Affiliate.

Since 1986, the affiliate has developed four chapters to better serve the 200,000 people with diabetes in the area. Governed by a 39-member Board of Directors, the affiliate today continues the fight against diabetes through education, patient services, research, funding, and a summer camp for children.

In honor of its founders, the affiliate has established a $30,000 Research Fellowship in the name of Clarence Rice and the Protas Award for the Outstanding Affiliate Director or Member.

Florida Affiliate

In the Sunshine State, efforts to fight diabetes are recorded as far back as 1970. At that time the fight was being carried out by the Florida Diabetes Association, under the leadership of Dr. George Heffner. But in just five years, this organization was to join the American Diabetes Association, establish an office in Jacksonville, and set the ambitious goal of achieving an operating budget of $100,000.

This affiliate's history, however, is not without elements of strife. In the late 1970s, a former chairman of the Board left the affiliate to organize a competing association in south Florida, a move that stirred up turmoil among volunteers and much confusion among the public. It was 1985 before this group was dissolved by a federal court order. Another incident that interrupted this affiliate's growth was the printing of a large order of cookbooks—the affiliate's first major fund-raising push—without Board approval. This error threatened the affiliate with bankruptcy and its projected $100,000 budget became a more elusive dream.

A complete reorganization was in order and leaders of this affiliate took the bull by the horns. Under the leadership of Patricia Schultz, R.N., as president (1978–80), the affiliate was brought from $20,000 in debt, two pending lawsuits relating to the cookbooks, no staff, no office. . . to a viable, healthy, growing, and most promising affiliate. In the midst of all this, the "units" and "lay societies" were certified as chapters and the affiliate initiated sound financial management through centralized accounting. By 1987, the

Florida Affiliate's total income had increased to about $1.3 million.

Georgia Affiliate

Founded as the Georgia Diabetes Association in 1957, the name was changed in 1966 to the ADA Georgia Affiliate, Inc. Today the affiliate serves over 4,500 members.

Over the years, fund raising has been one of the successful activities of this affiliate. Among those activities is the "Bucket Bridgade to Battle Diabetes", a statewide roadblock conducted in November, during which volunteers collect donations and distribute diabetes warning signs flyers. Last year $25,000 was raised. The Annual Orient Express Gala, a black-tie dinner/dance, is another fund raiser that has raised over $30,000 for diabetes research in a single year. The Georgia Affiliate's Golf Tournament is a major fundraiser for the state and raised more than $100,000 for research in 1989.

Other recent accomplishments include producing a national award-winning patient education manual and monthly newsletter, creating a nationally used computer program, instigating a free comprehensive rural-based eye screening program, developing a "Wilderness Camp," and entering the 19th year producing "Camp Liwidia", a sleep-in camp for over 250 children.

During its history, the Georgia Affiliate has produced a cadre of excellent volunteers that have served the affiliate in key leadership roles and have distinguished themselves nationally as well. Some of the recent honorees include Dr. John K. Davidson, winner of the Best Award, Dr. Terry Golden, winner of the 1989 "Volunteer Service" Award, and Joseph Davis and William Mamrack, who have served as national chairmen of the Board.

Hawaii Affiliate

Twenty-one years ago the Hawaii Lay Diabetic Society, Hawaii's first diabetes organization, was established. Formation of support groups, the sponsorship of workshops and a youth camp, and statewide advocacy for diabetes issues were the agenda.

In order to expand the scope of quality of its services, the Society decided in 1978 to join the American Diabetes Association. Since this time, the Hawaii Affiliate has expanded its programs to all areas of Hawaii, as well as many of the islands in the Pacific Basin. In 1989, youth from the affiliate's camp were invited to represent the U.S. in Japan at the first Pacific Basin Friendship Camp.

This affiliate plans to expand its efforts in the coming years in the areas of minority education and early intervention, in particular. A school awareness program is currently being designed to target young minority populations with information about the seriousness of diabetes and the importance of proper diet and weight control.

Idaho Affiliate

A tiny band of five volunteers launched this affiliate in 1972 as the Idaho Diabetes Association. Three years later, with a volunteer Executive Director and a bankroll of just over $2,000, it joined the American Diabetes Association as an affiliate.

The relatively small size of this affiliate has not interfered with the loyalty of its members. In fact, the first three Presidents—Drs. C.C. Johnson, Ward Dickey, and George Baker—remain active. Total membership blossomed from 191 in 1979 to 887 in 1987. And the affiliate's cash-on-hand fund balance has tipped the scales nearly as high as $105,000 in its short history.

Affiliate presidents have included Drs. Duane Espeland, W.R. Kennedy, Jack Magdiel, Adelia Simplot, Blaine Lenon, Phillip DeWald, Sara Nolen, Paul Street, Roger Keithly, and Robert Seehusen.

Downstate Illinois Affiliate

In its 12-year history, this affiliate has grown from a loose coalition of individuals scattered across the Land of Lincoln into a strong association of 18 chapters comprising hundreds of volunteers. In its first year, this affiliate raised $1,762. In 1987, more than $280,000 was raised to help support ADA programs and research.

This affiliate's story begins with a Springfield physician by the name of Thomas Masters. In 1974, Dr. Masters could see that the need for programs and services for people with diabetes far exceeded what was available from hospitals and local doctors' offices. So, with the help of Dorothy Buchanan, of Jacksonville, mother of a child with diabetes, he sent out a call for unity to the many small diabetes groups throughout the region. At an October meeting, bylaws were adopted and Mrs. Buchanan was elected first president of the Downstate Diabetes Association. Incorporation and recognition as an affiliate of the American Diabetes Association came the following year. By 1976, this affiliate had five chapters.

Founding officers and Board members were Michael Baker, Dr. Robert Murphy, Karen Knutson, Ronald Markley, George Heroux, Kennedy Hill, Sharon Lyons, Carmon Samuel, Donna Stoner, and, of course, Dr. Thomas Masters and Dorothy Buchanan.

Northern Illinois Affiliate

It was 1949 when the Chicago Diabetes Association, incorporated just one year earlier, became the seventeenth affiliate of the American Diabetes Association. Over the next 20 years, this all-physician organization went on to sponsor scientific meetings, camps for children with diabetes, and detection drives, often working with an enthusiastic lay group known as its "Service Unit."

At its ninety-ninth Board meeting in 1969, the affiliate opened its doors to lay members and went on to expand its geographic boundaries. From the Chicago Diabetes Association, it grew into the Greater Chicago Diabetes Association, and at last came to represent the entire northern region of Illinois. Its camping program prospered, professional and scientific programs developed, and an ambitious detection drive made the news.

Over the years, this affiliate has provided a record number of national ADA Presidents—five to be exact. They include Drs. Arthur A. Colwell, Sr., Henry T. Ricketts, James B. Hurd, Norbert Freinkel, and Donald I. Bell. (Dr. Colwell's son, Dr. John Colwell, also served as a national ADA President.)

Currently, the Northern Illinois Affiliate serves 10,000 members and has an annual budget in excess of $1 million.

Indiana Affiliate

Indiana doctors, including Drs. James Ashmore, William Kirtley, and Mary Root, who shared an interest in diabetes formed a professional society in 1950, the Indianapolis Diabetes Association. Under the direction of an executive secretary, Julia Shakel, the society undertook detection drives and camping programs for youngsters with diabetes across the Hoosier State.

During the late 1960s, the association began to expand and embarked on a gradual transition to a voluntary health organization. In 1972, the organization changed its name to the Indiana Diabetes Association and kicked off its own fund-raising campaign under the direction of Executive Director Tom Iozzo. Drs. John Galloway, Charles M. Clark, Jr., and Daniel Gillespie were instrumental in founding the organization. In 1975, it became the ADA Indiana Affiliate.

The first Board of Directors included Drs. J.H.

Warvel, C.L. Rudesill, J.O. Ritchey, Franklin B. Peck, Helen Van Vactor, Marion Shafer, Laura Hare, Frank Dailey, Ralph W. Showalter, and Georgia Hess.

Iowa Affiliate

A band of people interested in fighting diabetes in Iowa first met on January 24, 1967, at the Iowa Methodist Hospital in Des Moines. This group struck out on its own, establishing a camp for children with diabetes, holding educational meetings, conducting detection drives, and building chapters across the Hawkeye State.

In 1973, fund-raising drives were initiated and as the organization gained momentum, it began to hire staff members. On January 1, 1975, the American Diabetes Association gained this strong array of volunteers and programs when the organization became the ADA Iowa Affiliate.

Today, headquartered in Des Moines, this affiliate has eight chapters and 12 support groups. In 1989 the affiliate launched its first annual Kiss-A-Pig contest, and this new and exciting event will become a state-wide event, in addition to Bike Ride Plus.

The affiliate's "honor roll" includes Dr. Ronald D. Eckoff, Dr. Edward R. Hertko, Ann Hupp, A.K. Jernigan, Lloyd R. Nelson, and L.G. Snodgrass.

Kansas Affiliate

It was just one year after the birth of the Kansas Diabetes Association in 1972 that the organization's leaders applied for status as an ADA affiliate. Before the end of 1974, it was official: the organization was known as the ADA Kansas Affiliate.

The earliest and most successful of this affiliate's programs was Camp Discovery, for children with diabetes. Staffed by the youngsters' parents, the first camp hosted 33 children and nine junior counselors. Camp Discovery was held at various sites across the Sunflower State from 1973 to 1979. In 1979, a permanent home for the camp was found at the WaShunGa Area of Rock Springs Ranch. By 1989, there were 183 campers.

This affiliate has also emphasized professional education programs over the years. Other activities have included a bike-a-thon fund-raiser, first organized in 1974. With pledges totaling more than $12,000 on the first try, the bike-a-thon was quickly declared a success and became an annual tradition. Annual pledges have exceeded $70,000. The affiliate has raised even more for diabetes programs and research—from $20,000 to

$30,000—with the "Defeet Diabetes" run, which is held each year.

Kentucky Affiliate

Founded in 1961, the Kentucky Diabetes Association, Inc. was a professional society determined to improve the general welfare of persons with diabetes. The Jefferson County lay society was formed as a component to the Association. Although the organization has functioned as the ADA Kentucky Affiliate since 1980, the name was not legitimized until 1984.

Kentucky's staff has a challenge with a 3 percent higher incidence rate than the rest of the nation and an estimated 100,000 Kentuckians who are unaware they have diabetes. An emphasis on education is evident in the speakers bureau, displays, distribution of literature and films, media announcements, newsletters, and participation in the American Diabetes Alert and National Diabetes Month. This affiliate serves as an informational and referral resource for patients, provides support groups across the state, offers an annual accredited camp to 72 children aged 7 to 15, and publishes and distributes literature to inform those with diabetes and their families of the care and treatment currently available.

For professionals, the Kentucky Affiliate offers seminars, furnishes literature on current practices, and supports research efforts. Three clinical education programs were produced in 1989.

This affiliate is proud of its instrumental role in forming a coalition which introduced Pooled Risk Health Insurance legislation in Kentucky which, if passed, will give access to those who have been previously denied coverage because of a pre-existing condition.

Louisiana Affiliate

It was quite a merger in the late 1970s when the Greater Baton Rouge Diabetic Association, the Greater New Orleans Diabetes Association, the Northwest Louisiana Diabetes Association, and the Tri Parish Diabetic Unit combined forces to fight their common enemy. This conglomerate started with an income of just over $13,000 in 1978, but was producing more than $290,000 annually within 10 years.

Among the projects carried out by this affiliate are a Diabetes Alert Program, informing police about the special concerns diabetes raises, and the Whole Family Outing, a two-day mini-camp for families of children with diabetes. The affiliate also produces the *Creole*

Cookbook and sponsors an extensive camping program that involves more than 230 children with diabetes each summer. The affiliate's first statewide fund-raiser, "Bike, Hike and the Like," held in 1987, enlisted the support of Terry Bradshaw (former Pittsburgh Steeler quarterback) and raised $22,000.

The ADA Louisiana Affiliate now has 14 chapters and more than 3,300 members. An "honor roll" of original organizers pays tribute to those people responsible for this growth: James Ber, Sam Gallo, Dr. Morton Levy, Dr. Jerome Ryan, Dr. Sol Stern, Kate Wright, Etheleen Broomes, Dr. A.A. Herold, Jr., Frances Hazzard, R.D., Fred McCall, and C. Edwin Meador.

Maine Affiliate

Incorporated in 1972 and run entirely by volunteers for the first ten years, the Pine Tree Diabetes Association initiated numerous patient and professional educational activities.

The first staff was hired and retired in 1983. Full-time staff was not in place until the affiliate received a development grant from the National Service Center in 1986. Since that time, the affiliate has developed rapidly with staff and volunteers working together to help those with diabetes.

Currently, the Maine Affiliate has four chapters throughout the state and a fifth chapter under development. The affiliate has a very active Youth Services and Camping Committee and Program Committee, both of which are responsible for the numerous patient, public, and professional educational programs in the state.

Maryland Affiliate

In the Free State, efforts to help people with diabetes began with a summer camp. Looking to help the many Baltimore-area children with diabetes, Dr. Abraham A. Silver set up Camp Med-Chi at a rented campsite in 1952. With the help of various volunteers and support from local businesses, the camp prospered and began drawing children from as far away as Washington, D.C.

Soon, 44 acres of prime wooded land were purchased and the camp had a permanent home. Beginning in 1960, Dr. Silver and his supporters became involved in more diverse activities designed to help people with diabetes by incorporating and becoming the ADA Maryland Affiliate. Dr. Wilson Grubb was the first president and served with Executive Director Walter Thomas.

Camp Glyndon, as it came to be called, flourished. Even devastating vandalism that required significant rebuilding failed to dampen the spirit of ADA volunteers in Maryland. Along with Dr. Silver, the following people played an instrumental role in making the camp and the Maryland Affiliate a success: Carroll Markowitz, Nathan Silverstein, Herman Lissy, Gladys Goldstone, William Finlayson, Henry Irr, Gordon Salganik, Robert Black, Marcy Ehudin, James E. Swartz, Mary Busch, Dr. Clarence Rice, Melvyn Goodman, Tom Scrivner, William Wilkie, Morton Macks, DeWitt Delawter, Dr. Wilson Grubb, Dr. Julian Read, Eli Pinnerman, Dan Gohagan, Betty Hamburger, Theodore McKeldin, and Dr. Thaddeus E. Prout.

Massachusetts Affiliate

Much like their colonial ancestors, the people of Massachusetts looked to their New England neighbors for support when they knew it was time to fight. But in the late 1930s and early 1940s, the fight was against diabetes. As their numbers grew, a group of doctors established the New England Diabetes Association in 1942. For 30 years, this organization focused solely on furthering physician education. During the late 1960s, the physician members debated intensely whether to change course, admit non-physician members and start fund raising. Then, in 1972, not only did the association open its membership to other health professionals and lay persons, it also became an ADA affiliate.

The idea of changing over from a professional society to a voluntary health association was greeted with skepticism by some, but sensing the enthusiasm taking hold at the national level, they soon abandoned their fears. The first meeting of the ADA New England Affiliate was held in the town of Seekonk. Dr. George Welch, who had presided over meetings of the professional society, turned over his gavel to the new President, Dr. Ronald A. Arky.

In the late 1970s, the northern New England states broke away, and the Commonwealth of Massachusetts acquired its own affiliate. By the mid-1980s, the ADA Massachusetts Affiliate's budget topped $200,000.

Among this affiliate's founding members were Drs. Elliott P. Joslin, Howard Root, Harry Blotner, Frank Allen, and Priscilla White. Volunteers who helped make the change to a voluntary health association included Myrtis McSweeney, R.N., Richard Ryan, and Marjorie Cotton.

Michigan Affiliate

What began in 1948 as a group of medical professionals, affectionately called the "Detroit Sugar Club," grew into a state-wide voluntary health organization by 1965. The merger of medical and lay workers provided the fight against diabetes in Michigan with tremendous strength. Patient and public education emerged as top priorities in the beginning, and later, a major emphasis was placed on intensified diabetes research.

To encourage state and federal aid for diabetes research, a public affairs committee was formed. This committee was later to put Michigan in the national spotlight with its statistical reevaluation that emphasized the seriousness of the disease and helped to obtain additional funding. This same public affairs committee helped to push the diabetes act of 1974 through Congress.

For the ADA Michigan Affiliate, the 1980s have been marked by ever-increasing youth involvement. In 1981, the first edition of "Injection Connection," a quarterly publication geared toward children, was published. Camp Midicha, for children with diabetes, continues to prosper, having drawn more than 6,000 campers since 1954. The first youth was elected to the Board of Directors in 1986 and, that same year, the Board approved its $1 million budget. In 1987, revenues reached a new high, exceeding the $1 million mark.

Minnesota Affiliate

The first official organization for people with diabetes in Minnesota was developed in the Minneapolis/St. Paul area in 1954. It was called the Twin Cities Diabetes Association. In the beginning its primary focus was professional and patient education. One of the first major projects initiated by the Twin Cities Diabetes Association was a resident camping program for children with diabetes. Camp Needlepoint is still in operation today and continues to have a vital role in the Minnesota Affiliate. Day camping for younger children was added in 1986.

In the 1960s, the organization developed a major diabetes detection program. A mobile van, funded by the United Funds of Minneapolis and St. Paul, made diabetes highly visible in the community, and the organization focused on public awareness projects. The association received a renewed impetus in the 1970s as parents of children with diabetes became involved. A new group called the Parents of Young Diabetics assumed a leadership role throughout the entire organization. This group of volunteers was very interested in raising funds for research, because the Twin Cities Diabetes Association was hampered by agreements with local United Ways to not engage in fund raising. The entrepreneurial group incorporated an auxiliary organization, the Diabetes Research Fund, Inc. With restrictions no longer a factor, fund-raising projects blossomed—bike-a-thons, craft bazaars, garage sales, direct mail, and holiday card sales. These efforts resulted in the formation of what has proven to be the largest single ongoing fund-raising effort of the American Diabetes Association—the National Holiday Sales Program.

In 1974, the American Diabetes Association established a statewide affiliate, which operated with the Twin Cities Diabetes Association. In 1975, the Diabetes Research Fund merged with the new ADA affiliate. This newly organized affiliate assisted volunteers throughout the state in developing educational programs and raising funds to support the fight against diabetes. Thanks to a joint statewide educational effort called the Team Project, the number of chapters in Minnesota grew dramatically during the latter part of the 1970s.

The early 1980s began with the merger of the Minnesota Affiliate and the Twin Cities Diabetes Association. After several months of negotiation among volunteer leaders in both organizations, an official agreement was signed in February 1981. The name of the combined organization became the ADA, Minnesota Affiliate, Inc. Since that time, public support for the merged organization has grown from $328,000 to $800,000, and the affiliate has been a leader in the development of new programs in social services and government relations. These have been added to the traditional services in patient, professional, and public education. Since 1970, Minnesota has provided financial support for research, both locally and nationally.

Through the years, Minnesota has been fortunate to have had many dedicated volunteers who have helped build its program. Many went on to become active at the national level of the American Diabetes Association. Affiliate volunteers who have served on the national Board of Directors include: Donald Moberg, Donnell Etzwiler, M.D., Harlan Hanson, Norman Rickeman, Florence Ruhland, R.N., Virginia Hanson-Ullom, Carelyn Fylling, R.N., M.S., Marion Franz, R.D., Douglas Lund, and Bruce Zimmerman, M.D.

Mississippi Affiliate

Under the leadership of Karleen C. Neill, M.D., the

Mississippi Affiliate formed in 1958 as a professional medical society. Seven years later it was incorporated, and in 1969, it became a part of ADA to include both lay and professional members.

Key leadership in the affiliation with ADA included not only Karleen Neill, but Alton Covv, M.D., and Terry Beck. The affiliate endured some unstable times over the next 12-14 years, but 1983 marked a year of stabilization. Under the direction of Terry Odom, M.D., and Estelle Owens, R.N., a full time Executive Director was hired.

Since that time, this affiliate has grown and prospered. It contributes to the national research program and provides quality diabetes education to professionals, patients, and the public.

Missouri Affiliate

The Show-Me State Affiliate is showing its citizens greater and more effective service since three affiliates merged in 1987. Strong volunteerism of the Heart of America Affiliate in Kansas City, excellence in fund raising and youth services of the Greater St. Louis Affiliate, and the continuous patient education and support groups of the Missouri Regional Affiliate in Columbia are the hallmarks of the Missouri Affiliate which is now headquartered in Jefferson City.

The combined strength of these three former affiliates and their volunteers results in service to over 9,000 members in Missouri, as well as members in the metropolitan Kansas City, Kansas area and the St. Louis metro area including some counties in Illinois.

This affiliate is proud of its history of steadfastly supporting national research programs and its leadership in encouraging funding for research.

1990 marks the first year in the young ADA affiliate's history in which the Delegate Council will elect the Board of Directors, and the affiliate looks forward to continued financial stability.

Today the Show-Me State affiliate maintains regional offices in St. Louis, Kansas City, Columbia, and Springfield; and services 17 chapters.

The first slate of officers elected to head the new affiliate included Kristin K. Offutt, Dr. Philip E. Cryer, Dr. Charles E. Johnson, D.D.S., Laura A. Ross, and Charles H. Kopke, who has been the only president since the merger.

Montana Affiliate

A screening program and a camp for children with diabetes were the first order of business for the newly-elected officers of this affiliate in 1970. All affiliate business was carried out by lay volunteers in those days, but it wasn't long before a staff emerged, starting with a Field Representative in 1974, an Executive Director in 1978, and a Secretary the following year. Two Field Representatives worked out of offices in Billings and Missoula.

In 1979, the affiliate's current office in Great Falls was opened. At that time, membership totaled 90. Today, there are 1,200 ADA members in the Treasure State and several hundred volunteers, who help carry out the affiliate's programs. The Montana Affiliate's programs include 29 support groups, Camp Diamont for children with diabetes, and an annual Teen Retreat.

1988 marked an important change for both this affiliate and the Wyoming Affiliate. The Board of Directors voted to support the Wyoming Affiliate with field staff because the Wyoming Affiliate was struggling. Today, both remain separate affiliates but work together to educate people with diabetes and provide programs for them.

Nebraska Affiliate

This affiliate was incorporated in Nebraska in 1946 as the West Central Diabetes Association of Omaha. Nearly 10 years later, the name was changed to the Nebraska Diabetes Association and finally, in 1978, it became the ADA Nebraska Affiliate. At that time, the organization was headquartered at 819 Dorcas Street in Omaha. However, in 1987, the office was moved to its current location at 2730 South 114 Street.

Among the first officers of this affiliate were Dr. Lowell Dunn, Dr. A.S. Rubnitz, Dr. M. Grodinsky, Dr. A.L. Cooper, Alvin Johnson, Leta Holdrege, John A. Farber, and the Rev. Thomas Niven.

Nevada Affiliate

Founded in 1972 as the Nevada Diabetes Association, this affiliate joined the American Diabetes Association in 1975. In the early years, workers operated out of a city park building providing education programs and a campership program for children to attend summer camp. In the next few years, the ADA office changed location several times, but continued to provide services through the work of a small group of volunteers.

In 1983, a new surge in membership and growing professional seminars and patient education meetings breathed new life into the affiliate. Growth of the Nevada Affiliate continued with the addition of a full time Executive Director in 1988.

Today two healthy chapters and a state affiliate provide services to the people of Nevada. Providing more services throughout Nevada, several more chapters are beginning in rural areas. In 1989 the first summer camp for Nevada's children with diabetes became a reality with 30 children attending camp in Lake Tahoe.

New Hampshire Affiliate

Since a group of health-care professionals established it in 1977, the New Hampshire Affiliate has been providing patient education and support groups to the 50,000 people in the state with diabetes, their families, and friends. Affiliate volunteers and staff have created a network of chapters and support across the state which bring ADA programs into communities statewide.

This affiliate is especially proud of Camp Carefree, a residential camp for children aged 8 to 15 with diabetes. Medical volunteers started Carefree in 1979 to provide a healthful, educational, and recreational residential camping experience for children. Through the years, the camp's popularity has grown such that 110 children from all over New England are expected to camp during the 1990 season.

Two outstanding NH volunteers who have dedicated themselves to the work of ADA are William E. Dudley, II, M.D., of Dover, and Evelyn Holmes from Epsom.

Dr. Dudley, as the founder and moving force for Camp Carefree and a past president of the affiliate, has been an inspiration and example for all those who have associated with the camp and the affiliate.

As a person who has had diabetes for 58 years, Evelyn Holmes is an example of courage for the population with diabetes in the state. She brings her positive message of living a full active life with diabetes to support groups and chapters across the state. She is also a committed fund raiser for the ADA who works tirelessly to support affiliate programs.

New Jersey Affiliate

The New Jersey Diabetes Association had a long history of fighting diabetes even before it signed on as an ADA affiliate. From the beginning, this organization worked toward patient and professional education to help people with diabetes living in the Garden State. Then, in 1974, the ADA New Jersey Affiliate emerged.

In 1982 the affiliate was reorganized and, its headquarters was moved from Hackensack in Bergen County to a more central location in Bridgewater.

From a one room office, the affiliate has grown to include four regional chapter offices to better serve the needs of all New Jerseyans. Since its reorganization, the affiliate's budget has grown from $167,000 to 1.5 million.

The affiliate research commitment has included the funding of more than a dozen diabetes researchers at the University of Medicine and Dentistry of New Jersey.

Some outstanding fund-raising programs include the annual Golf Invitational which has raised more than $750,000; community service banquets honoring outstanding business and political leaders have raised in excess of $160,000; and Hoop LA, a basketball roast of state and national basketball coaches has raised $150,000 in two years.

Active programs for minorities, the Corporate Wellness Program for industry, and clinical education programs for health-care professionals have also grown successfully.

The affiliate honor roll of dedicated volunteers includes Wilton T. Barney; Martin G. Blechman, M.D.; Ira C. Mitchell, III; Rita M. Nemchik, R.N., M.S.; Arthur Krosnick, M.D.; Earle T. Holsapple, Jr.; John E. Beers; Robert A. Fuhrman, M.D.; and John L. Dugan, Jr.

New Mexico Affiliate

A classified advertisement in the Albuquerque newspapers in 1965 put this affiliate on the map. Some 20 or 30 people interested in fighting diabetes responded to that ad and attended the first meeting of the Albuquerque Diabetes Club. Although the group started off as a patient support group, it wasn't long before the need for a professional, medical point of view was felt and ADA membership was explored.

By 1971, this part-time Albuquerque club had blossomed into a statewide organization known as the ADA New Mexico Affiliate. Besides launching educational programs, the affiliate began raising funds and soon had opened a summer camp for children with diabetes. By 1987, Camp Triple D was drawing some 100 campers and counselors and had become a cornerstone of the affiliate's work.

In addition to the camping program, bike-a-thons and diabetes screening programs have become vital to this affiliate's activities. Currently, staff and volunteers are working to increase diabetes awareness among the state's diverse ethnic population, including Native Americans and Hispanics, who tend to have high rates of diabetes.

New York Downstate

In 1932 the Depression occupied the present and clouded the future. A decade had passed since insulin therapy first saved the life of a person with diabetes. The new facts about diabetes were spreading far too slowly, both among patients and professionals.

To make the most modern methods of diabetes care available to the greatest number of people, a small group of physicians and public health workers at the New York Academy of Medicine established the Committee on Diabetes, part of the Committee on Public Health Relations. The Committee on Diabetes soon became the New York Diabetes Association, Inc., (NYDA) the second such organization in the world.

Over the next few years, NYDA created professional education programs for medical students, doctors and nurses. Diabetes clinics opened with a NYDA committee to oversee their adherence to high standards of operation. For people with diabetes, Camp NYDA was founded in 1936, and patient education literature was produced and distributed.

With the end of World War II, NYDA added two major components to give the organization greater balance and strength: the Lay Society brought in non-medical volunteers to expand programs and fund-raising activities, and the Camp NYDA Service Group devoted itself to the growth and support of the camp. Since 1946, this affiliate has seen over 40 years of steady growth highlighted by several milestones.

Among those milestones are the world's first formal Vocational and Counseling Service for people with diabetes, started in 1961; Humanitarian Award dinners honoring former President Ford, Lee Iacocca, and actress Dina Merrill; the Annual Clinic Society Symposium established in 1963, which is the area's most comprehensive program on care and research; and the 50th Anniversary in 1983 of the Association's continuous service to professionals and patients.

The affiliate's three chapters today serve 14,000 members and fill more than 30,000 requests for information each year. The Clinical Society itself has nearly 700 members, including physicians and health-care professionals. NY Downstate works with the NY Upstate Affiliate on advocacy issues, such as insurance and employment discrimination, in the state legislature.

New York Upstate Affiliate

The first meeting of this affiliate took place in September 1982. It included ADA workers in Rochester, Buffalo, Utica, and Syracuse who came together in order to fight their common enemy: diabetes.

As a loose federation of diabetes organizations, these New York volunteers had raised a total of $133,000 in 1980. Today, calling on resources from every corner of the upstate region, this affiliate is a million-dollar corporation.

The affiliate, which started off with a membership of 2,000 in 1982, now serves more than 7,000 people with diabetes and their families. (The Rochester and Buffalo organizations became chapters but retained their autonomy until 1987.)

People responsible for the growth of this affiliate include Dr. Joseph P. Armenia, Dr. Edward B. Bradley, Roger W. Shaver, David A. Frye, Henry J. McCormick, Allen R. Bivens, Wyntha T. Boothe, Robert G. Campbell, Gerald B. Curtis, Dr. Robert DeCarlo, Jane D. DeCory, Dr. Mark L. Fruiterman, Kathleen N. Hausner, Charlotte Hillsberg, Sylvia M. Hough, Dr. Joseph L. Izzo, Gerardus S. Jameson, Stephen N. Marshall, Judith S. Pearson, R.N., Dr. Joel J. Schnure, Asa J. Smith, the Rev. William S. Smythe, Beverly J. Somerville, Robert L. Walker, and John S. Coombs.

North Carolina Affiliate

This affiliate's roots are in a regional medical program funded through a federal grant to the state to organize activities for people with diabetes in the 1960s. Dr. T. Franklin Williams led the program, and during the first few years he emphazied training nurses as diabetes educators. With renewal of the grant, the emphasis shifted to strengthening the work of the staff and others so that the organization could continue when federal funding was discontinued.

In 1971, the North Carolina Diabetes Association was incorporated as the North Carolina Affiliate, Inc. A staff of five and a Board of Directors with 23 members serve over 5,300 person with diabetes and healthcare professionals across the state. Twenty active chapters hold monthly patient education meetings, host support groups, and form the base for fund-raising efforts in towns throughout the state.

To educate people with diabetes, the North Carolina Affiliate offers members a variety of programs. Among them are a one-week residential camp for youth aged 8 to 15, Duke Diabetes Day, which is held in conjunction with Duke University Medical Center, for youth with diabetes and their families, a statewide patient education program as well as two professional education programs, and a State Youth Leadership Conference. Periodically, the affiliate publishes a newsletter to keep members abreast of activities within the state and on the national level.

Continuing current programs and searching for new avenues of service for the community with diabetes and health-care professionals are the primary goals for the future at the North Carolina Affiliate.

North Dakota Affiliate

For anyone living in North Dakota with a stake in the fight against diabetes, 1975 was a banner year. That was not only the year North Dakota's physicians-only ADA affiliate opened its doors to the public, but it was also the first year in which North Dakota celebrated November as "Diabetes Month." Before the year had drawn to a close, the state had its own poster child. In addition, Dr. E.A. Haunz was named outstanding clinician of the year by ADA national leaders. In short, the North Dakota Affiliate started off with a bang.

Since then, the affiliate's annual budget has swelled from $1,000 to close to $350,000, and membership has climbed from 150 to more than 1,000. In 1976, the first chapter was organized. There are currently 18 chapters throughout the state conducting diabetes education, raising funds for research, and helping to support Camp Sioux, one of only three free summer diabetes camps in the nation.

Among this affiliate's many accomplishments are two publications: one a free newsletter for the general public, the other a newsletter to health professionals.

The North Dakota Affiliate's first state-wide Board of Directors included Dr. Daniel W. Goodwin, Dr. E.A. Haunz, Mary Ann Keller, R.N., State Sen. Chuck Goodman, Judge Kirk Smith, Rep. Art Raymond, Dorothy DeHaan, R.D., Marlene Kuhl, R.N., Dr. Robert Warner, Mitchell Mahoney, Adrea Johnson, Pat Lukach, Dr. Ralph Dunnigan, Arlene Mack, R.N., W. Van Heuvein, Dr. Dean Strinden, Janet Matthews, R.N., Dorothy Revell, R.D., Dr. George Johnson, Dr. Fred Hofeldt, Kenneth Topp, and Jenell Oberlander, R.N.

Ohio Affiliate

The Buckeye State was served by four ADA affiliates until 1984. That year, the Greater Ohio, Cincinnati, Dayton, and Akron Area Affiliates joined forces to strengthen fund-raising efforts and increase contributions toward diabetes research programs. The merger provided many Ohioans with greater access to ADA programs and services.

Today, the ADA Ohio Affiliate serves 21 counties and speaks with one strong voice to state legislators.

Among this affiliate's honor roll of organizers are the following dedicated volunteers: Tim McGuckin, Clint Prettyman, Sanford Garfield, Dale Gehring, Vernon Grund, Angie Hagely, Emmy Hann, Phil March, Laura Lee Mostow Garfinkel, Edwin Sypolt, Marylouise Yonker, Stephanie Behrle, Phyl Heilbrun, Eric Laubach, Sue Monsell, Joe Robinson, Rosalie Stevens, David Weinberger, Jack Dougherty, O. Peter Schumacher, Bill Baxter, and T. Harrison Bryant.

Oklahoma Affiliate

In the Sooner State, east met west in 1983, and it meant great things for the fight against diabetes. That was the year that ADA's eastern and western Oklahoma chapters merged to become a full-fledged affiliate. Volunteers from Tulsa to the east and Oklahoma City to the west had a long history of meeting in Stroud, the half way mark on the highway that connects the two cities. But in the early 1980s, it became clear they could accomplish more together.

With the merger, two regional offices were established and before too long, this affiliate had 20 chapters. One of its first, all-volunteer efforts included screening 17,000 people for diabetes; a research program, a minority initiative program, and various youth programs followed.

The honor roll of affiliate organizers includes: Dr. Don P. Wilson, Dr. Piers Blackett, James F. Hirlinger, Adeline Yerkes, R.N., Debbie Burroughs, Dr. John Holcombe, Ann Richards Ketcham, Mike Camp, Dr. C. Alton Brown, Dr. Robert K. Endres, James Fenwick, Clydella Hetschel, Tommy Keen, Dr. John S. Muchmore, Dr. Steven Newell, Cooke Newman, Betty Raulston, Jim Rogers, Leonard Kindred, S. Douglas Dodd, Dr. Charles Rost, and Mr. and Mrs. William K. Warren.

Oregon Affiliate

With an interest in the cause of diabetes and a desire to improve the treatment of diabetes, several Oregon physicians founded this affiliate in the 1950s, and in 1962 the association was incorporated. Then, in 1975, under the direction of its president, John Stephens, M.D., the organization opened its doors as the Oregon Affiliate of the ADA. The affiliate flourished and by July the organization already had three chapters. At the end of the first year nearly $14,000 had been raised through bike-a-thons under the leadership of Executive Director Rita Dewart. The affiliate continued to grow and in 1987 celebrated its twenty-fifth anniversary.

Today, headquartered in Portland, the ADA Oregon Affiliate has 21 chapters and conducts several state-wide fund raisers including Bike Ride Plus, Daffodils for Diabetes, a Corporate Campaign, Holiday Auction and Summer's End Run. The affiliate boasts strong support of both national and local research projects. In addition, it provides programs including "Living Well With Diabetes" for people with diabetes, the Scientific Session for health-care professionals and "Growing Well With Diabetes" for young people with diabetes.

The original 1962 Board of Directors included Drs. Rudolph M. Crommelin, Robert L. Hare, Blair Holcomb (former national ADA president), Huldrick Kammer, Otto C. Page, John Partridge, John W. Stephens, Robert W. Schneider, and William Richey Miller.

Greater Philadelphia Affiliate

Clara Woodward became Executive Secretary of the Delaware Valley Diabetes Association at the time of its incorporation in 1940 as the "Philadelphia Metabolic Association," nine years after its 1931 founding.

Greater Philadelphia is proud of its rich history. Among the many activities of the Association, they published "Diabetic Digest," the first magazine for people with diabetes in the country and the predecessor to *Diabetes Forecast*.

Today, this affiliate serves over 3,500 general members and 200 professional members within a five county area of Pennsylvania. Activities include the Jubilee Ball, a black tie dinner dance held each November, at which the American Achievement Award is granted to a humanitarian, and an active camping program. Each year the camp hosts two-week camping sessions for campers aged 6-15 at Camp Firefly in Spring Mont. In addition, the affiliate hosts the Diabetes Update annually to discuss topics such as research, diabetes management, and complications.

Since last year, the affiliate has expanded its sporting events to include the annual Bar/Packard 10K Run, the Charity Cup Bodybuilidng Competition, and the Chris Short/ADA All-Star Golf Classic with support from the Philadelphia Phillies.

Mid-Pennsylvania Affiliate

In 1975, seven separate diabetes organizations—some of which had been fighting diabetes since the 1940s—banded together to serve residents of the 36 counties in central and northeastern Pennsylvania. Once this union was established, the Mid-Pennsylvania Affiliate was on a roll.

The establishment of 11 chapters and one branch in the affiliate has meant that patient and public information have been made available throughout the area. The chapters also maintain support groups for senior citizens, children, and parents of children with diabetes.

In 1979, a camp for children with diabetes was established and operates today as Camp Setebaid. The following year, a memorial award honoring affiliate volunteer Joanne Haines was established as a national award for selfless dedication and outstanding contributions to the cause of diabetes.

The 1980s have seen retreat weekends for affiliate planning, both Teen and Adult Weekends for recreation and sharing, the start of a government relations program, and frequent Clinical Education Programs for physicians and seminars for diabetes educators. Fundraising activity has also increased, and fiscal year 1986-87 saw a record income of more than $530,000.

Among this affiliate's first Board of Directors were Pat Douts, Jack Haaz, Eleanor Oneil, Mrs. Jerome Kaplan, Mr. and Mrs. James McGinn, Dorothy Smoke, Helen McCreary, R.N., Dr. David Lawrence, Patricia C. Stoppi, R.N., W. Robert Hay, Dr. William Hanisek, Joseph Savarese, Donna Arbott, Dr. John F. Craemer, Beverly Kanig, Mrs. George Nicodem, Dr. Melvyn Wolk, Nancy Aberman, Dr. James Voss, and Dr. Neal Zweig.

Western Pennsylvania Affiliate

This affiliate had its start as a group of parents trying to raise children with diabetes. Anxious not only to learn more about the disease, but to share common problems and keep abreast of the latest in research, they approached Dr. Allan Drash of Children's Hospital for help in organizing. In 1974, the group was accepted as a chapter of the Lehigh Valley Diabetes Association, already an ADA affiliate, and began working towards affiliate status.

This dream was realized just two year later, when the Pittsburgh Chapter was recognized as an ADA affiliate. With a staff of two, and a membership that totaled 168, the affiliate operated out of two rooms in an old church, raising some $27,000 a year. Today, the affiliate covers the 26 western-most counties of Pennsylvania, has 10 chapters, a membership of nearly 5,000, and raises more than $430,000 a year to help support ADA programs and research.

Founding members include: Dr. Allan L. Drash, Dr. David Finegold, Dr. Jerome Aarons, Dr. Dorothy Becker, Dr. James Field, Herc and Lucie Pappas, Nancy Aberman, Jane Kohlman, Dr. Neal Zweig,

Patricia Gerney, Dr. Jerome Wolfson, Rose Holman, Joanne Kampas, Charles and Gail Weisberg, Anita Bart, Alvin and Barbara Ring, Dr. and Mrs. James Voss, James A. Sliger, Millie Moeller, Claire Weinbaum, and Sally Kaufmann.

Puerto Rico

Among the youngest of the ADA affiliates is the Puerto Rico Affiliate. On February 27, 1988 the affiliate was born. Dr. Gildred Colon, president of the Puerto Rican Society of Endocrinology and Diabetology, led the effort of a group of lay and professional persons to form an affiliate.

Through television presentations, newspaper articles, monthly radio programs, and educational seminars, the affiliate launched its patient education campaign to meet the greatest deficiency in Puerto Rico. Since October 1988, the affiliate has continued to host educational programs for both patient and professional members.

In January 1989, the affiliate held "National Diabetes Day," to screen people for diabetes and distribute educational materials. The effort was so successful that a similar activity was held in February 1990.

Priorities for this developing affiliate include fund raising, publishing Spanish education materials, and establishing at least nine chapters in Puerto Rico and the Virgin Islands. In addition, an island-wide census is in the planning process to determine the number of people with diabetes in the region.

Professional education has met with excellent results. In conjunction with the Puerto Rican Society of Endocrinology and Diabetology and the Diabetes Association of the Caribbean, the First Congress of Diabetes in the Caribbean was held in October of 1989. Other education programs have been scheduled for 1990.

Rhode Island Affiliate

This affiliate started as a chapter of the Association's one-time New England Affiliate in 1972. Founder and first President Gladys Longo held the reins for eight years as the organization found its footing and started to grow. The Honor Roll of Original Organizers of the affiliate include: Gladys N. Longo, Dr. Jean M. Maynard, Dr. Dennis Krauss, Richard Ryan, Barbara Ryan, M.P.H., R.D., Russell H. Maynard, and Maurice E. Lague, O.D.

In 1980, with a part-time Executive Director, Sara Slate; an office located in a volunteer's home, and an annual budget of $20,000, the Rhode Island Chapter became the Rhode Island Affiliate. Two years later, a store-front office was opened to help foster public accessibility and a full-time executive director and a secretary/bookkeeper were hired.

Until 1986 the affiliate struggled financially with the demand for services exceeding its ability to raise money. The organization had a low profile in Rhode Island and relied on "Mom and Pop" type fund raising.

In the last four years this affiliate has managed a dramatic and successful turn-around. The Board of Directors has many corporate, civic and medical leaders as members. The budget has tripled to $175,000 and the staff has doubled in size. The agency is now located in a professional office complex, Fund raising now includes a corporate campaign, fashion shows, roasts of community leaders, golf tournaments and a mystery dinner called Dining for Diabetes-Flavors of Providence. Many outstanding professional and patient education programs are held yearly, and public awareness has increased with a Providence advertising agency taking the affiliate on as a *pro bono* client.

A typically Rhode Island slogan boasts: "We are the biggest little affiliate in the union."

South Carolina Affiliate

Chartered as the South Carolina Diabetes Association in 1967, this organization was headed by President Hulda J. Wohltmann. Ten years later, it became a part of the American Diabetes Association.

The original focus of the affiliate was on patient education and a diabetes camp for children. In its early years, the affiliate engaged in marginal fund-raising activities, but received significant income from the Combined Federal Campaign.

In the early 1980s, the affiliate was relocated from Greenville to the capital city of Columbia. In the years to follow, there was a growth in development of local chapters state-wide, and an emphasis was placed on developing annual fund-raising activities. Both of these trends continue today.

In 1989, the affiliate developed its own long-range plan based on the long range plan of the national organization. Activities being established now include expanded development of self-perpetuating chapters, a grass roots fund-raising plan, and new community services.

South Dakota Affiliate

When Volunteer Margaret Moore held a style show in Rapid City that raised over $10,000, she set the stage for the establishement of the South Dakota Affiliate. Ms. Moore sent the donation to the National Service Center, and NSC encouraged her to use the funds to develop the affiliate. Chartered in 1977, the office was established in Rapid City.

In the last 13 years, the South Dakota Affiliate has had some lulls in activity. Nevertheless, highlights include a Governor's Roast, Geranium Sales, publication of a South Dakota Cookbook, and a camping program at Camp Teepeetonka, formerly Camp Haunz. Volunteers throughout the state are gearing up for a number of events including bike rides, parent/youth retreats, a professional symposium, and continuation of the residential camping program, geranium sales, and roasts.

Now headquartered in Sioux Falls, the affiliate has only forward to go in its fight against diabetes.

Tennesee Affiliate

What better place for the American Diabetes Association to set up an affiliate than Tennessee—the Volunteer State!

It was during the annual meetings of the Tennessee Medical Association in the early 1950s, that several physicians interested in diabetes began seeking each other out. At informal meetings of their own, they discussed developments in diabetes treatment and research. Then, in 1963, they established the Tennessee Diabetes Association as an educational and scientific organization for physicians only.

But the physicians also took great interest in the Tennessee Camp for Diabetic Children, and over the years, this bond stirred interest in lay participation. In the early 1970s, however, an effort to convert the association into a voluntary health agency failed. This resulted in a split that left a host of satellite groups throughout the state for the remainder of the decade.

Nevertheless, the early 1980s were marked by mergers, and by 1985, the American Diabetes Association Tennessee Affiliate emerged as the consolidation of these groups. Today the affiliate has 26 chapters served by Regional Resource Centers in Johnson City, Knoxville, Chattanooga, Nashville, and Memphis.

The early founders of this affiliate include: Drs. Addison Scoville, Jean Hawkes, Bob Ackerman, Phillip Livingston, Sol Solomon, Abbas Kitabchi, and Oscar Crofford.

Texas Affiliate

The early history of the diabetes effort in Texas is not well documented, but professional groups existed in Dallas and Houston as early as the 1940s. In 1973 the Dallas Diabetes Association became an ADA member and was registered as the North Texas Affiliate, while the Houston Area Diabetes Association, formed in the 1950s and now recognized as the oldest chapter in continuous service in the state, joined the Association in 1975 as the South Texas Affiliate.

The 1970s saw several important developments for the North and South Texas Affiliates. More lay volunteers became involved and began to serve as directors, and staff persons were hired to direct activities in fund raising and program services in offices in Houston, Corpus Christi, San Antonio, Midland, Austin, Dallas, and Fort Worth.

A group of volunteers from both affiliates decided in 1981 that the state could be best served with a single corporate entity, and the merger of the organizations was begun. By February 1982, the Texas Affiliate was officially recognized.

In 1990, the affiliate has 12,000 members, 22 chapters, 50 support groups, six day camps, and an annual budget of 1.5 million. The affiliate has conducted 34 Clinical Education Programs for primary care physicians since 1984, and was a leader in the formation of the Texas Diabetes Council, designed to develop and carry out a state-wide plan to combat diabetes. In addition, Texas has been a leader in initiatives to bring public awareness to the problems of high risk groups, especially Blacks and Mexican-Americans.

This affiliate appreciates the dedication of the many lay and professional volunteers and staff who created the foundation of the Texas Affiliate.

Utah Affiliate

Programs for people with diabetes varied and spanned over 10 years before the Utah Affiliate was formed. In 1962, the Utah Diabetic Foundation was established to plan and implement a summer camping program for children with diabetes. Previously, the closest camp site was in Colorado.

In 1971, the University of Utah's Intermountain Regional Medical Program provided funding to establish the The Diabetes Center, an ambulatory diabetes education and treatment facility in Salt Lake City which served the intermountain region.

Three years later, that funding was discontinued, and efforts were underway to locate private funding sources to continue the Center's programs. It was decided to expand the purposes of the Utah Diabetic Foundation and change the name to Utah Diabetes Association.

After the American Diabetes Association approached the Utah Diabetes Association, it became an affiliate of the ADA in 1975. When an office was opened in 1976 in conjunction with the Utah Arthritis Foundation, a volunteer agreed to man the office for half a day. By September of 1977, a full-time Executive Director was at work.

Today the Utah Affiliate has 11 chapters and four staff members to serve 90 percent of the state's population.

Vermont Affiliate

This affiliate was founded in 1975 by a small group of volunteers led by Dr. George Welsh. Originally a chapter of the New England Affiliate, Vermont achieved ADA affiliate status in 1978. Five years later, the affiliate hired its first Executive Director.

Vermont now has more people than cows due to the federal whole-herd buy-out program, but it still has only half a million citizens, of whom over 800 are members of the national Association. The Vermont Affiliate is not wealthy in terms of dollars, but it is known nationwide for innovative services to people with diabetes and their families.

Some of this affiliate's rich activities include a Winter Weekend program for New England adolescents, summer camp scholarships, basic patient education series, professional education, and a variety of support groups enabling people with diabetes to share information and gain emotional support. The most recent endeavor, Person-to-Person, is a program whereby people with diabetes are trained to assist patients and their families in adjusting to diabetes, newly diagnosed or not.

Vermont Affiliate members have provided the national Association with a variety of research studies as well as publications for people with diabetes, including *The Other Diabetes* and *Diabetes: Reach for Health and Freedom*. Since 1976, several affiliate members have served in positions of leadership on the ADA National Board and on the National Diabetes Advisory Board. In 1988, the editorship of *Diabetes Care* came to Burlington.

It is clear that the affiliate presence attracts, trains and enables members to serve on the national scene. With great pride we welcome Vermont Affiliate member Edward Horton, M.D., who will become president of the American Diabetes Association in 1990– our 50th Anniversary year.

Virginia Affiliate

In Richmond, on April 15, 1949, Dr. William R. Jordan, Dr. H. St. George Tucker, and Dr. Robert Bailey, Jr., signed the necessary documents that created the Virginia Diabetes Association. The board of trustees, which had 10 members, accounted for the association's total membership at that time.

For years, this group concentrated on public diabetes education and hosted several professional education conferences. Then in 1974, the first fund-raising efforts got underway so that the association could hire an executive director. In 1976, the group became an ADA affiliate and by the end of that decade, this affiliate had an office in Virginia Beach, several chapters, and a growing base of volunteers.

Today this affiliate's membership is more than 4,100, and there are 15 chapters. They achieved their first $500,000 fund-raising budget in 1987, and leaders are hopeful of surpassing $700,000 in 1990 for the third consecutive year.

Today, the affiliate office is located in Charlottesville, and there are regional offices in Roanoke and Newport News.

Washington Affiliate

Lester Palmer, M.D., was a pioneer of sorts. He was instrumental in getting some of the first supplies of insulin to patients in the Northwest through the Virginia Mason Clinic. From there, he took the lead in establishing the Washington State Diabetes Association, Inc., in 1946—the first organization in the United States to achieve affiliate status.

Dr. Palmer held that lead for 13 years. Patient education seminars, as well as scholarships and camping programs for the young, were part of the program right from the start. Nurse Margaret "Brownie" Brown helped the group expand its programs to reach people with diabetes living in Alaska.

Dr. Palmer played such an integral role in the association that upon his death in 1959, a lull in activities ensued for the next 10 years or so. Then in the early 1970s, Dr. Robert Nielson, despite the lack of funds, decided it was time to get the organization back into operation. With the help of a part-time executive secretary, Joy Koski, an army of volunteers was mustered and, once again, funds began to materialize.

In 1974, the association became the Washington Affiliate of the American Diabetes Association. Many of Dr. Palmer's programs are alive, and there are many, many more in operation today. The affiliate has raised over $1 million for local research over the past 15 years, has over 20 chapters, and conducts over 50 support groups.

West Virginia Affiliate

This affiliate was incorporated in August 1950 as the West Virginia Diabetes Association. Even before this time, a clinical society of interested physicians had been working throughout the state. In the 1940s, under the sponsorship of Ralph H. Nestmann, M.D., and several of his colleagues in Charleston, a lay diabetes society was formed. This Charleston Diabetes Association actively served people with diabetes in the Charleston area. At the suggestion of the national office, a decision to merge the Charleston Diabetes Association with the West Virginia Diabetes Association was made. Shortly thereafter, an application for affiliation with the American Diabetes Association was prepared and filed. Richard N. O'Dell became the first president.

Wisconsin Affiliate

On November 22, 1949, four doctors—Maurice Hardgrove, Francis D. Murphy, Bruno Peters, and Harlen W. Kelley—formed the Wisconsin Diabetic Association. For the next 15 years, this association devoted itself mostly to professional education.

In 1964, the group began sending children with diabetes to a local summer camp and a tradition of diabetes education began. That same year, the association began enlisting lay volunteers in its fight against diabetes, independent support groups across Wisconsin were recruited to become members and chapters, and the association was awarded its first research grant in the amount of $500.

Today, this affiliate, which took the ADA name in 1976, has 15 chapters. The Wisconsin Affiliate is proud of several major accomplishments. In 1980 Wisconsin became the first state to mandate, by state law, health insurance coverage of diabetes supplies, equipment and education. For the past two years volunteers have met with legislators at Legislative Alert Day to discuss diabetes concerns and have worked with the Department of Transportation to revise procedures for drivers licenses.

The Wisconsin Affiliate is also very involved with youth services. Children with diabetes now have extended summer camp opportunities at a camp owned and operated by the affiliate. Annually, four youth delegates are selected to represent the affiliate at the National Youth Leadership Congress, and a mentor system is being developed to help these youth participate in chapter activities upon their return home.

The affiliate supports local research programs, sponsors an Annual Diabetes Educators Conference, cosponsors Upjohn's Clinical Education Program for primary physicians, and is developing a minority outreach program.

The Wisconsin Affiliate takes pride in having three board members, Sharon Maby, M.D., Jerid Kirt, and Edward Ehrlich, M.D., who have served in positions on the ADA national Board of Directors as well.

Wyoming Affiliate

This organization has a very young relationship with the American Diabetes Association. In 1981, Marlin Roberts of the National Service Center, assisted a small group of individuals from across the state in adopting bylaws and electing Bob Clizbe as president. He served for a year and was followed by Ralph Owen.

Under his direction, the Montana Affiliate agreed to work with the Wyoming organization for financial, population, and geographic reasons. In March 1988, the two affiliates signed an agreement that has allowed them to develop many educational and fund-raising activities. In the last two years, Wyoming has organized an effective board with an active Fund Raising Committee, as well as an Awareness Committee.

Camp Hope, the youth camp located in Casper, has been serving juveniles mainly through the efforts of Steve and Nancy Johnson. Through the turbulent years of the affiliate, the Johnsons spent much personal time trying to keep the camp open and available to the youth.

Dr. Eric Wedell is the current president and has also been involved with the affiliate since its inception in 1981. Currently chapters are organized in Cheyenne and Casper, and there are over a dozen active support groups.

Epilogue:
The Journey Continues

The history of the American Diabetes Association is first and foremost a history of people. Lamentably, the legions of those who have contributed to the growth and development of the Association are far too numerous to catalog completely in these pages. Yet, their contributions are visible in the strength and vitality of the American Diabetes Association as we move into the 1990s.

In compiling this history, past and current officers, volunteers, and staff members were asked two questions: What is the Association's greatest strength? and What is its greatest weakness?

Answers to the first question were unanimous: "Our programs in research and education and our human resources." To the second question, the replies struck a familiar chord: Impatience. "It takes too long to get things done."

While ADA's structure, with its yearly change in officers and its committees, creates a certain lack of continuity, this is more than offset by the annual infusion of "new blood," which provides growth and vitality. As one volunteer said so succinctly, "Everything in ADA takes time. . . . but we do get things done eventually." This is evident in the Association's wide ranging efforts in the areas of diabetes education, public awareness, advocacy, standards of health-care delivery, minority initiatives, and funding for diabetes research.

In the past, certain opportunities went unrecognized, and decisions were sometimes slow in coming. This is regrettable but understandable, because decision by consensus takes time. However, in all the debate over issues, the mission and good will of the Association have never been compromised.

There is no doubt that the greatest wealth of the Association lies with its thousands of dedicated volunteers all across the country. A list of past presidents reads like a *Who's Who* in the field of diabetes. A review of officers, board, and committee members who have served over the years reveals the inestimable wealth of time and talent expended on ADA programs. Credit for the recognized high quality of ADA patient, professional, and scientific programs goes to these volunteers.

Lay volunteers have made the same commitment, generously giving their time and expertise. From 1973 to 1990, the Association has benefited from the able leadership of Board chairpersons Gail Patrick Velde (Jackson), Wendell Mayes, Jr., Myles Tanenbaum, Benjamin Greenspoon, Harlan Hanson, Gordon Stulberg, Joseph Davis, Henry Rivera, Sam Gallo, S. Douglas Dodd, William Mamrack, and Sterling Tucker. To this list must be added the thousands of volunteers and staff in the more than 50 affiliates who work in tandem with their leaders to get the job done.

In addition to its human resources, the Association has one other distinct asset that has contributed to its success. It is a concerned organization. Chairman of the Board Wendell Mayes, Jr., (1974-77) described the Association as "an organization in which people demonstrate love for one another. Not an abstract or inanimate love, but the love of concern. Concern for others who share the same cause. This love is shown in the research laboratory, in a hospital emergency room, in a patient education program, at a budget committee meeting or in a door-to-door residential appeal on a cold wintry day. Concern for one another gives the Association a unity of purpose and makes consensus possible when dealing with controversial issues."

"In the rush of events, we should never forget why we are here," a former ADA president said. The purpose of the Association was set forth by Dr. Cecil Striker, first president and founder, and has been echoed by all ADA presidents and chairmen of the Board since that time. We are here because the American Diabetes Association has a mission, a commitment to all those touched by diabetes.

Our mission is to prevent and cure diabetes and to improve the lives of all people affected by diabetes. Our dream is of a world without diabetes. We will be here until our journey to the realization of that dream is at an end.

Appendix 1

American Diabetes Association
Constitution
As adopted June 12, 1940

Article I
Name
This Association shall be a membership corporation, and its name shall be "American Diabetes Association."

Article II
Purpose
The objects of this Association are:
1. To disseminate among physicians information relative to the diagnosis and treatment of diabetes by means of meetings, bulletins, publications of papers in scientific journals, and through a central office which would at all times make available information concerning various aspects of diabetes.
2. To educate the laity in the early recognition of diabetes and in the realization of the importance of medical supervision.
3. To secure and coordinate the active cooperation of associated groups acceptable to the Council in the educational and organization phases of the Association.
4. To make and publish statistical surveys of diabetes.
5. To encourage and support clinical, experimental, sociological, and statistical studies by means of grants.
6. To encourage the adequate treatment of diabetics and the establishment of summer camps for children.

Article III
The membership of the Association shall consist of four classes:
1. Active members
2. Associate members
3. Honorary members
4. Corporate members

Only active members in good standing shall have the right to vote.

Any physician with proper qualifications may be elected an active member of the Association by a majority vote of the Council. Active members shall pay stipulated annual dues.

All those interested in the aims and purposes of the Association, whether physician, scientists, statisticians, dieticians (sic), nurses, social workers, or laymen, may become associate members upon election of the Council, and upon payment of stipulated annual dues.

Honorary membership may be conferred by the Council on those individuals who have rendered distinguished services in medical or other fields related to diabetes.

Associated medical and welfare organizations, civic or educational groups, and insurance companies, may be elected to corporate membership of the Association in recognition of the auxiliary services which they may render to the Association.

Article IV
The Council
The affairs of the Association shall be governed by a Council of at least six and not to exceed fifteen elected from among any of the groups holding active membership in the Association. The officers of the Association shall serve ex-officio as additional Council members. Members of the Council shall be elected at the Annual Meeting of the Association for a period of three years. The first election should be so arranged that in the future only a third of the Council will come up for election at every Annual Meeting. The members of the Council, as well as officers, shall serve without compensation. The Council shall do such proper and needful things as in their judgment will tend to promote the usefulness of the Association and to carry out the purposes for which it has been organized and shall be responsible for determining its policies and activities. The Council shall meet at least once a year and five members shall constitute a quorum.

Article V
Officers
The officers of the Association shall consist of the President, First Vice-President, Second Vice-President, Secretary, and Treasurer. The officers shall be elected annually at the meeting of the Association. The President shall also be the Chairman of the Council and shall preside over the Annual and other meetings. He shall conduct the affairs of the Association and appoint all the committees of the Association. The duties of the other officers are the usual duties associated with their respective titles. The term of the office of the President shall be limited to one year.

In their discretion the Council may appoint a salaried executive officer and staff to attend to the business of the Association and its various committees, under the direction of the President.

Article VI
Committees
Annually the President shall appoint the following committees:
1. The Nominating Committee of not less than three active members to present nominations for officers and members of the Council at the Annual Meeting.
2. The Finance Committee of not less than three active members whose function it shall be to secure funds as well as to advise with the Treasurer concerning payments, deposits, and investments.
3. The Membership Committee of not less than five active members whose duty shall be to arouse interest in the Association and to pass on the qualifications of the candidates for active membership, associate membership, honorary membership, and corporate membership.
4. Special Committees in respect to any particular matter or for any particular purpose may be appointed by the President on the vote of the Council.

Article VII
Meetings
1. Annual Meeting.
   At least one annual meeting shall be held. The site and date of this meeting shall be determined by a quorum of the Council.
2. Special Meetings.
   The holding of any special meetings shall be determined by a quorum of the Council.

Article VIII
Amendments
These By-laws may be altered, amended or repealed by a two-thirds vote of the members of the Council present at a meeting of the Council, provided that the proposition to amend, repeal or alter has been presented in writing at a previous meeting of the Council and that subsequent to such presentation twenty days' notice in writing has been given of the proposed amendment in the call for the meeting.

Appendix 2

American Diabetes Association Presidents

Cecil Striker, M.D.	1940-41
Herman O. Mosenthal, M.D.	1941-42
Joseph T. Beardwood, Jr., M.D.	1942-44
Joseph H. Barach, M.D.	1944-46
Russell M. Wilder, M.D.	1946-47
Edward S. Dillon, M.D.	1947-48
Charles H. Best, M.D.	1948-49
Howard F. Root, M.D.	1949-50
Lester J. Palmer, M.D.	1950-51
Arthur R. Colwell, M.D.	1951-52
Frank N. Allan, M.D.	1952-53
Randall G. Sprague, M.D.	1953-54
Henry B. Mulholland, M.D.	1954-55
Henry T. Ricketts, M.D.	1955-56
Frederick W. Williams, M.D.	1956-57
John A. Reed, M.D.	1957-58
Alexander Marble, M.D.	1958-59
Francis D.W. Lukens, M.D.	1959-60
Franklin B. Peck, Sr., M.D.	1960-61
Blair Holcomb, M.D.	1961-62
Jerome W. Conn, M.D.	1962-63
Thomas P. Sharkey, M.D.	1963-64
Rachmiel Levine, M.D.	1964-65
Thaddeus S. Danowski, M.D.	1965-66
Laurentius O. Underdahl, M.D.	1966-67
Edwin W. Gates, M.D.	1967-68
Harvey C. Knowles, Jr., M.D.	1968-69
Robert C. Hardin, M.D.	1969-70
James B. Hurd, M.D.	1970-71
Stefan S. Fajans, M.D.	1971-72
William H. Grishaw, M.D.	1972-73
Addison B. Scoville, Jr., M.D.	1973-74
Max Ellenberg, M.D.	1974-75
George F. Cahill, Jr., M.D.	1975-76
Donnell D. Etzwiler, M.D.	1976-77
Norbert Freinkel, M.D.	1977-78
Fred W. Whitehouse, M.D.	1978-79
Ronald A. Arky, M.D.	1979-80
Donald I. Bell, M.D.	1980-81
Oscar B. Crofford, M.D.	1981-82
Irving L. Spratt, M.D.	1982-83
Allan L. Drash, M.D.	1983-84
Karl E. Sussman, M.D.	1984-85
Harold Rifkin, M.D.	1985-86
Daniel Porte, Jr., M.D.	1986-87
John A. Colwell, M.D., Ph.D.	1987-88
Charles M. Clark, Jr., M.D.	1988-89
Sherman M. Holvey, M.D.	1989-90

Appendix 3

American Diabetes Association
Chairmen of the Board

Gail Patrick Jackson (Velde)	1973-74
Wendell Mayes, Jr.	1974-77
Myles H. Tanenbaum	1977-79
Benjamin Greenspoon	1979-81
Harlan L. Hanson	1981-83
Gordon T. Stulberg	1983-84
Joseph H. Davis	1984-85
Henry M. Rivera	1985-86
Sam A. Gallo	1986-87
S. Douglas Dodd	1987-88
William A. Mamrack	1988-89
Sterling Tucker	1989-90

Appendix 4

American Diabetes Association
Executive Directors/Executive Vice Presidents

J. Richard Connelly, Executive Director, 1949-73

Ernest M. Frost, Ed.D., Executive Vice President, 1973-76

John L. Dugan, Jr., Executive Vice President, 1977-1980

Robert S. Bolan, Ph.D., Executive Vice President, 1980-

Appendix 5

Guest Editorial
by Edward S. Dillon, M.D., President
from first issue of *ADA Forecast*, Vol., I, No. 1, January 1948

The American Diabetes Association

To the readers of the *A.D.A Forecast* the American Diabetes Association extends cordial greetings.

The membership of the American Diabetes Association at the present time is composed chiefly of about one thousand doctors who are specialists in diabetes or who have an especial interest in diabetes. There are many scores of medical magazines for doctors, but very few for laymen.

There are certain characteristics of diabetes which make it unique among diseases and which seem to make a magazine for diabetics highly desirable. In the first place, the number of diabetics is enormous, estimates run as high as 2,000,000 people, though half of them may be unrecognized. Secondly, it should be emphasized that diabetes is a chronic, dangerous disease and should never be lightly regarded, even though a particular case is mild. Unlike almost all other chronic, dangerous diseases, diabetes can be completely controlled. For this control there is, of course, a cost of time, money, effort and especially of a will to succeed. But the reward far exceeds the cost, and diabetics, therefore, are entitled to hope and good cheer.

To control diabetes the patient himself should have knowledge of his disease and cooperation with his doctor much more than that usually required in other diseases. In sponsoring *A.D.A. Forecast*, a magazine for diabetics and all others interested in diabetes, the American Diabetes Association plans to broadcast as widely as possible accurate information about diabetes. It plans to encourage the individual diabetic to take care of his disease, to banish fears, and at the same time to point out dangers and pitfalls, especially to the careless.

Appendix 6-A

Report of the Treasurer [1941]

The report of the financial status of the Association as of May 26, 1941, is as follows:

Income	$2,079.50
Expenditures	860.64
Balance	$1,218.86

Income:
Contributions—Union Central Life Ins. Co.	$ 500.00
Eli Lilly and Co.	1,000.00
Dues	397.00
Other Income	182.50
Total	$2,079.50

Expenditures:
Charter	$ 25.00
Organization Expenses	177.00
Secretarial Expenses	90.00
Office Expenditures	448.64
Meetings	120.00
Total	$ 860.64

Appendix 6-B
Report of the Treasurer [1950]

The finances of the American Diabetes Association, Inc. have been reviewed by your Treasurer periodically during the last year and the financial statement for the fiscal year ended May 31, 1950, as submitted by our auditors A. R. Taylor & Company, has been carefully considered.

Preliminary remarks of the annual auditors' report relative to transfer of funds and other matters have been studied. At this time I wish to call your attention to the deposit, with the Boston Safe Deposit & Trust Company of Boston, Massachusetts, of $100 to establish the Research Fund of the American Diabetes Association, which is a parent fund for the Nordisk Insulinfond Foundation for the Elliott P. Joslin Fellowship. The Foundation is a $50,000 gift from the Nordisk Insulinfond of Copenhagen, Denmark. The income from the Insulinfond Foundation during the lifetime of Elliott P. Joslin is to be applied to the study of diabetes as he shall direct, and thereafter applied to that purpose as may be directed by the Advisory Committee of the Research Fund of the American Diabetes Association, Inc., subject to certain requests of the donor and provisions of the trust agreement.

Summary of Cash Receipts and Disbursements
For the Fiscal Year Ended May 31, 1950

Receipts
Membership dues	$13,788.48
General contributions	28,398.00
Subscriptions to *A.D.A. Forecast*	31,572.64
Sale of books and pamphlets	7,194.53
Sale of *Proceedings*	1,115.27
Diabetes Detection Fund contributions	16,001.00
Clinical and Research Fund contributions	5.00
Total receipts	$98,074.92

Disbursements
General Scientific Fund	$11,643.35
A.D.A Forecast Activities Fund	53,624.00
Diabetes Detection Fund	11,912.12
Total disbursements	$77,179.47
Excess of Receipts over Disbursements	$20,895.45
Balance, May 31, 1949	78,115.89
Balance, May 31, 1950	$99,011.34

Appendix 7-A

Banting Medal For Distinguished Scientific Achievement

The Banting Medal honors meritorious career achievement in the field of diabetes research and is the highest scientific award of the American Diabetes Association. Recipients deliver a lecture at the Annual Scientific Sessions.

1941—Elliott P. Joslin, M.D.
  "Diabetes Yesterday, Today and Tomorrow"
1942—William Muhlberg, M.D.
  "An Analysis of Statistics Bearing On Diabetes Mellitus"
1943—Fred W. Hipwell, M.D.
  "Memories"
1944—Leonard G. Rowntree, M.D.
  "The Challenge of Diabetes to Banting; and Today"
1945—No meeting due to war
1946—Bernardo A. Houssay, M.D.
  Hans C. Hagedorn, M.D.
  R. D. Lawrence, M.D.
  Eugene Opie, M.D.
  Sydney Smith
1947—George H.A. Clowes, Ph.D.
  "Banting Memorial Address"
1948—Rollin T. Woodyatt, M.D.
  "Foundations of the Conception of Acidosis"
1949—Herbert M. Evans, M.D.,
  "The Search for the Diabetogenic Principle of the Anterior Hypophysis"
  Frederick M. Allen, M.D.
1950—F.G. Young, D.Sc.
  "The Endocrine Approach to the Problem of Diabetes"
1951—C.N.H. Long, M.D.
  "Endocrine Control of the Blood Sugar"
1952—R.R. Bensley, M.D.
1953—Shields Warren, M.D.
  "An Interpretation of Diabetes in the Light of its Pathology"
  Walter R. Campbell, M.D.
  A. Almon Fletcher, M.D.
  (Drs. Campbell and Fletcher of University of Toronto, Faculty of Medicine, were the first physicians to clinically administer insulin.) *ADA Forecast* July/August 1953.

1954—Sir Henry Dale
"Hormones of the Posterior Lobe"
1955—Carl F. Cori, M.D., Lecturer
"Influence of Epenephrine and Glucagon on Enzyme Systems in Muscle and Liver, Recent Advances in Insulin Research"
Eugene F. Dubois, M.D.
1956—William C. Stadie, M.D., Lecturer
"Recent Advances in Insulin Research"
1957—DeWitt Stetten, Jr., M.D., Ph.D., Lecturer
"Certain Aspects of the Metabolism of Glycogen"
John R. Murlin, Ph.D., D.Sc.
1958—Jerome W. Conn, M.D., Lecturer
"The Prediabetes State in Man"
William H. Olmsted, M.D.
1959—George W. Thorn, M.D., Lecturer
"The Adrenal and Diabetes"
E.T. Bell, M.D.
1960—Priscilla White, M.D., Lecturer
"Childhood Diabetes: Its Course and Influences on the Second and Third Generations"
J.P. Collip, M.D.
1961—Rachmiel Levine, M.D.
"Concerning the Mechanism of Insulin Action"
1962—A. Baird Hastings, Ph.D.
"Ah, Sweet Mystery"
1963—Bernardo Houssay, M.D., Lecturer
"Hormonal Factors of Diabetes Ketosis"
Garfield G. Duncan, M.D.
1964—Francis D.W. Lukens, M.D., Lecturer
"Insulin and Protein Metabolism"
Moses Barron, M.D.
Professor Joseph P. Hoet
Leland S. McKittrick, M.D.
Peter J. Moloney, Ph.D.
David A. Scott, Ph.D.
Ernst Wertheimer, M.D.
1965—Solomon A. Berson, M.D., Lecturer
"Some Current Controversies in Diabetes Research"
I. Arthur Mirsky, M.D.
1966—Robert H. William, M.D.
"Secretion, Fates and Actions of Insulin"
1967—Alexander Marble, M.D.
"Angiopathy in Diabetes: An Unsolved Problem"
1968—Arthur R. Colwell, Sr., M.D.
"Fifty Years of Diabetes in Perspective"

1969—Earl W. Sutherland, M.D., Lecturer
"The Biological Role of Cyclic AMP and its Relation to Carbohydrate Metabolism"
Robert L. Jackson, M.D.
1970—Paul E. Lacy, M.D.
"Beta Cell Secretion—From the Standpoint of a Pathobiologist"
1971—George F. Cahill, Jr., M.D., Lecturer
"Physiology of Insulin in Man"
William R. Kirtley, M.D.
1972—Dorothy C. Hodgkin, Ph.D.
"The Structure of Insulin"
1973—Arnold Lazarow, M.D., Ph.D.
"Selective Islet Differentiation in Organ Culture and Islet Transplantation"
1974—Albert Renold, M.D.
"Spontaneous and Induced Hypofunctions of Endocrine Pancreas"
1975—Roger H. Unger, M.D.
"Diabetes and the Alpha Cell"
1976—Donald F. Steiner, M.D.
"Insulin Today"
1977—David M. Kipnis, M.D.
"Protein Turnover"
1978—Stefan S. Fajans, M.D.
"Etiology and Clinical Heterogeneity of Idiopathic Diabetes Mellitus"
1979—Charles R. Park, M.D.
"Control of Hepatic Glucose Output"
1980—Norbert Freinkel, M.D.
"Islet Metabolism and Secretory Performance"
1981—Lelio Orci, M.D.
"Macro- and Micro-Domains in the Endocrine Pancreas"
1982—Jesse Roth, M.D.
"Evolutionary Organs of Insulin and Other Intercellular Messenger Molecules: Implications for Human Biology"
1983—Arthur Rubenstein, M.D.
"Proinsulin and C-peptide: Interaction of Clinical and Basic Research"
1984—Daniel W. Foster, M.D.
"From Glycogen to Ketones—and Back"
1985—Bjorn Nerup, M.D.
"Studies on the Pathogenesis of Insulin-Dependent Diabetes Mellitus"
1986—Albert I. Winegrad, M.D.
"Does a Common Mechanism Induce the Diverse Complications of Diabetes?"

1987—Joseph Larner, M.D., Ph.D.
"Insulin Signaling Mechanisms—Lessons from the Old Testament of Glycogen Metabolism and from the New Testament of Molecular Biology"
1988—Gerald M. Reaven, M.D.
"Role of Insulin Resistance and Hyperinsulinemia in Human Disease"
1989—Ora Rosen, M.D.
"Structure and Function of the Insulin Receptor"

Banting Medal for Service

Each year, this award is presented to the outgoing ADA President. The medal reads "This medal is awarded . . . for distinguished service in the interest of doctor and patient." (For a listing of Banting Medal for Service recipients, see the list of ADA Presidents, Appendix 2.)

Additionally, in 1979, Professor Rolf Loft was presented the Banting Medal for Service to the International Diabetes Federation.

Appendix 7-B

Charles H. Best Medal For Distinguished Service In the Cause of Diabetes

The Charles H. Best Award was established to honor service by a nonphysician; however, this has been modified to include physicians who are being honored for achievements not associated with their professional expertise.

1974—Senator Gale W. McGee
1974—Senator Richard Schweiker
1975—Ray A. Kroc
1976—Oscar B. Crofford, M.D.
1977—Representative Louis Stokes
1978—Wayne Newton
1979—President Gerald R. Ford
1980—Jim (Catfish) Hunter
1981—David M. Kipnis, M.D.
1982—The Daniel T. Gillespie Family
1983—J. William Flynt, M.D.
1983—President Ronald Reagan
1984—James M. Fowler, D.D.S.
1984—Everett J. Grindstaff
1985—Keatha K. Krueger, Ph.D.
1985—Nina Berlin
1985—Jean F. Curran
1985—Hon. Governor Robert T. Graham
1985—Lee Iacocca
1985—Dorothea F. Sims
1985—Lester B. Salans, M.D.
1986—John H. Davidson, M.D., Ph.D.
1987—Neil W. Pettinga, Ph.D.
1987—Senator Lowell Weicker
1988—Richard Verville
1988—Joan Foran
1989—Lions Clubs International

The Charles H. Best Medal for Service

This award honors service by the outgoing ADA Board Chairman.

1974—Gail Patrick Velde
1978—Wendell Mayes, Jr.
1979—Myles H. Tanenbaum
1981—Benjamin Greenspoon
1983—Harlan L. Hanson
1984—Gordon Stulberg
1985—Joseph H. Davis
1986—Henry Rivera
1987—Sam A. Gallo
1988—S. Douglas Dodd
1989—William A. Mamrack

Appendix 7-C
American Diabetes Association Award Winners

Outstanding Affiliate Service Award
Sponsored by Squibb-Novo since 1983
This award was established to honor volunteers for meritorious service to an affiliate association.

1956—Alice P. Hoover
1957—C. Paul and Addie Lou Tiley
1958—Louise Hayes Williams
1959—Anna Smrha
1960—Edith Jenkins
1961—Carolyn J. Spiegel
1962—Mrs. Alan J. Arthur
1963—Wilma Van Der Beek
1964—Pauline Steigerwald
1965—Helen Turner Whitney
1966—Frances Vroom
1967—Peter S. Kaufman
1968—Lloyd C. Pray, Ph.D.
1969—Mrs. Robert E. (Dorothy) Childs
1970—Mrs. Henry A. Friedman
1971—Lowell Echard
1972—Jon W. Hall
1973—Dina Merrill
1973—Dorothy Child
1974—Ruth Hanson
1975—Beverly Holman
1975—Samuel M. Shrilberg
1976—Gordon P. Sprague
1977—Harvey and Karen Carafiol
1978—Sydelle Feinman
1979—Jane Zarish
1980—Nettie Richter
1981—Gilbert Marks
1982—Todd and Connie Leigh
1983—G. F. (Joe) DeCoursin
1984—Sandra Lewis
1985—David Grier
1986—Timothy J. McGuckin
1987—Harriet Silverberg
1988—Clydella Hentschel
1989—Terry Golden, M.D.

Outstanding Scientific Achievement Award by an Investigator
Sponsored by Eli Lilly & Co.

1957—Solomon A. Berson, M.D.

1958—James B. Field, M.D.
"Studies of the Antagonist to Insulins"
1959—Marvin D. Siperstein, M.D.
"Fat Metabolism"
1960—Albert E. Renold, M.D.
"The Delayed or Adaptive Effect of Insulin in the Liver, the Metabolism of Fructose and Sorbitol, and on the Metabolism of Adipose Tissue"
1961—Rosalyn S. Yalow, Ph.D.
"The Development of a Sensitive Technique for Determinationof Insulin in Biological Materials"
1962—Harry N. Antoniades, Ph.D.
"The State, Transport and Regulation of Insulin in Blood"
1963—James M.B. Bloodworth, Jr., M.D.
"The Pathology of the Microangiopathy of Diabetes"
1964—Roger H. Unger, M.D.
"Studies of the Physiologic Role of Glucagon"
1965—George F. Cahill, Jr., M.D.
"The Role of Adipose Tissue in Normal Metabolism"
1966—Norbert Freinkel, M.D.
"Insulin Homeostasis During Pregnancy and 'Alcohol Hypoglycemia' "
1967—David M. Kipnis, M.D.
"The Physiology of the Intracellular Transport, Regulation, and Phosphorylation of Glucose, Insulin, and Growth Hormonein Relation to Carbohydrate and Lipid Metabolism"
1968—Robert G. Spiro, M.D.
"Enzymes Involved in Microchemical Changes in the Outer Wall of Small Blood Vessels"
1969—Donald F. Steiner, M.D.
"The Physiology of the B Cell Leading to the Discovery of Proinsulin and its Characterization"
1970—Oscar B. Crofford, M.D.
"The Mechanism of Insulin Action"
1971—Daniel Porte, Jr., M.D.
"The Relationship Between Catecholamines and Insulin Secretion in Humans"
1972—John H. Exton, Ph.D.
"Regulation of Glucose Metabolism by the Liver at the Cellular and Molecular Levels"
1973—Arthur H. Rubenstein, M.D.
"Circulating Proinsulin and C-Peptide"

1974—Jesse Roth, M.D.
"Secretion of Growth Hormone and Proinsulin, and the Assessment of Blood Levels of Proinsulin"
1975—Pedro Cuatrecasas, M.D.
(accepting the award for Dr. Cuatrecasas was Dr. Dean Lockwood)
1976—Philip Felig, M.D.
"Insulin and Glucagon in Normal Phyiology and Diabetes"
1977—Peter H. Bennett, M.D.
"Natural History of Diabetes Mellitus in the Pima"
1978—J. Denis McGarry, Ph.D.
"New Perspecties in the Regulation of Ketogenesis"
1979—Leonard S. Jefferson, Ph.D.
"Role of Insulin in the Regulation of Protein Synthesis"
1980—Jerrold M. Olefsky, M.D.
"Insulin Resistance and Insulin Action: An In Vitro and In Vivo Perspective"
1981—C. Ronald Kahn, M.D.
"A Pathophysiologic View of Insulin Receptor Structure and Function"
1982—Michael P. Czech, Ph.D.
"Symbiotic Relationship Among Hormone Receptor Systems"
1983—Howard S. Tager, Ph.D.
"Abnormal Products of the Human Insulin Gene"
1984—Alan D. Cherrington, Ph.D.
"Regulation of Glucose Supply for the Liver"
1985—Steven J. Jacobs, M.D.
"Insulin Receptor: Structure and Function"
1986—George S. Eisenbarth, M.D., Ph.D.
"Genes, G.O.D., Glyconjugates and Autoimmune Beta Cell Insufficiency (Type I Diabetes)"
1987—Ralph A. DeFronzo, M.D.
"The Triumvirate—B-Cell, Liver, Muscle: A Collusion Responsible for Type II Diabetes Mellitus"
1988—John E. Gerich, M.D.
"Glucose Counterregulation and Its Impact in Diabetes Mellitus"
1989—Richard N. Bergman, Ph.D.
"A Physiologic Approach to Understanding Glucose Tolerance: The Minimal Model Method"

Annual Award for Outstanding Contribution to Diabetes in Youth
Sponsored by Boehringer-Mannheim Diagnostics
This award recognizes exceptional contributions of those who work with young people with diabetes.

1973—Aaron Fox Foundations
1973—Harlan L. Hanson
1973—Joyce Kortman
1973—Fred Wolinsky
1974—Melvyn Coldman
1974—Robert Jackson, M.D.
1974—Patricia McAlister
1975—Priscilla White, M.D.
1975—Caroline Sanders
1976—Barbara Cavanaugh
1976—Mary Connolly
1976—Donnell D. Etzwiler, M.D.
1976—Abraham Silver, M.D.
1976—Matthew Steiner, M.D.
1977—Sheila Garvey, R.N.
1977—Mary Olney, M.D.
1977—Howard Traisman, M.D.
1978—Ronald B. Youngquist
1979—Samuel M. Wentworth, M.D.
1980—Luther B. Travis, M.D.
1982—Charlene Bandurski
1983—Frank Robles, R.Ph.
1984—Linda M. Siminero, R.N., M.S.
1985—Kathleen Wishner, M.D., Ph.D.
1986—Nettie Richter, M.S.
1987—Robert K. Endres, M.D.
1988—Marilyn Moore
1989—Dorothy Becker, M.B.B.Ch.

The Addison B. Scoville, Jr., Award for Outstanding Volunteer Service
The Addison B. Scoville Award was established in 1974, and is given for outstanding service by a board or committee member.

1974—Addison B. Scoville, M.D.
1975—Ernest M. Frost, Ed.D.
1977—Wendell Mayes, Jr.
1981—Alvin Z. Levine
1984—Robert L. Kroc, Ph.D.
1986—Annette Schapiro
1987—Oscar B. Crofford, M.D.
1988—Virginia Hanson-Ullom
1989—Sandra Segal Polin, J.D., M.P.A.

Outstanding Physician Educator in the Field of Diabetes

Sponsored by The Upjohn Company
This award was established to stimulate, acknowledge, and reward outstanding education efforts by physicians in the field of diabetes.

1975—Alexander Marble, M.D.
1976—Leona V. Miller, M.D.
1977—Philip W. Felts, M.D.
1978—Frederick C. Goetz, M.D.
1979—John K. Davidson, M.D.
1980—Leo P. Krall, M.D.
1981—John W. Runyan, M.D.
1982—Ann Lawrence, M.D., Ph.D.
1983—Donnell D. Etzwiler, M.D.
1984—H. St. George Tucker, Jr., M.D.
1985—Charles R. Shuman, M.D.
1986—J. Stuart Soeldner, M.D.
1987—Ronald A. Arky, M.D.
1988—Daniel W. Foster, M.D.
1989—Oscar B. Crofford, M.D.

Outstanding Clinician in the Field of Diabetes

Sponsored by Roerig, a Division of Pfizer Pharmaceuticals
This award was established to stimulate, acknowledge, and reward outstanding clinicians in the field of diabetes.

1975—Edgar A. Hauntz, M.D.
1976—David Hurwitz, M.D.
1977—Henry E. Oppenheimer, M.D.
1978—Priscilla White, M.D.
1979—Marvin E. Levin, M.D.
1980—Harold Rifkin, M.D.
1981—James M. Moss, M.D.
1982—George P. Heffner, M.D.
1983—Harvey C. Knowles, Jr., M.D.
1984—Alan L. Graber, M.D.
1985—Burritt L. Haag, M.D.
1986—Holbroke S. Seltzer, M.D.
1987—O. Peter Schumacher, M.D.
1988—Allan L. Drash, M.D.
1989—Fred W. Whitehouse, M.D.

Outstanding Health Professional Educator in the Field of Diabetes

Sponsored by Miles, Inc., Diagnostics Division
This award was established to stimulate, acknowledge, and reward outstanding educational efforts by health professionals in the field of diabetes.

1977—Rita M. Nemchik, R.N., M.S.
1978—Barbara M. Prater, M.S., Ph.D.
1979—Diana Guthrie, R.N., Ph.D.
1980—Carelyn P. Fylling, R.N., M.S.
1981—Barbara Christman Adair, R.N., M.S.N.
1982—Myrtis A. McSweeney, R.N.
1983—Maria Alogna, R.N., M.P.H.
1984—Margaret C. Yarborough, R.Ph.
1985—Marion Franz, R.D., M.S.
1986—Deborah A. Hinnen, R.N., M.N.
1987—Madelyn L. Wheeler, M.S., R.D.
1988—Phyllis R. Crapo, R.D.
1989—R. Keith Campbell, R.Ph.

Outstanding Contribution to Camping and Diabetes Award

Sponsored by Becton Dickinson Consumer Products
This award acknowledges an individual who has made an exceptional contribution to the camping program.

1979—Donnell D. Etzwiler, M.D.
1980—Vivian Murray, R.D.
1981—Samuel Eichold, M.D.
1982—Ronald B. Youngquist
1983—Kathleen Krauser, R.N., M.N.
1984—Jerome R. Ryan, M.D.
1985—Robert K. Endres, M.D.
1986—Paul Madden, M.D.
1987—Luther B. Travis, M.D.
1988—Martha Leigh Spencer, M.D.
1989—Campbell P. Howard, M.D.

Youth Leadership Award

Sponsored by The NutraSweet Company
This award recognizes a young adult's leadership within the ADA and the community.

1985—Kara Vereault
1986—Tom Casey
1987—Susanna Maiuri
1988—John Nawrocki
1989—Joby Jobson

Wendell Mayes, Jr., Award

This medal is awarded to a non-health-professional volunteer for outstanding service in the cause of diabetes.

1986—Wendell Mayes, Jr.
1987—Benjamin Greenspoon
1988—Dorothea Sims
1989—Lee Iacocca

Fund Raising Volunteer Recognition Award
Sponsored by George Rice & Sons
This award is given to recognize and stimulate exceptional leadership among volunteers working in the area of fund raising.

1989—Bruce Furness

Rachmiel Levine, M.D. Award
Established in 1989, this award will honor the ADA's Senior Vice President upon leaving office.

1989—Linda S. Hurwitz, R.N., M.S.

Kelly West Award
The Kelly West Award, established in 1989, is given in memory of Kelly West, widely regarded as the "father of diabetes epidemiology." The award is sponsored by the Council on Epidemiology.

1989—Harry Keen, M.D.

Appendix 8

Research Symposia, 1962-1985

1962—Cellular Metabolism in Relation to Cell Structure
1963—The Microangopathy of Diabetes
1964—Insulin Synthesis, Storage, Release, Transport and Antagonism
1965—Glucose, Fatty Acids and Diabetes
1966—Glucagon
1967—Diabetes, Pregnancy and the Newborn
1968—Growth Hormone: Secretory Control, Endocrine Interrelationships, Metabolic Effects and Bearing upon Clinical Diabetes
1969—Glucogenesis and its Controlling Mechanisms
1970—Synthesis and Release of Insulin
1972—Cell Membranes
1973—Ketosis and Ketogenesis
1974—Transplantation of Pancreatic Islets and the Histocompatibility of Endocrine Tissues
1975—Perspectives in Current Diabetes Research
1976—Current Topics in Diabetes Research
1977—Current Trends in Diabetes Research
1978—Biology of the Islets and Metabolic Regulation
1979—New Concepts in the Etiology of Diabetes, Mechanism of Insulin Action, and Regulation of Protein
1983—Diabetes and Exercise
1984—Recent Advances in the Pathogenetic Mechanism and Treatment of Insulin-Dependent Diabetes Mellitus
1985—Obesity and Non-insulin Dependent Diabetes Mellitus
1986—Research and Therapeutic Issues in Diabetes: Biology of Metabolic Regulation; Etiopathogenesis of Diabetes Mellitus; Metabolic Physiology and Pathophysiology; Clinical Diabetes Mellitus
1987—The Immunology of Diabetes
1989—Diabetes, Lipoproteins, and Atherosclerosis (March)
Pancreatic B-Cell Ion Channels: Role in Diabetes Pathogenesis and Therapy (October)
NOTE: No programs in 1971, 1980, 1981, 1982, 1988.

Appendix 9

American Diabetes Association Annual Meetings
On June 12, 1940, 26 physicians held a meeting and elected officers. The Association was founded by 31 physicians and incorporated on August 27, 1940.

1) 1941 Cleveland, Ohio
2) 1942 Atlantic City, New Jersey
3) 1943 New York, New York
4) 1944 Chicago, Illinois
5) 1945 no Annual Meeting due to war
6) 1946 Toronto, Canada
7) 1947 Atlantic City, New Jersey
8) 1948 Chicago, Illinois
9) 1949 Atlantic City, New Jersey
10) 1950 San Francisco, California
11) 1951 Atlantic City, New Jersey
12) 1952 Chicago, Illinois
13) 1953 New York, New York
14) 1954 San Francisco, California
15) 1955 Atlantic City, New Jersey
16) 1956 Chicago, Illinois
17) 1957 New York, New York
18) 1958 San Francisco, California
19) 1959 Atlantic City, New Jersey
20) 1960 Miami Beach, Florida

21) 1961 New York, New York
22) 1962 Chicago, Illinois
23) 1963 Atlantic City, New Jersey
24) 1964 San Francisco, California
25) 1965 New York, New York
26) 1966 Chicago, Illinois
27) 1967 Atlantic City, New Jersey
28) 1968 San Francisco, California
29) 1969 New York, New York
30) 1970 St. Louis, Missouri
31) 1971 San Francisco, California
32) 1972 Washington, D.C.
33) 1973 Chicago, Illinois
34) 1974 Atlanta, Georgia
35) 1975 New York, New York
36) 1976 San Francisco, California
37) 1977 St. Louis, Missouri
38) 1978 Boston, Massachusetts
39) 1979 Los Angeles, California
40) 1980 Washington, D.C.
41) 1981 Cincinnati, Ohio
42) 1982 San Francisco, California
43) 1983 San Antonio, Texas
44) 1984 Las Vegas, Nevada
45) 1985 Baltimore, Maryland
46) 1986 Anaheim, California
47) 1987 Indianapolis, Indiana
48) 1988 New Orleans, Louisiana
49) 1989 Detroit, Michigan
50) 1990 Atlanta, Georgia

Appendix 10: American Diabetes Association's Nationwide Comprehensive Long-Range Plan Synopsis

Revised Mission Statement
The mission of the American Diabetes Association is to prevent and cure diabetes and to improve the lives of all people affected by diabetes.

Nationwide Five-Year Goals
Fund-Raising Services
Fund raising of the American Diabetes Association will emphasize public support and maintain revenue income, which will enable the Association to carry out its activities and services.
Goal 1: Increase annual public support income by at least 12 percent per year.
Goal 2: Conduct broad-based, fund-raising activities and services coordinated and implemented on a nationwide basis independent of other diabetes organizations.
Goal 3: Establish new sources of funding with emphasis on the need for diabetes research.
Goal 4: Increase annual revenue income by 10 percent every year from relevant, appropriate, and carefully selected products and services that further the Mission of the Association. Approximately 90 percent of revenue income shall be generated at the National Service Center.
Goal 5: Every volunteer shall support fund-raising activities and functions.

Research Activities
Nationwide research activities of the American Diabetes Association lead to the prevention and cure of diabetes, and provide research information for use by scientists and practitioners to improve the lives of people affected by diabetes.
Goal 1: Allocate 15 percent of nationwide unrestricted public support income, plus 100 percent of nationwide research-restricted income, to research awards and grants, which would constitute a total of nearly 30 percent of total public support.
Goal 2: Support only the highest quality research by reviewing and funding research programs at the national level or through nationally approved affiliate research programs.
Goal 3: Maintain current high-quality, broad-based research activities and develop new initiatives in areas of identified need.
Goal 4: Cooperate with organizations that fund diabetes research.

Public Activities
Nationwide public activities of the American Diabetes Association improve the lives of people affected by diabetes by making the general public aware of diabetes and its implications and through advocating effective public policy decisions.
Goal 1: Increase the proportion of the American population that is aware of diabetes and its seriousness by at least 10 percent per year to a goal of at least 75 percent and raise the proportion of Americans aware of the American Diabetes Association to at least 50 percent by 1993.
Goal 2: Increase the number of people reached through American Diabetes Alert activities by at least 10 percent each year as determined by an independent polling organization.

Goal 3: Play the leading advocacy role on behalf of constituencies interested in diabetes policies.
Goal 4: Maintain regular contact with 50 percent of federal and state legislators and appropriate federal and state regulatory agencies.
Goal 5: Encourage reimbursement for inpatient and outpatient medical care, education, counseling, and materials necessary in the treatment of diabetes by establishing legislative and organizational liaisons and sharing standards with government bodies and insurance carriers.
Goal 6: Plan and implement comprehensive public education program aimed at individuals and groups whose functions have a direct impact on the lives of people with diabetes.

Professional Activities
Nationwide professional activities of the American Diabetes Association improve the lives of people affected by diabetes by educating health-care providers on the diagnosis and treatment of diabetes and its complications and by establishing high-quality standards for diabetes health-care delivery.
Taken as a whole, professional education programs at all levels of the organization must be self-supporting to the greatest extent possible.
Goal 1: Develop and disseminate standards and criteria for the proper treatment of people with diabetes.
Goal 2: Continue to be the leader in the publication of quality professional materials and journals for health-care professionals throughout the world.
Goal 3: Reach 50,000 primary-care health providers (physicians, nurses, dietitians, and others) with professional education programs based on care standards.
Goal 4: Continue to conduct internationally renowned annual scientific and medical postgraduate meetings and programs.
Goal 5: Improve access to and delivery of health care.
Goal 6: Assess and evaluate existing and emerging technology for diabetes care.

Patient Activities
Nationwide patient activities of the American Diabetes Association improve the lives of people with diabetes by informing people about diabetes and its care, by operating support groups and camps for people with diabetes, and by establishing, reviewing, and updating standards for diabetes education programs.
Goal 1: Identify 3 million people who have diabetes and provide them with comprehensive information about their disease.
Goal 2: Promote availability of high-quality diabetes patient education, support, and information programs.
Goal 3: Ensure that elderly, underserved, and minority people with diabetes are reached with diabetes information.
Goal 4: Provide for the special needs of youth and their families by designing and conducting comprehensive programs and services.

Management Services
Management services of the American Diabetes Association organize the human, financial, and information resources of the Association into a structure that allows the Association to be effective and efficient in carrying out its activities and services.
Goal 1: Develop guidelines to encourage standardization of administrative operations such as financial management procedures, minimum and maximum fund balances, long-range plans, and personnel policies and procedures.
Goal 2: Expand the scope of memberships in the Association.
Goal 3: Recruit, train, and retain volunteers to set policy and to work with staff to implement the goals and objectives of the Association.
Goal 4: Hire, train, and retain staff to work with volunteers to implement the goals and objectives of the Association.
Goal 5: Through affiliates, organize chapters to reach 75 percent of the populated area within the affiliates' territories.

Long-Range Planning Process
Through an organized process of long-range planning, the American Diabetes Association is able to review, evaluate, and revise the long-range plan at all levels and in all components of the organization.
Goal 1: Clarify the intent and impact of the long-range plan.
Goal 2: Maintain an annual process for review, evaluation, and revision of the long-range plan.

Index

Abbott Laboratories, 70
Accounting procedures, 112, 128
Acidosis
 emergencies, 21–22
ADA/ADA Family Cookbook, 199
ADA Forecast, (renamed *Diabetes Forecast*,) 39–41, 51–52, 68–70
Adler, Sidney, 6
Advertising Committee (ADA), 69
Affiliate Builder, 97
Affiliate Volunteer Leadership Conference (ADA), 281
Age
 diabetes and, 5, 102
 and drug effectiveness, 87–88
Ahern, JoAnn, 202
Airlie meeting, Financing Quality Health Care, 229–30
Alabama Affiliate, 287
Alaska Affiliate, 287–288
Albert, Carl, 184
Aldose reductase inhibitors, 244
Allan, Frank N., 72
Allen, Frederick, 2, 76
Allen, James H., 16
Allen, Steve, 231
Alpert, Louis K., 67, 292
Altshuler, Samuel S., 3, 6, 8, 23–24
Amaranth, Order of the, 192–193, 228
American Association of Diabetes Educators (AADE), 153–154, 181, 196, 202, 222–223
American Camping Association, 53
American Catholic Hospital Association emergency instructions for diabetes, 22
American College of Obstetricians and Gynecologists, 92
American College of Physicians, 3, 9
American Contract Bridge League, 194
American Diabetes Alert, 266
American Diabetes Association (ADA). *See also specific committees*.
 affiliates, 42, 50–52, 65–68, 90–91, 97, 106, 110–112, 127–133, 151–152, 154, 187–188, 194, 196–197, 220–221, 224, 226, 233, 267, 275, 281, 287–319
 and animal research, 279–281
 annual meetings, 332–333
 Assembly of Delegates, 67, 100
 Award winners, 329–330
 beginnings, 1–18
 budget planning, 172–173, 188–191, 282–283
 chairmen of the board, 325
 Constitution and Bylaws, 7–8, 73, 106, 113, 136–137, 154, 168, 181–182, 236–237, 323–324
 as cosponsor of film, 44
 as cosponsor of gestational diabetes workshop, 92
 emblem, 82
 executive director/executive vice presidents, 325
 first Annual Meeting, 9–10,
 fund-raising activities of. *See* Fund-raising
 growth activities, 23–24, 52–54, 77–79, 95–97, 109–113, 141–143, 151–152, 185–187, 203–204, 236–237, 281–282
 guest editorial, 325
 and health-care financing, 230
 insurance activities, 46–47, 93–94, 116–117, 167–168
 Hiram Hamster symbol, 140–141
 income growth, 187–191
 incorporation as non-profit organization, 7
 international programs, 248
 long range plans, 170, 184–185, 221, 226–227, 333–334
 marketing strategy for, 89
 membership policies, 24–25, 72–73
 minority activities, 263–265
 National Service Center, 251–252
 patient education, 193, 217, 228–229, 252–253, 271–274
 position statements, 259
 postgraduate course, 77, 133, 142–143, 146, 263
 presidents, 324
 product endorsement, 95
 professional education programs, 94–95, 112, 132, 176, 223, 240–241, 270–271
 professional councils of, 221, 224, 262–263
 publications, 12–13, 23, 36, 39–41, 46, 51–52, 59–61, 68–70, 187, 270–274
 public awareness/relations activities, 113–116, 191–194, 230–233, 265–268
 relocation of, 221
 research activities of, 5, 35–57, 73–75, 116, 129, 141–148, 160–167, 226–228, 274–276, 229–281
 reorganization, 59–82, 127–137
 resource allocation, 258–259
 silver anniversary of, 119
 tax exemption, 20
 treasurers' reports, 325–326
 as voluntary health agency, 126–137, 151
 volunteer activities, 135–136, 156–158, 217, 220, 321–322, 238–239, 248, 267
American Dietetic Association, 10, 199
American Heart Association, 196
American Hospital Association emergency instructions for diabetes, 22
American Pharmaceutical Association, 201
American Red Cross, 22
American Society of Hospital Pharmacists, 201
Ames (Company) Laboratories
 award sponsor, 183
 Dextrostix, 106
 solid phase blood testing system, 146
 supplier of urine test equipment for camp, 209
Anderson, George E., 6, 24, 51–52, 17
Angiotensin converting enzyme (ACE), 286
Animal research, 54, 279–281
Antoine, Tex, 115
Arizona Affiliate, 288
Arkansas Affiliate, 288–289
Arky, Ronald A., 123, 142, 183, 189, 192–193, 196–197, 207, 239, 299
Armed services and diabetes treatment, 23

Arquilla, Edward R., 207
Arteriosclerosis and diabetes, 2, 56
Ashe, Benjamin I., 6
Assan, R., 243
Atkins, Christopher, 251–252
Atkinson, Mark A., 285
Atlas Powder Company, 63

Baio, Scott, 231
Baker, Howard H., Jr., 173
Ball, Michael F., 142
Banting, Frederick G., 1, 6–9, 11–12, 20, 37–39, 77, 95, 158
Banting, Lady, 158
Banting Memorial Lectures, 12, 15, 26, 74, 88, 101, 103, 126, 148, 158
Banting Memorial Medal, 38–40, 92, 103, 110, 326–328
Barach, Joseph H., 7–8, 34, 38–39, 73
Baran, Mary Ellen, 213
Barr, Patricia, 255
Bauer, W. W., 60
Beardwood, Joseph T., Jr., 3, 7–8, 21, 23, 60, 117
Bearskin Meadow Camp, 51
Becker, Richard, 243
Becton Dickinson, 69–70, 183, 331
Beef as source of insulin, 277
Behrman, Sr. Maude, 207–208
Bell, Donald I., 198, 202, 224–25
Bell, E. T., 80
Benedict's test, 5, 81
Benjamin, Samuel, 51
Benko, George, 160–161
Berg, Paul, 216
Berlin, Nina, 252
Berson, Solomon A., 60, 89, 158
Best, Charles H., 6–9, 11–12, 20, 32, 38–39, 41–42, 63, 73–74, 77, 95, 102, 110, 127–128, 156, 158, 173–174, 208–209
Best (Charles H.) Birthplace Trust, 127–128
Best (Charles H.) Medal for Distinguished Service, 173, 236, 328
Best, Mrs. Charles H., 158
Beta cells
 studies, 175–176, 244
 64K autoantibody and, 285
 transplantation of, 213
Betschart, Jean, 131–132
Biguanides. See Metformin
Bike-a-thons, 155–156, 255, 282
Birney, David, 251, 266, 277
Birney, Meredith Baxter, 251, 266, 277
Blacks and diabetes, 263
Blaine, Belford C., 7
Blood analysis
 to detect diabetes, 36
 radioimmunoassay test for insulin, 60
Blood glucose, 254
 determination/monitoring of, 65, 106, 202, 220, 284
 drugs for lowering of, 84, 87–88, 244, 285–286
 implantable device for sensing, 286
 self-monitoring, 217, 220, 224–225, 284
 tolerance tests, 36, 243
Blood sugar elevation. See Hyperglycemia.
Blood vessel disease, as complication, 175–176, 244
Blue Cross/Blue Shield, 217
Board Mentor Program (ADA), 281

Boehringer Mannheim, 183, 330
Bolan, Robert S., 190–191, 217, 219–220, 232, 242, 256
Bolduan, Charles F., 3–6
Bolduan, Mrs. Charles F., 117
Boshell, Buris R., 161, 166
Bowen, Gurin, Barnes, and Roche, 129
Boyd, Julian D., 16
Brink, Stuart, 254
British Conference on Diabetes and Pregnancy, 101
British Medical Research Council, 101
Brownlee, Michael, 285
Bryan, John, 110
Bullock, Robert, 162
Burroughs Wellcome & Company, Inc., 69
Bustamante, Albert G., 264–265
Butterfield, Alfred, 44

Cahill, George F., Jr., 153, 161, 166, 178, 192–193, 210, 241
California Affiliate, 289–290
Camerini-Davalos, R. A., 175
Campbell, Walter R., 158
Camp Firefly. See Pennsylvania Camp for Diabetic Children
Camping programs, 5, 50–53, 123, 208–209
 fund raising techniques for, 90
Camp NYDA, 69
Camp Seale Harris, 52
Carbohydrates and diabetes, 39, 96, 239–240
Carbohydrate values, 48–49
Cardiovascular disease and diabetes, 2
Carlson, Bill, 226
Carter, Tim Lee, 165
Cavanaugh, Barbara, 163
Center for Economic Studies in Medicine, 270
Center for Health Statistics, 47
Centers for Disease Control, 92
Chick, William L., 173, 176, 243
Child, Dorothy, 132
Childs, Mrs. Robert E., 142–143
Children. See also Youth activities
 diabetes in, 56, 76, 122
 educational activities for, 241–242
Chlorpropamide, 88
Cholesterol
 and diabetes, 81
Christ Child Society Farms for Convalescent Children, 51
Chute, Andrew L., 77
Citizen's Arrest sporting event, 282
Civilian defense and emergency medical care, 59–60
Clara Barton Birthplace Camp, 51
Clark, Charles M., Jr., 237, 264, 267–268, 295
Clarke, Bobby, 156
Classifications and Diagnosis of Diabetes and other Categories of Glucose Intolerance, 212
Cleveland Book, 94
Clinical and Research Fund, 63, 73
Clinical Diabetes, 187
Clinical Diabetes Reviews, 270
Clinical education program, 240–241
Clinical Research Grant Program (ADA), 275
Clowes, George H. A., 26
Cobb, Sidney, 176
Collip, James B., 7–9, 11, 95
Colorado Affiliate, 290

Colwell, Arthur R., 60–61, 65–66, 71, 126, 276
Colwell, John A., 237, 241, 271
Combined Federal Campaigns, 130
Combined Health Information Databank, 94–95
"Comedy Crusade Against Diabetes," 268–270
Committee on Affiliate Associations (ADA), 132, 190
Committee on Camps (ADA), 53
Committee on Clinics (ADA), 31
Committee on Development (ADA), 158
Committee on Diabetes Detection (ADA), 41
Committee on Diabetes in Youth (ADA), 171, 208–209
Committee on Education of Juvenile Diabetics (ADA), 242
Committee on Emergency Medical Care (ADA), 59
Committee on Employment (ADA), 92
Committee on Family Behavior (ADA), 196
Committee on Finance (Budget and Finance) (ADA), 71, 170, 189–190
Committee on Food and Nutrition (NRC), 17, 196
Committee on Food Values (ADA), 48–49
Committee on Foundation of Local Societies (ADA), 23–24
Committee on Function and Structure (ADA), 236–237
Committee on Insulin Syringe Unification (ADA), 27–28
Committee on Interstate and Foreign Commerce (House of Representatives), 165
Committee on Long Range Plans (ADA), 170
Committee on Materials and Therapeutic Agents (ADA), 201, 210
Committee on Nostrums. *See* Committee on Scientific and Medical Programs (ADA)
Committee on Patient Education (ADA), 193, 196–197, 217
Committee on Planning and Organization (ADA), 189–90, 242
Committee on Professional Education (ADA), 143
Committee on Public Affairs (ADA), 162, 164–165, 206
Committee on Public Education (ADA), 113
Committee on Purposes and Policies (ADA), 54, 60, 71–72
Committee on Research (ADA), 141, 172
Committee on Scientific and Medical Programs (ADA), 50, 99–100
Committee on Scientific Evaluation (ADA). *See* Committee on Scientific and Medical Programs (ADA)
Committee on Standards For Admission to Membership (ADA), 24–25, 53
Committee on Statistics (ADA), 102–103
Committee on Teaching Dietetics to Medical Students (ADA), 47–48
Committee on the Employment of Diabetics (ADA), 44
Committee on Voluntary Health Agencies (ADA), 111
Committee on Youth (ADA), 196–197
Committee on Youth and Parents Groups (ADA), 227
Committee on Youth Services (ADA), 227
Committees on Diabetes, 79
Committee to Study Functions and Structure (ADA), 110–111, 127–130
Compound 860. *See* Sulfonylureas
Con Edison of New York, 45
Cone, Lawrence, 144
Conn, Jerome W., 60, 101, 116, 141
Connaught Laboratories (Toronto), 8
Connecticut Affiliate, 290–291

Connelly, J. Richard, 42, 47, 52, 61, 73, 78–79, 91, 110, 130–131, 151–152, 169–170, 182
Cookbook for Diabetics, 89, 197, 199
Cori, Carl F., 158
Corwin, E. H. L., 7
Council on Complications, 262
Council on Diabetes in Pregnancy, 285
Council on Education, 228, 262
Council on Epidemiology and Statistics, 221
Council on Exercise, 262
Council on Foot Care, 262
Council on Health Care Delivery and Public Health, 221, 228
Council on Nutritional Science and Metabolism, 221, 224, 255
Council on Pregnancy and Diabetes, 224
Crampton, Joseph H., 117
Crapo, Phyllis, 239, 254–255
Crick, F. H. C., 106
Crofford, Oscar, 166, 172, 184, 221, 225–227
Crosby, Bing, 114
Cross, Frank B., 6
Cunningham, Linda, 158
Cunningham, Tom, 158
CURE campaign, 249, 283
Curran, Robert, 132
Cyclamates, 132, 137–138
Cyclosporin, 213, 216, 243–244
Czech, Michael P., 243

Danowski, Thaddeus S., 127, 143
Dave's Diary, 68–70
Davidson, Jaime, 264
Davidson, John K., 161–162, 166, 167, 198–199
Davis, Joseph H., 191, 237, 242, 258–259, 321
Davis, Mary, 51
Death from diabetes, 15, 35–36, 80
  age and, 76
  insulin role in prevention, 55–56
DeFronzo, Ralph A., 241
Degenerative disease and insulin therapy, 57
Delatour, Beechman J., 6
Delaware Affiliate, 291
Denmark
  clinical trials on diabetes, 81
  sponsorship of diabetes research, 73–74
Dextrostix, 106
Diabetes, 13, 59–60, 63, 69
Diabetes '83, 187
Diabetes Abstracts, 12–13, 23, 36, 52, 69
Diabetes Care, 187, 270
Diabetes Control and Complications Trial (DCCT), 196, 220–221, 284, 253
Diabetes control programs, 196, 203, 220–221
Diabetes Detection Drive, 40–42
Diabetes Educator, 201
Diabetes Forecast (successor to *ADA Forecast*), 41, 52, 171–172, 201, 233–234
Diabetes mellitus,
  "carriers" of, 102–103
  causes of, 176, 216
  complications, 2, 21–22, 32, 55, 80, 121, 175, 194–197, 212, 220–221, 284–286
  consumer publications on, 272–274
  cookbooks, 89, 197, 199, 273–274
  costs, 270–271
  detection of, 35–57

diagnostic procedures for, 36, 67–68, 243
education on. *See* Educational programs
heredity and. *See* Genetic studies
juvenile, 56, 76
latent, 101
legislation, 160–167, 203–204, 263–265, 277–281
life expectancy and, 1–2, 15,
long-range plan to combat, 165, 333–334
long-term study of, 80, 220–221
mass screening programs for, 211. *See also* National Diabetes Detection Week, National Diabetes Month
morbidity statistics, 36
mortality statistics, 15, 36
and neuropathy, 174, 244
and pregnancy, 55, 80, 91–95
specialists in, 13
transmission by parents, 34
Diabetes Prevention Act, 265
Diabetes Program Directors Workshop, 95
Diabetes Related Literature Index, 94
Diabetes Research and Training Centers (DRTC's), 162, 165, 178
Diabetes Research Fund, Inc., 157
Diabetes Spectrum, 271
Diabetes Supplement 1, Index Medicus, 94
Diabetic Guidebook for Physicians, 88
Diabetologist as medical specialty, 13
Diabinese. *See* Chlorpropamide
Diagnosis of diabetes, 3, 35–57, 67–68, 243
Diagnosis Related Groups, 216
Dickinson, Angie, 231
Diet, 32
  diabetes and, 5, 15–17, 23–24, 33, 43
  exchange lists, 37–38, 47–50
  "free," 75
  and obesity in diabetics, 34
  starvation, 2, 11, 76
  sucrose and, 239–240, 255
Dietitians
  in ADA, 73
  and carbohydrate use, 240
  and educational programs, 223
Dillon, Edward S., 7, 51, 325
District of Columbia Affiliate, 291–292
Dixon, G. H., 122
DNA studies
  and human insulin production, 207–208, 244
  Nobel Prize for, 106
  synthetic, 126
Dodd, S. Douglas, 166, 276, 321
Douglas, Mike, 231
Downie-Maryniuk, Melinda, 239
Doyle, Dane, Bernbach, 191
Drash, Allan L., 225, 311
Drew, George, 37
Dreypack for diabetes diagnosis, 67–68
Drivers' licenses, 119
Drugs. *See specific drug names*
Dublin, Louis I., 45
Ducat, Leatrice, 152–153, 166
Dugan, John L., Jr., 128, 186–187, 189, 191, 199
Dunkley, Eric, 189
Dunn, H. L., 47
Dupre, J., 243
Durrett, J. J., 20–21

Edison, Thomas Alva, 3–4
Educational programs
  on nutrition, 47–50, 197–200, 254–254
  for patients, 193, 217, 228–229, 252–253, 271–273
  for professionals, 77, 94–95
  public, 4–5, 43–44, 61, 212
  self-study for affiliates, 221
  standards for, 252
Egypt, summer camp in, 209
Eichold, Samuel, 52–53
Eisenbarth, George, 244–245
Eisenhower, Dwight D., 60
El-Beheri, Barbara, 199
Eli Lilly and Company, 7–8, 12, 21, 201, 227
  glucagon preparation, 81
  highly purified insulin, 243
  Outstanding Investigator Award, 88–89, 329
  NPH insulin, 69
  Research Laboratories, 33
Ellenberg, Max, 110, 121, 133–134, 153, 174
Emergency medical care, 105
Employment agencies' involvement, 45–46
Employment equity. *See also* Workplace
  and diabetes, 44–46, 92–93, 117–119, 148–149, 235, 278–279
Encore, 96–97
Endocrine Society Liaison Committee (ADA-), 271
Engdahl, John, 158
England
  effects of war on diabetes in, 32
  government provisions during war, 21
Engle, Frank, 65
Eskimos, low diabetes incidence in, 145
Established Investigator Program, 172
Etzwiler, Donnell D., 110, 153, 166, 171, 183, 186, 205–210, 221
Exchange Lists for Meal Planning, 37–38, 47, 49–50, 89, 131, 197–199, 240, 254–255
Exercise in diabetes control, 216

"Facts About Diabetes," 68
Fajans, Stefan S., 153, 158, 160–161, 169
Farley, Barbara, 111
Farm Animal and Research Facilities Protection Act of 1989, 281
Farquarson, Ray F., 77
Federal Aviation Administration, 235
Federal Rehabilitation Act of 1973, 148–149
Federal Security Administration, 20
Federal Security Agency, 43–44
Federal Trade Commission Medical Advisory Division, 20–21
Felig, Philip, 173, 212, 225
Fellowship programs
  in ADA, 24–25, 132
  USPHS, 63, 65
Ferguson, William, 130, 154–155, 186
Fetal cell transplants, 285
Field, Frank, 232
Field, Pamela, 232
Film premiers for fund raising, 192–193, 242
Films on diabetes, 231–232
Finch, Robert, 137
First-aid instructions for diabetes complications, 22
Fishbein, Morris, 9
Florida Affiliate, 292–293

Flynt, J. William, 166, 203–204
Food and Cosmetic Act, Delaney Clause, 206
Food, Drug, and Cosmetic Act, certification of insulin by, 30–31
Food rationing and diabetes during World War II, 19
Ford, Gerald, 161, 166, 167, 173, 178, 192
40 Commonly Asked Questions About Type II Diabetes (NIDDM), 241
Fowler, James, 227–228
Franz, Marion, 225, 239, 254–255
Fredericks, John R., 98
Freinkel, Norbert, 182, 191, 198, 207, 210, 260, 262–263
Frey, Donald N., 170
Froesch, E. R., 65
Frost, Ernest M., 151–152, 186, 188, 191
Funding, federal, 277
Fund raising, 70–72, 84, 89–91, 109, 112–113, 128–132, 154–156, 188–189, 191–194, 232–233, 242, 282–283
Fund Raising Manual for Affiliate Diabetes Associations 90
Fund Raising Volunteer Recognition Award, 332
Fundus photography, 217

Gallo, Sam A., 237, 321
Galloway, John, 295
Gambert, Steven, 271
Gangrene as diabetes complication, 32
Ganim, Joseph N., 7
Garn, Jake, 274–276
Garn, Sue, 274–275
Gastineau, Clifford F., 146, 171
Gates, Edwin W., 132, 127–128
Genetic studies, 1–2, 34, 56, 101, 106, 144, 285
   genetic engineering, 207–208, 211
George Rice & Sons, 183
Georgia Affiliate, 293
Germany, 84
Gestational diabetes, 92, 145, 243, 260–261
Gibbs, C.B.F., 3, 117
Gibson, Dolores, 264
Gibson, Jessie O., 159
Gilbert, Walter, 216
Gillespie, Daniel, 295
Givers Guide to National Philanthropies, 97
Glenn, John, 231
Globin insulin with zinc, 30, 69
Glucagon, 121, 144
   and pancreas functions, 175
   preparation and studies of, 81, 101
Glycemic control, 196, 240
Glycemic index, 216
Glycohemoglobin tests, 211, 217
Glycosuria and diet, 76
Goals for Diabetes Education, 270
Gohdes, Dorothy, 166, 254, 264
Goldberg, Morton F., 176
Goldsmith/Jeffrey, 191
Gordon, Gamal, 209
Goulet, Robert, 231
Government Relations Committee (ADA), 204, 281
Grace Hospital Diabetic Camp, 50
Graham, John H., IV, 220
Great Depression, 7
Greater Philadelphia Affiliate, 310

Greene, Susan, 158
Greenspoon, Benjamin, 189–190, 197, 224, 237, 321
Grishaw, Dorothy, 172
Grishaw, William, 115, 122, 168, 172
Guest, George M., 76
Guidebook for ADA Affiliates in Conducting a Bike-a-thon, 155–156
Guidebook for Professionals: The Effective Application of Exchange Lists for Meal Planning, 198
Guillemin, Roger, 211
Gullickson, Bill, 231
Gurin, Maury, 170
Guthrie, Diana, 223, 225

Hagedorn, Hans C., 1, 39, 56, 74
Haist, R. E., 11
Hall, Jon W., 167
Hamwi, George J., 121
Handbook for Physicians, 42, 69
Handicapped, legislation for, 148–149
Haney, Carol, 95
Hansen, Barbara, 254
Hanson, Harlan, 156, 158, 227, 321
Hanson-Ullom, Virginia, 156, 158
Hardin, Robert C., 133, 139–140
Harris, LaDonna, 264
Harris, Seale, 8
Havens, James, Jr., 11–13
Hawaii Affiliate, 293–294
Hazzard, Frances O., 47–48
Health care delivery, 228–230
   by private sector, 216
Health care professionals, 222–223
   study programs for, 143
Health-care teams, 126
Health insurance. *See* Insurance
"Healthy Food Choices," 255, 272
Heart-lung machine, 82
Heffner, George, 164–165
Heflin, Howell T., 280
Hemoglobin A1c test, 220
Henabery, Joseph E., 44
Heredity and diabetes, 2, 56
Heselton, John, 78
High blood pressure and diabetes, 56
High technology and diabetes, 281–283
Hijikata, Sandra, 158
Hill, Dana, 226
Hill, Wendy, as subject of film, 43
Hinton, Deborah, 227, 253
Hiram Hamster as ADA symbol, 140–141
Hirsch, Ed, 123
Hirsch, Gloria, 123
Hirsch, Irl, 123
HLA antigens role in diabetes, 216
Hodgkin, Dorothy C., 106, 145, 158
Holcomb, Blair, 87, 113, 310
Holiday sales program, 156–158, 232–233
Holler, Harold, 255
Holvey, Sherman M., 241, 268
Ho Mita Koda camp, 50–51
Hoover, Joan, 159
Hope, Bob, 114, 230
Hormone therapy in pregnant women with diabetes, 101
Horne, Lena, 242
Horton, Edward S., 241, 254, 317

Hospital for Sick Children, 77
House, Lawrence, 144
House Committee on Interstate and Foreign Commerce, 77–79
Houssay, Bernardo, 39, 158
Hoyer, Steny, 166
Hunter, Catfish, 230
Hunt, Sara, 132
Hurd, James, 132, 148
Hurwitz, Linda, 222, 253, 271
Hyperglycemia, 56
  and blood vessel diseases, 175
  and diet, 76
  studies, 16–17
  sucrose and, 239–240
Hypoglycemia. *See* Insulin, shock

Iacocca, Lee, 169–170
Idaho Affiliate, 294
IDF Directory, 261
Illinois Affiliate, Downstate, 294–295
Illinois Affiliate, Northern, 295
Immunosuppresive drugs. *See* Cyclosporin
Indiana Affiliate, 295–296
Indian Health Care Amendment Act, 263–264
Industrial Hygiene Foundation, 46
Insulin, 55–56, 102, 158–160, 200–203
  concentration preference, 159, 175, 200–203
  discovery, 1–2, 6–9, 37–39, 144
  early use, 1–3, 11–13
  highly purified, 243
  human, 207–208, 211, 216, 244
  implants, 210
  mixtures of, 28, 30, 56–57, 80
  molecular structure of, 145
  nasal, 243
  NPH, 56–57, 69, 80
  preparation in Europe, 81
  proinsulin, 144–146
  protamine zinc, 1, 15, 28, 30, 39, 56–57
  pumps, 212, 217, 225–226, 243, 284
  radioimmunoassay blood test, 60
  reserve supplies during wartime, 105
  resistance to, 60
  "second messenger" of, 243
  shock, 44, 121
  structure studies, 158
  supply and demand, 21, 26–27
  synthetic, 122
  synthetic human-like, 211
  syringes. *See* Syringes
Insulin-reactive diabetes, 2
Insurance and diabetes, 25, 46–47, 93–94, 116–117, 125, 167–168, 217, 228–230, 277–278
International Conference on Camping, 208
International Diabetes Federation, 73–74, 109–110, 118, 122, 248, 260–261
"International List of Causes," 47
International Workshop/Conference on Gestational Diabetes, 92, 260–261
Intestinal wall studies, 144
Iowa Affiliate, 296
Islands of Langerhans and diabetes, 39
Islet cell
  implants, 210
  microencapsulation, 243
  transplants, 213, 244, 253, 284

Jackson, Gail Patrick, 161, 168–169, 172–174, 236, 322
Jackson, Robert L., 16
Jacobson, Dorothy, 158
January, Lewis E., 134
Janz, William, 43–44
Jefferson, Leonard, 173
Jenkins, David, 239, 254
Jenner, Bruce, 230
John, Henry, 8, 51, 53, 76
Johnsson, Sven, 121
Joslin Diabetes Center, 171, 210
Joslin Diabetes Foundation, 143
Joslin, Elliott P., 2, 8, 11, 15–16, 32, 33, 36, 73, 75–76, 87–89, 92, 102, 113.
Joslin (Elliott P.) Fellowship, 73
Joslin (Elliott P.) Research and Development Award, 123, 141–142
Joslin (Elliott P.) Medal, 159
Joslin Pregnancy Clinic, 93
"Journey and the Dream," 242
Juvenile Diabetes Foundation (JDF), 152–154, 201, 227

Kaadt Diabetic Institute, 99–100
Kahn, C. Ronald, 210
Kahn, Richard, 220
Kansas Affiliate, 296
Kaplan, Dorothy, 171
Katsoyannis, Panayotis G., 122, 158
Kaufman, Michael, 159
Keiding, Niels Ried, 74
Keller, Mary Ann, 94
Kennedy, Edward, 206
Kennedy, John F., 114
Kentucky Affiliate, 297
Kenyon and Eckhardt, 191
Kidney dialysis machine, 82
Kidney transplantation, 274–275
Kid's Corner, 194–195
King, Harry E., 57
Kirtley, William M., 110, 295
Kissebah, Ahmed, 254
Knowles, Harvey C., 110, 132–133, 225
Koch, Ed, 266–267
Kornberg, Arthur, 253
Kortman, Joyce, 160–161
Krall, Leo, 171, 207, 233–234
Kreisberg, Robert, 271
Kroc, Ray, 155, 194, 233, 236
Kroc, Robert, 194
Kroc Collaborative Study group, 195–196, 284
Kroc Foundation, 194–195
Krosnick, Arthur, 234

Labeling of oral hypoglycemic drugs, 140
Labor-HEW Appropriations Act, 166
Labor unions' involvement, 46
Lacy, Paul, 166, 176, 178, 213, 284
LaFave, Diane, 158
Lamont-Havers, Ronald, 162
Lapham, Larry, 172
Larner, Joseph, 173
Larsson, Dr., 76
Laser treatment for retinopathy, 212, 217
Lasichak, Andrea, 255
Lawrence, Patricia, 182–183, 196, 271

Lawrence, R. D., 39
Lea, Clarence F., 30
Lebovitz, Harold E., 241
Lee, G. Rodney, 154–155
Legislation for diabetes, 160–161, 203–204, 263–265, 277–281
Lente insulin, 81, 101
Levin, Charles M., 7
Levin, Marvin, 253
Levine, Rachmiel, 95–97, 117, 119, 144, 158, 176, 197
Levy, Philip, 234
Lichtenstein, Dr., 76
Life insurance. *See* Insurance
Lilly. *See* Eli Lilly and Company
Lions Clubs International sponsorship of research activities, 227–228, 274–275
Lipton, Bronna, 264
Lobbying activities, 134–135
Lofquist, Barbara, 37–38
Long-term study of diabetes, 80, 220–221
Louisiana Affiliate, 297–298
Lukens, Francis D.W., 60, 84–85, 97–99, 112

McDonald's Corporation, 155, 194, 236
McGee, Gale, 115, 134, 162, 164, 173, 204
Maclaren, Noel, 285
Macleod, J. J. R., 6–9, 11
McLoughlin, Christopher J., 113
McNeil Laboratories, 92
McNutt, Paul D., 20
Mae, Louinia, 166–167
Mahler, Richard J., 142
Maine Affiliate, 298
Mamrack, William, 259, 264, 321
Management Letter, 97
Manufacturers' Life Insurance Company, 47
Marble, Alexander, 76–77, 110, 140–141
Margolin, Morris, 24
Martin, Donald B., 207
Mary Foley Camp, 51
Maryland Affiliate, 298–299
Maschak-Carey, Barbara, 22
Massachusetts Affiliate, 299
Mason, Cynthia, 281–283
Matschinsky, Franz, 173
Mayer, Eric D., 237
Mayes, Wendell, Jr., 166, 168, 174, 182, 186, 188, 236–237, 321–322
Meadows, Audrey, 231
Medical Student Research Fellowship Program (ADA), 275
Medicare/Medicaid, 125, 217
 reimbursement for shoes, 277–278
Membership issues, 24–25, 72–73
Mentor-Based Postdoctoral Fellowship Program, 275
Merimee, Thomas J., 142
Merrill, Dina, 171, 192
Metformin, 285–286
Metropolitan Life Insurance Company, 10, 45
Metzger, Boyd, 263
Mexican Americans and diabetes, 263
Michigan Affiliate, 300
Miles, Inc., 183, 331
Miller, Max, 139
Minnesota Affiliate, 300–301
Minnesota Highway Department, 119

Minnesota Research Dinners, 156
Minority Initiative (ADA), 265
Minority programs, 263–265
Mintz, Daniel H., 244
Mirsky, I. Arthur, 6, 23
Mish, J. Hammond, 51
Mississippi Affiliate, 301–302
Missouri Affiliate, 302
Mitchell, J. West, 7, 117
Montana Affiliate, 302–303
Montgomery, R. D., 46–47
Moore, Mary Tyler, 95, 157, 192
Morris, Walter, 132
Mosenthal, Herman O., 3, 5–6, 8, 16, 19–20, 32
Mrazek, Robert, 280
Muhlberg, William, 7–8, 25, 113
Mulholland, Henry B., 67, 79
Mullann, Elizabeth M., 68
Murphy, Patrick, 152, 171

Nadig, Perry, 243
Najarian, John, 210
Natcher, William, 166
National Academy of Sciences/National Research Council
 Committee on Food and Nutrition, 17
 review of cyclamates, 138
 review of saccharin, 205
National Bike-Ride Plus, 251
National Coalition for Recognition of Diabetes Patient Education Programs (NACOR), 252
National Commission on Correctional Health Care, 115–116
National Commission on Diabetes, 166, 178
 Committee on Research, 178
National Conference on Teaching and Research in Diabetes, 95
National Diabetes Advisory Board, 94, 178, 185, 252
National Diabetes Data Group (NDDG), 203, 263
National Diabetes Detection Week, 41–42, 52, 96, 113–114
National Diabetes Information Clearinghouse, 94–95, 203
National Diabetes Mellitus Research And Education Act, 165, 178, 203, 221
National Diabetes Month, 42, 191, 268–269
National Diabetes Program, 164
National Diabetes Research and Education Act of 1974, 94, 134, 149
National Health Council
 accounting requirements, 128
 ADA membership in, 22, 142
 public awareness program for research, 277
 standards and ethical guidelines, 142
National Health Survey, 36, 102–103
National Holiday Sales Program, 156–158, 232–233
National Institute of Arthritis, Metabolic and Digestive Diseases, 95, 220, 252–253
 expansion of activities, 162–163
 renaming of, 160–161
National Institutes of Health, 92, 165, 227, 220–221, 251–253
National Library of Medicine Literature Analysis Project, 94
National Media Awards for Excellence in Journalism, 232
National Medical Research Day, 277

341

National Office of Vital Statistics, (NOVS), 47
National Pituitary Agency, 253
National Society for the Prevention of Blindness, 212
National Standards for Diabetes Patient Education, 253
Nationwide Comprehensive Long-Range Plan, 256–258, 283
Native American Indians
    diabetes research and control programs for, 204, 263–265
    incidence of diabetes in, 145
Nebraska Affiliate, 303
Neill, Karleen C., 301–302
Nelligan, William D., 166
Nemchik, Rita, 253
Nephropathy and diabetes, 76, 121, 122
    angiotensin converting enzyme and, 286
Neuropathy and diabetes, 174, 176, 244
Nevada Affiliate, 303–304
Newburgh, Lewis H., 8
New Hampshire Affiliate, 304
New Jersey Affiliate, 304–305
New Mexico Affiliate, 305
News and Views, 142–143
Newton-John, Olivia, 231
Newton, Wayne, 192
New York Academy of Medicine, 7
New York Downstate Affiliate, 306
New York Upstate Affiliate, 306–307
New York Diabetes Association, 5, 7, 51
Night clinics, 45
Nirenberg, Marshall W., 253
Nixon, Richard M., 165, 173
Nobel Prize in Chemistry
    for DNA structure studies, 216
    for structure of biochemical compounds, 106
Nobel Prize in Physiology and Medicine
    for anti-viral vaccines, 60
    for discovery of insulin, 1, 8–9
    for DNA studies, 106
    for hormone studies, 148, 211
    for insulin studies, 216
Non-physician health professionals
    in ADA, 73, 223
    educational programs for, 112, 132, 175
Nordisk Insulinfond, 73–75
Nordisk-USA, 243
North Carolina Affiliate, 307–308
North Dakota Affiliate, 308
Novo insulin preparations, 81, 243
Novo Nordisk, 183
NPH-50 insulin, 56–57
Nuclear threats. *See* Civilian defense
Nurses in diabetes care, 202. *See also* Team approach
    educators in ADA, 73
NutraSweet Company, 183, 227, 331
Nutrition. *See also Exchange Lists*
    guidelines, 197
    high-fiber diets, 216
    importance for diabetes control, 47–50
Nutritional Recommendations and Principles for Individuals with Diabetes Mellitus, 254–255
Nutrition Guide for Professionals, 271
Nuttall, Frank, 239, 255

Obesity
    diabetes and, 145
    and diet in diabetes, 34

insulin effectiveness and, 56
Office of Civilian Defense, 22
Office of Price Administration (OPA), 26–27
Ohio Affiliate, 308–309
Oklahoma Affiliate, 309
Olefsky, Jerold M., 241
Olmsted, William H., 49
Olney, Mary B., 51
Omnibus Reconciliation Act, 216
O'Neill, Thomas P. (Tip), Jr., 165
Opie, Eugene, 39
Oral drugs
    contraceptives, 144–145
    for diabetes treatment, 84, 87–88
    high-potency, 216
    second-generation, 244
Orci, Lelio, 176
Order of the Amaranth, 192–193, 228
Oregon Affiliate, 309–310
Orinase. *See* Sulfonylureas
Outstanding Affiliate Service Award, 329
Outstanding Clinician in the Field of Diabetes, 183, 331
Outstanding Contribution to Camping and Diabetes Award, 52, 183, 331
Outstanding Contribution to Diabetes in Youth Award, 183, 330
Outstanding Fund Raising Volunteer Award, 183
Outstanding Health Educator Award, 223
Outstanding Health Professional Educator in the Field of Diabetes, 183, 331
Outstanding Investigator Award. *See under* Eli Lilly and Company
Outstanding Layman Award, 142
Outstanding Physician Educator in the Field of Diabetes, 331
Outstanding Service in the Field of Diabetes to a Physician Educator, 183
Owen, John A., Jr., 65
Owens, Louis B., 3, 8,

Palmer, Lester J., 61, 63, 91, 317
Pancreas
    from animals in insulin production, 30
    and beta cell secretions, 176
    relation to diabetes, 6, 39
    and glucagon level, 175
    transplants, 213, 217, 253
Pansky, Benjamin, 144
Panza, John, 165
Parents as diabetes transmitters, 34
Parents of Young Diabetics, 156
Parks, Tom, 268–269
Paulesco, N. C., 6
Paullin, James E., 8
Peck, Franklin B., 12, 33, 60, 109–110, 113, 115
Penile prostheses, 243
Pennsylvania Affiliate, Mid-, 310–311
Pennsylvania Affiliate, Western, 311–312
Pennsylvania Camp for Diabetic Children, 51
Penrose, L. S., 34
Peterson, Charles M., 225
Phenformin, 88, 210–211
Philadelphia Metabolic Association, 51
Physical examination form, non-discriminatory, 45
Physician's Guide to Insulin-Dependent (Type I) Diabetes, 271

Physician's Guide to Non-Insulin-Dependent (Type II) Diabetes (NIDDM), 241, 271
"Pigs Are Precious," 202
Pilot's license restrictions, 235
Pituitary glands and diabetes, 39
Pituitary growth hormone and diabetes research, 65
Ploman, Dr., 76
Polentz, Paul F., 7, 117
Police education program, 115
Polin, Sandra, 235
Policy on the Sale of Medical Equipment and Medicines, 224
Pollack, Herbert, 6
Pons, Juan A., 21
Porte, Daniel, Jr., 253, 271
Porter, Mariana, 155
Postgraduate courses, 77, 133, 142–143, 145, 176, 263
Poutas, John J., 46
Powers, Margaret, 255, 271
Pregnancy and diabetes, 55, 80, 91–95, 145, 225
Pressure groups, 45
Prestholdt, John, 158
Pricing of health care services, 224
Prison education program, 115
Proceedings, 12–13, 23–24, 52, 69
Product endorsement, 95
Professional Advisory Panel (ADA), 238
Proinsulin, 144–146
Prospective payment Plan, 216
Prostheses, 5
Protamine zinc insulin (PZI), 1, 15, 39, 56–57
  mixtures with unmodified insulin, 28, 30
Protas, Maurice, 292
Publications Committee (ADA), 23
Publications, 12–13, 23, 36, 39–41, 46, 51–52, 59–61, 68–70, 79, 187, 270–274
Public awareness programs, 113–116, 191–194, 217, 230–233, 265–268
Public Health Service Act, 264
Public Law 93-354. *See* National Diabetes Mellitus Research And Education Act
Puckett, Dorothea Webb, 166
Puerto Rico, insulin shortages during war, 21–22
Puerto Rico Affiliate, 312

Quackery
  in diabetes treatment, 97–100
  Federal control of, 20

Rachmiel Levine, M.D. Award, 332
Radioimmunoassay test for blood insulin measurement, 60
Raskin, Philip, 225
Reber, Howard J., 181
Recognition Program, 253
Reed, John, 47, 51, 61, 78, 90, 113
Renold, Albert E., 65, 96, 255–256
Research, 5, 80–81, 274–276
  animals in, 279–281
  conferences on, 194–195
  for diabetes detection, 36, 41–43
  funding for, 61, 84, 178–179, 226–228, 277
  legislation for, 160–167
  organizing for expansion, 63, 65, 116
  Symposia, 332
Reserve supplies for diabetes, 105–106
Retinopathy and diabetes, 75, 121, 176, 196, 212, 284

Reveno, William S., 3, 117
Reynolds, Burt, 230
Reynolds, P. Preston, 264
Rhode Island Affiliate, 312–313
Rice, E. Clarence, 51, 292
Rice, George, 332
Richter, Netti, 194–195, 227
Ricker, Alyne, 243
Ricketts, Henry T., 74, 84–85, 87–88, 110
Rider, Claire V., 45
Rifkin, Harold, 121, 233–234, 241, 261, 263
Riley, William, 285
Rivera, Henry, 321
Robert J. Brady Company, 187
Robinson, Jackie, 115, 159
Rockefeller, Nelson A., 184
Rogers, Paul G., 161, 163, 165
Roosevelt, Franklin D., 19
Root, Howard F., 41, 52, 60, 73–75
Root, Mary, 295
Roerig, 183, 331
Rose, Robert M., 176
Rosenhoover, Frank, 237
Rubenstein, Arthur, 173
Ruhland, Florence R., 225, 253

Saccharin, 132, 137–138, 205–207
St. Peter, Diana, 158
St. Peter, Peter, 158
Salans, Lester B., 166
Salk, Jonas, 60
Sanderson, Edward L., 207
Sanger, Frederick, 102, 158, 216
Sansum, W. D., 8
Santiago, Julio V., 225
Saturday House, 193–194
Saxl, Eva, 28, 30–31
Saxl, Victor, 28, 30–31
Scali, McCabe, Sloves, 191
Schade, David S., 225
Schally, Andrew, 211
Scharp, David W., 176, 284
Schecter, John S., 33
Scheidler, Leona, 4–5
Schmahl, Philipp J. R., 6
School personnel and diabetes awareness, 171
Schultz, Patricia, 222–223, 227, 237, 253, 292
Schumacher, O. Peter, 225
Schweiker, Richard S., 160, 163–164, 167, 172
Scientific Sessions (ADA), 263, 285
Scott, E. L., 6
Scott, James R., 8
Scott, Ralph, 6
Scoville, Addison B., Jr., 110, 152–153, 170, 173
Scoville, (Addison B.), Jr., Award, 174
Searle, G. D., 227
Segar, Laurence F., 3
Semilente insulin, 81
Service, Nancy Holina, 158
Sex and diabetes, 5, 123
Sharkey, Thomas P., 57, 109–110, 122, 127
Shelvin, Edmund L., 92
Shepardson, H. Clare, 8
Sherwood Medical Industries, 201
Shipman, Sidney J., 111
Shoes, therapeutic, 217, 277–278
Shuman, C. R., 243

Silver, Robert L., 243
Simonson, Louise O., 172
Sims, Dorothea, 166, 229, 252, 258
Skyler, Jay S., 153, 241
Small Grants Program, 132–133
Smith, Beverly Chew, 6, 9, 117
Smith, Sydney, 39
Smith, Ted, 158
Smith, Tom, 227
Solis, Carlos, 264
Somatostatin, 211
Soskin, Samuel, 95–96
South Carolina Affiliate, 313
South Dakota Affiliate, 314
Sprague, Randall G., 60, 71, 78, 110, 159, 161, 163–164
Spratt, Irving L., 211, 225, 227, 243–244, 253
Squibb, E.R., and Sons, 42, 201, 227
Squibb-Novo, 183, 244, 329
Staggers, Harley O., 165
Stars War on Diabetes, 231
Statistical studies, 15, 35–36, 122–123
    on prevalence of disability, 45
Steiger, William A., 160, 163
Steiner, Donald F., 144, 158, 207
Steiner, William O., 44
Stenholm, Charles, 280–281
Stephens, Anna O., 6
Stephenson, Richard M., 135
Stevens, Caroline, 187, 220, 237
Stokes, Louis, 166
Stoney, George F., 6
"Story of Wendy Hill" film, 43
Stress as a cause of diabetes, 176
Striker, Cecil, 3–10, 12–14, 20–21, 52, 110, 117, 208, 322
Suarez, Lillian Haddock, 166
Subcommittee on Health (Senate), 163–164
Subcommittee on Public Health and Environment (House), 161, 163–164
Sucrose and diabetes, 239–240
Sulfonamides, 84
Sulfonylureas, 84, 88, 138–139
Summer Camp for Diabetic Children (Egypt), 209
Summer camps. *See* Camping
Surveys
    on diabetes, 102
    on employment practices, 93
    of membership, 98, 112
Sussman, Karl, 183, 189–190, 221, 237, 242
Sutherland, Earl W., 148
Sycaryl, 70
Synthalin, 30
Syringes
    early difficulties with, 5, 26–27
    evaluation of, 50
    standards for, 27–31, 210
    for U100, 159, 175

Talbert, William, 132, 157–159
Tanenbaum, Myles, 161, 182, 321
Task Force on ADA Structure, 222, 237
Task Force on Nutrition and Exchange Lists, 254–255
Task Force on Resource Allocation, 258
Task Force on Sucrose, 239–240, 254
Team approach
    to diabetes treatment, 73, 126, 153, 222–223

Tennesee Affiliate, 314
Texas Affiliate, 315
Theiler, Max, 60
Third party reimbursements, 217, 228
Thompson, Leonard, 8
Thompson, Linda, 230
Thompson, Robert, 158
Thosteson, George C., 3, 117
Thymus gland studies, 144
Tierney, Thomas J., 170
Today Show and civilian defense announcements on diabetes supplies, 106
Todd, John A., 285
Tolbutamide. *See* Sulfonylureas
Tolstoi, Edward, 6, 32, 56, 117
Tom-Orme, Lillian, 264
Toxemia and diabetes, 55
Tranquada, Robert, 110–111
Travel restrictions during World War II, 19, 23
Trucco, Massimo, 285
Truman, Harry S., and diabetes treatment measures, 26–27
Tuberculosis Association, 4
Tucker, Sterling, 264, 321
Tuechter, J. L., 3

U100 insulin, 159, 171, 175
Ulene, Art, 231–232
Ullom, John, 158
Ultralente insulin, 81
Underdahl, Laurentius O., 110, 128
Unger, Roger, 144, 175
Uni-Betic Camp, 172
Union Life Insurance Company, 7, 10, 12
United Fund, 131
United Nations Committee on Caloric Value of Food, 48
University Group Diabetes Program, 138
University of California Diabetic Childrens' Camp, 51
University of Toronto, 6, 8, 11, 39
    Committee on Insulin, 30–31
Upjohn Company, 183, 242, 331
Urine testing to detect diabetes, 2, 5, 36, 41, 123
U.S. Bureau of Medical Devices, 210
U.S. Civil Service Commission, 46, 93
U.S. Department of Agriculture, 48
U.S. Department of Health, Education and Welfare, 95
U.S. Department of Transportation, 235
U.S. Food and Drug Administration, 30, 137–139, 201
U.S. Public Health Service, 36, 41–44, 49, 92, 95
    fellowships, 63, 65
    Rehabilitation Service, 46
    survey on diabetes, 102
U.S. Surgeon General, 60
U.S. War Production Board
    and diabetes treatment shortages, 21
Utah Affiliate, 315–316

Vander Jagt, Guy, 160–161, 163
Velde, Gail Patrick. *See* Jackson, Gail Patrick
Vermont Affiliate, 316–317
Verville, Richard, 204
Vinik, Aaron, 254
Virginia Affiliate, 317
Virginia Mason Clinic, Camp Banting, 51
Vitrectomy, 176, 217
Vivisection and public attitudes, 54

Volcker, Paul, 249
Voluntary health agencies, 61
von Eiff, Ted, 209

Wagener, Henry P., 34
Wakerlin, Dr., 112
Wallenstein, Willard, 6
Walt Disney Company, 192
Wang, K. Z., 158
Ward, Cathy, 191
Washington Affiliate, 317–318
Washington Diabetic Camp for Children, 51
Waters, Marie, 193
Watson, E. M., 34
Waxman, Henry, 166
Weiker, Lowell, 166
Weinberger, Caspar, 166
Wells, Frank, 188
Wendt, Leonard F. C., 50
Werner, Larry, 154–155, 168
West (Kelly) Award, 332
West Virginia Affiliate, 318
Whedon, Donald, 162
Wheeler, Madelyn, 255
White, Priscilla, 51, 56, 91–95, 103
Whitehouse, Fred W., 183, 198, 201, 207, 221
Whittlesey, McKinley, 167
Wilcox, Francis P., 135–136
Wilder, Russell M., 8, 17, 39
Wilkins, M. H. F., 106
Williams, Ellen, 13
Williams, Frederick W., 3, 6, 9, 68–70, 117
Williams, John, 11–13
Wilson, David K. (Pat), 170, 173
Winegrad, Albert I., 145, 161
Wisconsin Affiliate, 318–319
Wolf, James F., 256
Wolverton, Charles A., 78–79
Women as health professionals, 153–154
Woodward, Clara, 310
Woodyatt, R. T., 9
Workplace and diabetes, 276
World Book of Diabetes in Practice, 261
World Health Organization, 118
World Statistics on Diabetes, 122
World War II
    Britain's diabetes activities during, 21, 32
    effect on diabetes treatment, 19–34
Wylie-Rosett, Judith, 239, 255
Wyoming Affiliate, 319

Yalow, Rosalyn S., 60, 89, 158, 211
Young, W. Wayne, 225
Younger, M. Donna, 93
Youth activities, 171–172, 226–227. *See also* Children
Youth Coordinating Committee (ADA), 242
Youth Leadership Award, 183, 331
Youth Leadership Congress, 226–227

Zagoria, Robert, 235
Zahn, Helmut, 158
Zuelzer, George Ludwig, 6